EPILEPTOGENIC AND EXCITOTOXIC MECHANISMS

EPILEPTOGENIC AND EXCITOTOXIC MECHANISMS

Proceedings of the Advanced Course in Epileptology
Erice, Sicily, January 1992

Edited by
G. Avanzini, R. Fariello, U. Heinemann and R. Mutani

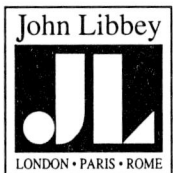

John Libbey
LONDON · PARIS · ROME

British Library Cataloguing in Publication Data

Epileptogenic and Excitotoxic Mechanisms
Proceedings of the Advanced Course in Epileptology
Erice, Sicily, January 1992
    I.   Avanzini, G.
    616.85

Current Problems in Epilepsy: 8
ISSN: 0950-4591
ISBN: 0 86196 386 5

Published by

John Libbey & Company Ltd, 13 Smiths Yard, Summerley Street, London SW18 4HR, England.
Telephone: 081-947 2777: Fax 081-947 2664
John Libbey Eurotext Ltd, 6 rue Blanche, 92120 Montrouge, France.
John Libbey - C.I.C. s.r.l., via Lazzaro Spallanzani 11, 00161 Rome, Italy

© 1993 John Libbey & Company Ltd. All rights reserved.
Unauthorised duplication contravenes applicable laws.

Printed in Great Britain by Whitstable Litho Printers Ltd., Whitstable, Kent.

Contents

	Foreword	vii
	Preface	ix
	Opening remarks	1
Chapter 1	Animal models of epilepsy *V. La Grutta*	5
Chapter 2	Basic mechanisms of focal epileptogenesis *David A. Prince*	17
Chapter 3	Generalized epileptogenesis *Giuliano Avanzini*	29
Chapter 4	Mechanisms of action of antiepileptic drugs *R.G. Fariello*	41
Chapter 5	GABA-mediated potentials and epileptogenesis *Massimo Avoli and Granger G.C. Hwa*	51
Chapter 6	Morphological aspects of neocortical maturation *Roberto Spreafico and Carolina Frassoni*	59
Chapter 7	Noradrenergic and peptidergic neurotransmission in hippocampal kindling *A. Vezzani, A. Monno, M. Rizzi, A. Galli, C. Bendotti and R. Samanin*	67
Chapter 8	Epileptogenesis in the hippocampus of the isolated guinea-pig brain maintained *in vitro*: a model for limbic seizures *Marco de Curtis, Denis Paré and Rodolfo R. Llinas*	79
Chapter 9	Ontogenetic models of epilepsy *Maria Rita de Feo and Oriano Mecarelli*	89

Chapter 10	Potassium homoeostasis and epileptogenesis in the immature hippocampus *U. Heinemann, D. Albrecht, H. Beck, E. Ficker, B. Nixdorf and J. Stabel*	99
Chapter 11	Postnatal development of EAA-mediated excitation in rat neocortex *S. Franceschetti, S. Buzio, F. Panzica, G. Sancini and G. Avanzini*	107
Chapter 12	GABA excites immature rat CA3 hippocampal neurones *Enrico Cherubini*	115
Chapter 13	Kindling in developing animals *L.S. Velíšek, E.F. Sperber and S.L. Moshé*	121
Chapter 14	Excitotoxicity and the developing brain *Claude G. Wasterlain and Raman Sankar**	135
	Author Index	153
	Subject Index	154

Foreword

In my opinion this book needs no introduction. The great interest of the subject and the well known scientific merit of the contributors warrant it as one of the most important recent accounts on basic mechanisms of the epilepsies with special emphasis on seizure-induced cellular damage in the developing brain.

It is my pleasure however, as President of the Lega Italiana contro l'Epilessia, to comply with the wish of my friend Giuliano Avanzini in introducing the book to everyone interested in the field of epileptology. It is my belief that diagnostic, clinical and therapeutic approaches to the epilepsies must be grounded on the information provided by the basic sciences. This can greatly contribute to strengthening our effectiveness in the management of the patient with epilepsy, which is our ultimate goal.

Raffaele Canger
President of the Lega Italiana contro l'Epilessia

Preface

This book arose from the proceedings of the Second Advanced Course in Epileptology of the Lega Italiana contro l'Epilessia (LICE), organized by the International School of Biophysics, Ettore Majorana Center for Scientific Culture, Erice (Italy) on January 15 – February 2, 1992. Here are collected the lectures from the first session devoted to the basic mechanism of epilepsy with special emphasis on seizure-induced cellular damage in the developing brain. Most of our present understanding of epileptogenesis comes from experimental studies carried out in animal models of some aspects of epilepsy, which are comprehensively reviewed here. A special section is devoted to the electrophysiology and behaviour of experimentally induced seizures in developing animals. The description of the anatomical, biochemical and functional aspects of the maturing brain is the object of a specific chapter.

Particular attention is given to the kindling phenomenon which is the subject of two specific chapters where the systems involved in this interesting example of epileptogenic plasticity in mature and immature animals are illustrated.

Electrophysiological features of the ictal and interictal discharges seen in animals with acute foci can be replicated in brain tissue maintained *in vitro*. As stated in Chapter 2 by David Prince, data obtained from *in vitro* tissue or cultured cells may provide an invaluable source of information providing they are carefully compared with preparations from intact animals and from man. Along this line the most important information on epileptogenesis and excitotoxic mechanism is systematically reviewed.

The following points are worth being emphasized. Focal and generalized epileptogenesis share common mechanisms but differ in some others, especially with regard to the involvement of thalamic structures. These latter play an essential role in the genesis of generalized epileptiform discharges of the petit mal type.

A depression of GABA-mediated inhibition results in focal epileptiform discharges in both hippocampus and neocortex. However, depending on the experimental conditions, epileptiform discharges can be seen also at a time when GABA may play an important role in cell growth and differentiation by raising intracellular calcium levels.

Excitatory amino-mediated responses also show significant age-dependent changes which may account for the peculiar phenomenology of infantile epilepsies. In particular NMDA receptor-mediated effects have been found in young animals to be less voltage-dependent than in adults, thus allowing more calcium to enter the postsynaptic neuron when glutamate is released.

Active and voltage-dependent transmembrane ionic exchanges are primarily or secondarily involved in epileptogenesis. Delayed maturation of Na-K-ATPase and glial cells results in immature ionic homoeostasis which may account for peculiar susceptibility of the young brain to epileptogenic agents.

Our present understanding of basic mechanisms of the epilepsies allows pharmacologists to design drugs with specific pharmacological action targeted on crucial epileptogenic factors. This approach has led to some promising results. A better knowledge of the fundamental steps of epileptogenesis in appropriate animal models, taking into account the influence of age-related factors, is a prerequisite for further progress in this direction.

The issue of excitotoxicity is widely discussed throughout the book and is specifically dealt with in the last chapter devoted to the developing brain. Several seizure-related factors lead to an intracellular rise of calcium, which can reach toxic concentrations in the cytoplasm. This risk is particularly high in the immature brain due to the overexpression and facilitation of the NMDA receptors, the depolarizing effect of GABA and the immaturity of the ionic homoeostasis. In spite of the existence of some protective factors such as better lactate transport out of the brain and immaturity of presynaptic glutamatergic terminals, neonatal seizures can thus result in brain damage and/or poor brain development. The results of the neurobiological studies of excitotoxicity in the developing brain may hopefully provide a basis for new strategies aimed to prevent the development of severe infantile epileptic encephalopathies and to alleviate their dramatic consequences.

The authors succeed in combining personal observations with a comprehensive review of the literature, thus providing the reader with an updated information on every topic.

The subsidy for publication by Wellcome Italia Spa is gratefully acknowledged.

We would like to thank the Publisher for the perfect and timely work. We also thank Mrs Maria Teresa Pasquali who collaborated in editing the manuscripts.

Giuliano Avanzini
Ruggero Fariello
Uwe Heinemann
Roberto Mutani

Opening remarks

V. La Grutta

Istituto di Fisiologia Umana G. Pagano, Palermo, Italy

Epilepsy is one of the commonest disorders of the nervous system, with an incidence, in Italy, of about 38 cases per 100,000 and an estimated prevalence of about six cases per 1000. These figures, in the first instance, give rise to complex actuarial considerations, and also, since the basic mechanisms and causes of the disorder are not completely known, remind us that an unequivocal and definitive therapeutic approach for all the various forms of epilepsy has not yet been devised.

In the last 20 years, great progress has been made in molecular genetics, neuroanatomy, biophysics, and neuroscience in general, which have made it possible to identify both specific neuronal relationships and many of the neurotransmitters and neuromodulators which are so important in the control of neuronal excitability and metabolism. These experimental findings have also turned out to be of great significance in the study of basic mechanisms of epileptic activity.

Convulsive activity in the brain does not diffuse in a non specific manner, but follows defined pathways. Particular subcortical circuits have been identified whose function is not only fundamental for the modulation and control of propagated convulsive activity, but also for their involvement in the mechanisms of action of anticonvulsant drugs. In this context, it seems worthwhile to recall some facts about nigro-striatal control of experimentally induced epileptiform activity, which have been derived from the experimental model known as 'focal hippocampal epilepsy'. Following localized threshold stimulation of the hippocampus by a convulsive agent, penicillin, regular and strictly focal spiking activity is obtained in the hippocampus. This model is extremely flexible and sensitive, allowing the observation of differential modulation as a result of electrical stimulation of specific structures or local injection of pharmacologically active substances. It is possible to observe inhibition (disappearance of spiking activity), moderate facilitation (increase in rate of spiking), or even a clear proconvulsivant action evidenced by diffusion and generalized seizures. In effect, spiking may be considered as the liberation of local circuits from control systems, for example GABAergic, with consequent predominance of the excitatory component (for example excitatory amino acids). Contrarily, electrical silence between spikes may be considered as a momentary predominance of inhibitory processes which oppose their generation and diffusion, for example by local GABAergic interneurons; I mean strategic structures within the circuit. Among the subcortical structures examined, the caudate nucleus exerts an effective inhibitory role against paroxysmal activity of hippocampal origin (La Grutta & Sabatino, 1988). This modulatory effect is brought about through GABAergic control of the medial septal nucleus, from which there is an efferent cholinergic projection. The globus pallidus, on the other hand, acting through the lateral habenula and the dorsal raphe nucleus, potentiates hippocampal epileptic activity. In particular, at the level of the raphe there is a synaptic mechanism which brings about a disinhibitory effect which is responsible for the facilitation of paroxysmal hippocampal activity induced from the pallidum and habenula. Pharmacological experiments have demonstrated the importance of excitatory amino acid neurotransmission between pallidum and habenula and between the latter and the raphe, emphasizing the fundamental role of excitatory amino acid antagonists, which are substances with anticonvulsant activity (Sabatino et al., 1991).

A series of experimental investigations has, furthermore, clarified the fundamental role of the substantia nigra as a centre of primary importance in the generation and diffusion of paroxysmal activity. Within the substantia nigra two components have been identified which can be distinguished from one another both by their afferent and efferent connections as well as by neurotransmitters involved. In particular, the pars reticulata, which is GABAergic in nature, sends projections to the thalamus and to the nuclei of the tectum and the superior colliculus. It modulates neocortical epileptic activity and its diffusion towards motor effectors. Recently, Karen Gale (1986) has also demonstrated the proconvulsivant action of the substantia nigra pars reticulata with respect to a localized area deep within the piriform cortex, which, because of its sensitivity to convulsivant agents, has been called the area tempesta. The pars compacta of the substantia nigra, on the other hand, uses dopamine as a neurotransmitter and sends its efferents to the striatum and limbic structures such as the hippocampus (Scatton et al., 1980). This nigral projection, together with the dopaminergic efferents from the ventral tegmental area (A10), controls the paroxysmal activity of the hippocampus (La Grutta & Sabatino, 1990). Furthermore, the crucial role played by the substantia nigra in the modulation of epileptic activity (for example, hippocampus and area tempesta) has finally been confirmed by biochemical studies which have shown an alteration in nigral transmission in animals which are genetically epileptic or have a long history of convulsive crises. In practice, it should be emphasized that the generation of epileptiform activity in neural structures depends on a local disturbance of neurotransmitter equilibrium, with diminution of inhibitory (e.g. GABA) and predominance of excitatory transmitters (e.g. excitatory amino acids). The final amplification of abnormal activity with diffusion to other structures, even if not to the motor target (cranial or spinal motoneurons), can be attributed to the activity of specific subcortical control circuits which modulate its propagation (Sabatino et al., 1988). It is evident that the individual chemical nature of receptors, together with specific sites of action of transmitters, is of considerable importance in terms of therapeutic potential, based on the use of molecules with agonist or antagonist activity in relation to the transmitters implicated.

In recent years, many sophisticated microphysiological neurochemical techniques have been employed to demonstrate the existence of neurochemical agents which are able to bring about long- or short-term changes in membrane ion flux, such as calcium, potassium, sodium, chloride and second messengers. These findings, together with those found as a result of experiments on excitatory amino acid transmission in the nervous system (Young & Faag, 1990), indubitably provide useful indications for a better comprehension of mechanisms which form the basis of the generation, diffusion, and maintenance of the epileptic discharge.

The study of genetic and environmental factors can also bring new contributions to the problem of the greater or lesser role of hereditary predisposition in determining the various forms of epilepsy. Presentations with new and surprising conclusions on the relationship between epileptogenesis and the development of the nervous system will be found to be particularly stimulating.

In conclusion, investigations on neuronal substrates, subcortical control circuits, basic biochemical mechanisms, the biophysical peculiarities of the epileptic neurons, and the findings of molecular genetics together constitute a valid basis for the attainment of better understanding in both the pharmacological and clinical fields, for the choice of antiepileptic therapy considered. It is worthwhile once again to emphasize, at this juncture, the value of basic research aimed at increasing our understanding of the clinical aspects of the condition.

References

Gale, K. (1986): Role of the substantia nigra in GABA-mediated anticonvulsant action. In: *Advances in neurology*, Vol. 44, eds. A.V. Delgado-Escueta, A.A. Ward, D.M. Woodbury & R.J. Porter, pp. 343–364. New York: Raven Press.

La Grutta, V. & Sabatino, M. (1988): Focal hippocampal epilepsy: effect of caudate stimulation. *Exp. Neurol.* **99**, 38–49.

La Grutta, V. & Sabatino, M. (1990): Substantia nigra-mediated anticonvulsant action: a possible role of a dopaminergic component. *Brain Res.* **515**, 87–93.

Sabatino, M., Ferraro, G. & La Grutta, V. (1991): Relay stations and neurotransmitters between the pallidal region and the hippocampus. *Electroencephalogr. Clin. Neurophysiol.* **78**, 302–310.

Sabatino, M., Gravante, G., Ferraro, G., Savatteri, V. & La Grutta, V. (1988): Inhibitory control by substantia nigra of generalized epilepsy in the cat. *Epilepsy Res.* **2**, 380–386.

Scatton, B., Simon, H., Le Moal, M. & Bischoff, S. (1980): Origin of dopaminergic innervation of the rat hippocampal formation. *Neurosci. Lett.* **18**, 125–131.

Young, A.B. & Faag, G.E. (1990): Excitatory amino acid receptors in the brain: membrane binding and receptor autoradiographic approaches. *TiPS* **11**, 126–133.

Chapter 1

Animal models of epilepsy

Roberto Mutani, Roberto Cantello, Maria Gianelli and Carlo Civardi

Department of Neurology, University School of Medicine, Novara, Italy

Summary

The paper is a review of some models of epilepsy, grouped according to their practical usefulness in studying specific epileptological problems. As far as basic mechanisms of focal epileptogenesis are concerned, there are models working through the blocking of inhibitory systems (mainly the GABA system) and the enhancement of excitatory systems (acetylcholine, excitatory amino acids). The cobalt and alumina models of chronic partial seizures are described. The iron model is a good model of post-traumatic epilepsy. Many models are of the generalized spike-and-wave pattern and they show that a leading role can be played by either subcortical or cortical or cortico-subcortical structures. Models of status epilepticus are reviewed. The kindling model is described from both the point of view of the possible relevance of kindling to human epileptogenesis and its usefulness for testing the antiepileptogenic and antiepileptic properties of new drugs.

Introduction

The present primary goals of animal models of epilepsy are the study of the basic mechanisms of epileptogenesis, a better understanding of the clinical epileptic seizures and syndromes, and the screening of potential new antiepileptic drugs. However, when the animal models were developed in the physiology laboratories in the last century, the goal was to get a better understanding of the function of the central nervous system. From this point of view, epilepsy can be considered, according to one of its smartest 'pupils', Wilder Penfield (1967), as 'the great teacher'. As Penfield wrote in 1954, 'the problems of epilepsy are the problems of the central nervous system . . . . It is as though the epileptic process were providing a demonstration of the function of the various parts of the nervous system'. For example, the observation in man of particular epileptic seizures, later called 'jacksonian' allowed Jackson to hypothesize the existence of motor cortical centres. But it was only later on that evidence of such centres was given by Fritsch & Hitzig (1870) who reproduced the seizures described by Jackson through the galvanic stimulation of the brain cortex in the dog.

With the discovery of the convulsant power of electrical stimulation the era of experimental epilepsy begins, and the brain, through the 'Rosetta stone of the stimulating electrode' (Purpura, 1953), has progressively revealed many of its secret functions. Through the microelectrode we learned to 'listen in on the private life of a single neuron' (Morrell, 1961). During the last three decades, the techniques of experimental epilepsy have multiplied and have been refined at an astonishing rate, along with the improvement of our knowledge of the basic events responsible for epilepsy and of the clinical epileptic syndromes, and with the appearance of new rationally developed antiepileptic drugs. It is through the models, and hopefully in the near future, that we will get a better understanding of the many and still unresolved epileptological problems. The present paper is intended not to be a long and boring list of models, but a review of some models from the point of view of their grouping in relationship to their practical usefulness in facing specific epileptical questions (Mutani et al., 1988).

Models for studying the basic mechanisms of focal epileptogenesis

The study of the basic mechanisms of epileptogenesis has represented and still represents the best utilization of the experimental models. When models are used for this purpose, the old problem of the ambiguous correlation between the experimental data and human epilepsy is, at least partially, overcome: actually there is no evidence that the basic mechanisms in a single neuron or a single neuronal aggregate involved in epileptogenesis are different according to the mammal species. From the models we learn that focal epileptogenesis can derive from two different types of mechanisms.

Blocking inhibitory systems

Impairment of GABA-mediated inhibition

GABA, synthetised in the brain from glutamic acid by glutamic acid decarboxylase (GAD) and metabolized by glutamic acid transaminase (GABA-T), is the major inhibitory neurotransmitter. It acts via $GABA_A$ receptors to open Cl^- channels and hyperpolarize the membrane, and via $GABA_B$ receptors to open K^+ or Ca^{2+} channels (Bormann, 1988). Impairment in the function of GABA neurons leads to seizures: compounds which diminish GABA synthesis through GAD inhibition (isoniazid, allylglycine) or which impair GABA receptor function (bicuculline, penicillin, picrotoxin, some beta-carbolines) induce epileptogenesis.

The model using penicillin topically applied to neocortex or injected in the medium of preparation *in vitro* has been the most widely used. In the cat, penicillin (a piece of gelfoam soaked with 50,000–100,000 U/ml of sodium penicillin applied to the pia) rapidly diffuses into the cortex; after a few minutes, when it reaches layers III–IV, interictal spikes begin to occur followed by ictal activity. The convulsive effect of penicillin topically applied to the cortex of monkey and man was reported by Walker et al. (1945).

Matsumoto & Ajmone-Marsan (1964) described the paroxysmal depolarization shift with burst firing as the microelectrode correlate of the EEG interictal spike. Wong & Prince (1979) showed that the effect of penicillin is due to a bicuculline-like block of GABA-mediated inhibition. The development of cobalt and alumina foci in neocortex is paralleled by a decrease of all aspects of GABAergic transmission (GAD activity, GABA levels and uptake) (Ribak et al., 1979; Ross & Craig, 1981a, b; Bakay & Harris, 1981). Ribak et al. (1989) provided an elegant demonstration that a selective decrease in the number of GABAergic cells occurs in monkeys with previous seizures implanted with alumina gel.

Though not confirmed by Sherwin & Van Gelder (1986), neurochemical findings indicate an alteration of GABAergic neurons in epileptic tissue specimens of refractory temporal lobe patients (Lloyd et al., 1984). The reported data, showing that focal epileptogenesis in acute and chronic models and in man is accompanied by the impairment of GABA-mediated inhibition, were the major factor pushing research towards new and rationally developed antiepileptic drugs capable of enhancing GABA transmission (e.g. gamma-vinyl-GABA) (review in Mutani et al., 1991).

However, as pointed out by Gale (1989), increased GABA transmission does not always result in inhibition of brain excitability. In some areas of the brain (e.g. caudate nucleus, superior colliculus), the increase of GABA transmission is actually proconvulsant. The fact that GABA-elevating drugs exert a net anticonvulsant effect suggests that actions at anticonvulsant sites outweigh the actions at proconvulsant sites. Two brain areas, substantia nigra and area tempestas, are examples of specific brain regions where increases of GABA can achieve an anticonvulsant effect. Substantia nigra output exerts a proconvulsant effect, lowering the convulsive threshold and facilitating discharge propagation, and is inhibited by GABA (Garant & Gale, 1987). The area tempestas participates in the triggering and initiation of seizures associated with limbic and forebrain circuits. GABA elevation in the area tempestas prevents seizures in various models (Piredda et al., 1987).

Impairment of glycine-mediated inhibition

Topical strychnine is the oldest chemical convulsant used to elicit seizures. In the dog, Baglioni & Magnini (1909) described the 'strychnic clonus' after application of strychnine to the motor cortex. This agent was used in the classic studies on reflex epilepsy by Amantea (1921) and Clementi (1929), and on the contralateral propagation of the epileptic discharge by Gozzano (1935) and Mc-Culloch (1949). Strychnine produces paroxysmal depolarization shifts and epileptiform firing patterns with topical administration in several species (Ajmone-Marsan, 1969). Strychnine, a relatively selective antagonist of the inhibition exerted post-synaptically by glycine in various brain and especially spinal areas, produces a blockade of inhibitory post-synaptic potential (IPSPs) through blockade of chloride conductance (Faber & Klee, 1974). Other proconvulsant effects of strychnine on membrane properties, ion conduction and neurotransmitter systems have been reported (review in Faingold, 1987).

Enhancement of excitatory systems

Acetylcholine

Convulsions due to potentiation of cholinergic transmission can be obtained by topical application of cholinesterase inhibitors (physostigmine, eserine), cholinomimetic agents (pilocarpine, acetylcarnitine) and muscarinic receptor agonists (carbachol) (review in Woodbury, 1980).

Excitatory amino acids

Systemic or topical application of Glu/Asp produces convulsions in animals (Johnston, 1972). Kainate, an excitotoxic analogue of Glu, induces prolonged status epilepticus (Ben Ari et al., 1979). Dodd & Bradford (1976) found excessive release of Glu in the brain rendered epileptic by topical application of cobalt. In the feline generalized penicillin epilepsy model and in the pre-epileptic period, Van Gelder et al. (1983) found a decreased brain content of Glu/Asp, interpreted as due to loss from the interneuronal compartment into the extracellular space. Glu has been found to be elevated in the serum of patients with absence seizures (Monaco et al., 1991). Increased levels of quinolate (Feldblum et al., 1988), an excitotoxic agent proposed as an endogenous N-methyl-d-aspartate (NMDA) receptor agonist, and controversial data on Glu/Asp levels (Van Gelder et al., 1972; Perry et al., 1975), have been reported in epileptic human brain tissue. The receptors for excitatory amino acids are currently divided into at least three categories: NMDA, kainate and quisqualate. Glu activates all three types of receptors, whereas Asp activates NMDA receptors selectively. NMDA receptors under baseline conditions are blocked by physiological concentrations of Mg^{2+}. This block is voltage-dependent and, when neurons are depolarized, they become responsive to NMDA agonists. Thus, it has been postulated that NMDA receptors may be more involved in epileptiform activity than in background synaptic activity (Dichter, 1989). Also, NMDA receptor activation plays a crucial role in long-term potentiation, learning and memory, and kindling. An excessive NMDA receptor activation with massive Ca^{2+} influx is thought to occur during repeated seizures and brain ischaemia (Meldrum, 1988), and would be responsible for neuronal damage and the long-lasting plastic changes reinforcing the epileptogenic conditions as seizures keep recurring (Gloor, 1989).

Impairment of excitatory amino acid transmission can be achieved by (i) inhibition of synaptic release; the novel anticonvulsant lamotrigine is a potent inhibitor of Glu release. (ii) Block of

NMDA receptors. Many NMDA receptor antagonists are presently under preclinical evaluation as anticonvulsant and cerebroprotective agents (review in Chapman & Meldrum, 1991).

Models of chronic partial seizures

The reproducibility of human partial simple seizures is fairly good. There is no relevant difference, for instance, between the clinical semiology of the jacksonian fit in the monkey and in man, apart from the more important foot clonic jerks in the monkey as a consequence of the greater extension of the corresponding somatotopic motor cortical area. The reproducibility appears strongly ambiguous, on the other hand, in the case of partial complex seizures involving brain structures implicated in affective-instinctive-mnesic integration. In the cat, amygdaloid seizures, for example, include motor automatisms, and it remains questionable if these feline automatisms are the equivalent of the automatisms of human partial complex seizures. In spite of these limitations, the models of chronic partial seizures have produced advances in the knowledge of the mechanisms implied in temporal lobe epilepsy (Gastaut et al., 1958) and in the propagation of the discharge (Jasper, 1969), of the biochemical changes associated with epileptogenesis (Emson, 1978), and of the facilitatory or inhibitory action exerted by other cerebral structures on the focus. Dow et al. (1962) and Mutani et al. (1969) described the cerebellar inhibitory influence on the cortical and rhinencephalic focus, with the subsequent controversial clinical applications (review in Cooper et al., 1974). The most widely used models for chronic partial seizures are the cobalt and the alumina ones.

Cobalt model

After the discovery of the convulsant effect of cobalt (Kopeloff, 1960), the partial seizures obtained in the cat by topical application of cobalt on the motor cortex and into rhinencephalic structures were described by Henjyoji & Dow (1965) and Mutani (1967a, b). In the cat, seizures begin a few days after implant and last for months. Cobalt epileptogenic action has been associated with decrease of brain monoaminergic, cholinergic and GABAergic activities, decrease of Glu/Asp and taurine, increase of glutamine and glycine. At the cellular level, cobalt would induce a blockade of chloride active extrusion mechanisms and of Ca^{2+}-activated potassium conductance (review in Craig & Colasanti, 1987).

Alumina model

Aluminium (Al) was the first metal demonstrated to be epileptogenic when applied directly to the cerebral cortex of monkeys (Kopeloff et al., 1942) in the form of Al cream or gel. It is epileptogenic in the rabbit, dog and cat but not in the rat. In the monkey, seizures develop many months after implant and are persistent throughout the lifetime of the animal. By contrast, convulsions develop in cats after 1 month but terminate after 2 months from the implant (review in Craig & Colasanti, 1987). Al epileptogenic action has been associated with the gliotic changes occurring at the implant area and the selective vulnerability of GABA interneurons to Al with subsequent decrease of all aspects of GABAergic transmission in monkeys with previous seizures (Ribak et al., 1989). Intracellular recordings of hippocampal slices, prepared from intracisternally $AlCl_3$ intoxicated rabbits, have provided evidence that Al exerts its epileptogenic action through multiple neurotoxic mechanisms involving membrane electrotonic shortening and blockage of Ca^{2+}-activated K^+ conductance (Franceschetti et al., 1990).

Models of post-traumatic epilepsy

In cats, rats and guinea-pigs intracortical injection of blood, heme compounds and $FeCl_2$–$FeCl_3$ produces a chronic epileptogenic focus (review in Willmore, 1990). This focus has pathological features similar to those of human post-traumatic focus and electrophysiological patterns of discharge similar to those of human foci (Reid & Sypert, 1980). The iron hypothesis of post-traumatic epilepsy (PTE) starts from the consideration that focal brain damage with blood extravasation into brain tissue is the main provocative factor of human PTE (Jennet, 1975). Red blood cell extravasation is followed by decompartmentalization of ferrous compounds from haemoglobin and deposition of iron into the lipid-rich environment of neural tissue.

Haber–Weiss iron-catalysed reactions at phospholipid membranes immediately form peroxidative agents such as $O_2^{\cdot -}$, H_2O_2 and $OH^{\cdot}$. These free radicals continue lipid peroxidation, generating a self-sustained reaction leading to more and more extensive neuronal membrane disruption up to cell death (Willmore & Dubin, 1982).

Though the specific cellular mechanism for the epileptogenic effect of iron remains unknown, theoretically any treatment designed to prevent lipid peroxidation should be effective in preventing iron epileptogenic injury. Antiperoxidant agents (such as tocopherol associated with selenium, deferoxamine, steroids, superoxide dismutases) should be given at the moment of the injury, in view of the immediate development of lipid peroxidation. Many antiperoxidant agents have been and are presently under evaluation for prophylaxis of iron epilepsy, and some of them are considered for prophylaxis of human PTE (review in Mutani et al., 1992).

Models of generalized spike-and-wave pattern

This is one of the most fascinating topics in experimental epilepsy. From the experiments of Jasper & Drooglever-Fortuyn (1946) to the feline generalized penicillin epilepsy of Prince & Farrell (1969) and the strain of Wistar rat inbred in the Strasbourg Centre de Neurochemie, the history of the attempts to reproduce the features of human petit mal epilepsy is rich with tens of different models of generalized SW pattern. Some of them are acute and therefore can be proposed as models of seizures rather than models of epilepsies. But, in any case, none of the chronic and genetic models can reproduce the complex of signs and symptoms which characterize the human syndrome, in view of the differences between man and models in terms of the anatomophysiological organization of the central nervous system. However, it is possible that species-related differences may lead to different expression of common pathophysiological mechanisms, which can be profitably investigated in animals (Avanzini & Marescaux, 1991). The models of generalized SW pattern show that, according to the specific model, a leading role can be played by subcortical, cortical and cortico-subcortical structures.

Subcortical structures

In cats, electrical stimulation of midline thalamic nuclei produces SW discharges (Jasper & Drooglever-Fortuyn, 1946) accompanied, in the unanaesthetized animal, by absence seizures (Hunter & Jasper, 1949). A similar picture was obtained by introduction of penicillin (Ralston & Ajmone-Marsan, 1956) and alumina cream (Guerrero-Figueroa et al., 1963) in the same nuclei. Bilateral SW patterns associated with myoclonic jerks were obtained by Cesa-Bianchi et al. (1967) by introduction of cobalt in the midline thalamic and lower brainstem structures of the cat.

Recently, in Wistar rats, the nucleus reticularis thalami (RTN) has been identified as a key structure in regulating SW discharges. RTN neurons are characterized by low-threshold Ca^{2+} conductances, which enables them to produce 6–8 Hz oscillatory activities (review in Avanzini & Marescaux, 1991).

Cortical structures

In cats, Marcus showed that it was possible to obtain generalized SW discharges by means of bilateral and symmetrical cortical foci, both acute (Marcus & Watson, 1966) and chronic (Marcus, 1972). Mutani et al. (1973) obtained a similar picture with asymmetrical chronic cortical foci. In this study evidence was presented for a major role played by corpus callosum in mediating bisynchrony of discharge.

Cortico-subcortical structures

In the feline generalized penicillin epilepsy model (Prince & Farrel, 1969) evidence has been given that SW discharges are due to cortico-subcortical interactions. Application to subcortical structures and ventriculo- cisternal perfusion of penicillin (Fisher & Prince, 1977; Gloor *et al.*, 1977) do not produce SW discharges. By contrast, this pattern is obtained by diffuse bilateral application of penicillin to the cortex (Fisher & Prince, 1977). This observation, associated with the finding that after parenteral penicillin the paroxysmal discharges first appear in the cortex (Gloor *et al.*, 1977), leads to the conclusion that parenteral penicillin produces a mild, diffuse epileptogenic state in the cortex (Quesney & Gloor, 1978); in response to afferent subcortical volleys (Quesney *et al.*, 1977) this would give rise to SW discharges. Intracortical and possibly interhemispheric mechanisms would play a major role in the synchronization of the rythms (Fisher & Prince, 1977). The corpus callosum plays a major role in mediating bisynchrony of discharge, which is disrupted by callosal split (Mutani, 1980).

Pharmacological models

Some direct GABA agonists such as (tetrahydroisoxazolopyridinol) THIP and muscimol can induce SW discharges in naive animals (Golden & Fariello, 1984) and enhance epileptic activity in models of absence seizures (feline generalized penicillin epilepsy, Wistar rats)(review in Avanzini & Marescaux, 1991). This is in agreement with the hypothesis that an increase in GABAergic transmission may be involved in the pathogenesis of generalized SW discharges (Gloor & Fariello, 1988).

Models of status epilepticus

Systemic administration of bicuculline produces a convulsive generalized status, while systemic administration of penicillin produces a nonconvulsive generalized status. Kainic acid is a structural analogue of glutamate with a powerful excitatory and neurotoxic action. Systemically administered, it penetrates well into the brain, and provokes a partial status epilepticus of multifocal, mostly limbic, origin, with and without secondary generalization (review in Faingold, 1987).

The models of status epilepticus have provided relevant data on the mechanisms of neuronal damage (review in Delgado-Escueta *et al.*, 1982). By means of the bicuculline model, it has been possible to clarify the role played by systemic (hyperthermia, hypoglycaemia, hypoxaemia, lactic acidosis) versus intrinsic brain (inhibition of protein synthesis, deficit of high energy substrates, vasogenic oedema) factors (Meldrum, 1983). The harmful intrinsic brain factors may cause serious permanent impairment when acting on the immature developing brain (Wasterlain & Dwyer, 1983). The kainic model has allowed precise investigations on the role of neuronal hyperactivity as a factor of metabolic damage. Meldrum (1983), following the observation of 'selectively vulnerable' neurons during the kainic-induced status, proposed the hypothesis of the excess of NMDA receptor stimulation with massive Ca^{2+} influx and subsequent metabolic derangement.

The kindling model

The term kindling (Goddard, 1967) refers to a phenomenon perhaps related to learning and memory (Majkowsy, 1989), in which the short, intermittent and subthreshold electrical stimulation of a brain structure induces a progressive and plastic increase in brain excitability. This is shown by the appearance of a longer and longer afterdischarge, with subsequent appearance of clinical ictal symptomatology, at first partial and then generalized. There is a graduation of kindling from stage 0 to stage 5 (Racine, 1972a, b), and when an animal is at stage 5, it is said to be fully kindled. This enhanced excitability is long-lasting, perhaps permanent. If an animal has reached stage 5 and is left unstimulated for 1 year, it will respond with a class 5 seizure when stimulated again.

Kindling can be also induced by repeated subthreshold application of chemical convulsants to a

particular brain structure (review in Wasterlain *et al.*, 1986). It can be initiated with a convulsant and concluded with another, or initiated electrically and concluded chemically. Interhemispheric transfer has been shown, i.e. kindling of the left amygdala is facilitated by previous kindling of the right amygdala.

The many and extensive reviews published on the cellular and molecular mechanisms of kindling (McNamara, 1986, 1987); Wasterlain *et al.*, 1986; Moshè & Ludwig, 1988), agree in considering these mechanisms still elusive and obscure. Long-term potentiation (LTP) may share with kindling some common underlying mechanisms, though LTP is not necessary to, and cannot completely account for, kindling (Cain, 1989). Though NMDA receptor activation seems to play a major role, many transmitters (GABA, norepinephrine, serotonine, acetylcholine) are probably involved in kindling (McNamara *et al.*, 1987). Sprouting, axonal growth and synaptic reorganization have been described in the kindled structure (Sutula, 1990). Plastic changes would involve second messenger systems, with action on the nuclear DNA (*C-fos* gene) and production of C-fos protein (Dragunow & Robertson, 1987).

Though there is no evidence of kindling occurrence in humans, the issue of the possible relevance of kindling to human epileptogenesis is still controversial. According to Fariello & Golden (1985), drawing a parallel between the two phenomena is 'a matter of faith rather than science'. These authors emphasize that: (i) there is no available evidence that the nature of the transition from the pre-afterdischarge to the afterdischarge phase has anything to do with human epileptogenesis; (ii) the ingravescent progression of epileptic events observed in kindling is only exceptionally encountered in clinical practice, and actually the opposite phenomenon is at least as frequently found. On the contrary, anecdotal observations by Stramka *et al.* (1977), after thalamic stimulation for pain relieving, and by Morrell (1979), in a patient with temporal lobe tumour, would raise the possibility of the occurrence of kindling in humans. According to Wasterlain *et al.* (1986) and Sutula (1990), kindling-like phenomena would take place in the silent period between a potentially epileptogenic brain insult and the development of epilepsy. Such a mechanism would possibly play a role in the development of post-traumatic epilepsy and temporal lobe epilepsy with mesial temporal sclerosis due to perinatal hypoxic-ischaemic brain injury. Despite our incomplete understanding of the basic mechanisms of kindling and the unproven occurrence of kindling in man, this model is recommended to test the antiepileptogenic and antiepileptic properties of new drugs. Conventional and new drugs do not necessarily show both actions (review in McNamara, 1989 and in Mutani *et al.*, 1991). A good action against both the development of kindling (antiepileptogenic) and the kindled seizures (antiepileptic) is shown by phenobarbitone, valproate, benzodiazepines, GABA-agonists including gamma-vinyl-GABA, and lamotrigine. Phenytoin and carbamazepine only have an antiepileptic action while, on the contrary, the NMDA receptor antagonist MK-801 and the alpha$_2$ agonist clonidine show a stronger antiepileptogenic action.

References

Amantea G. (1921): Über experimentelle beim Versuchstier infolge afferenter Reize erzeugte Epilepsie. *Pflugers Arch.* **188**, 287–297.

Ajmone-Marsan C. (1969): Acute effects of topical epileptogenic agents. In: *Basic mechanisms of the epilepsies*, eds. H.H. Jasper, A.A. Ward & A. Pope, pp. 102–140. Boston: Little, Brown and Co.

Avanzini, G. & Marescaux, C. (1991): Genetic animal models for generalized non-convulsive epilepsies and new antiepileptic drugs. In: *New antiepileptic drugs*, eds. F. Pisani, E. Perucca, G. Avanzini & A. Richens, pp. 29–38. Amsterdam: Elsevier.

Baglioni, S. & Magnini, M. (1909): Azione di alcune sostanze chimiche sulla zona eccitabile della corteccia cerebrale del cane. *Arch. Fisiol.* **6**, 240–249.

Bakay, R.A & Harris, A.B. (1981): Neurotransmitters, receptors and biochemical changes in monkey cortical epileptic foci. *Brain Res.* **206**, 387–408.

Ben Ari, Y., Trembley, E., Ottersen, O.P. & Naquet, R. (1979): Evidence suggesting secondary epileptogenic lesions after kainic acid: pretreatment with diazepam reduces distant but not local brain damage. *Brain Res.* **165**, 362–365.

Bormann, J. (1988): Electrophysiology of $GABA_A$ and $GABA_B$ receptor subtypes. *TINS* **11**, 112–117.

Cain, D.P. (1989): Long-term potentiation and kindling: how similar are the mechanisms? *TINS* **12**, 1–6.

Cesa-Bianchi, M.G., Mancia, M. & Mutani, R. (1967): Experimental epilepsy induced by cobalt powder in lower brain-stem and thalamic structures. *Electroencephalogr. Clin. Neurophysiol.* **22**, 525–536.

Chapman, A.G. & Meldrum, B.S. (1991): Excitatory aminoacids in epilepsy and novel antiepileptic drugs. In: *New antiepileptic drugs*, eds. F. Pisani, E. Perucca, G. Avanzini & A. Richens, pp. 39–48. Amsterdam: Elsevier.

Clementi, A. (1929): Stricninizzazione della sfera corticale visiva ed epilessia sperimentale da stimoli luminosi. *Arch. Fisiol.* **27**, 356–387.

Cooper, I.S., Amin, S., Gilman, S. & Waltz, J.M. (1974): The effect of chronic stimulation of cerebellar cortex on epilepsy in man. In: *The cerebellum, epilepsy and behaviour*, eds. I.S. Cooper & M. Riklan, pp. 119–171. New York: Plenum Press.

Craig, C.R., Colasanti, B.K. (1987): Experimental epilepsy induced by direct topical placement of chemical agents on the cerebral cortex. In: *Neurotransmitters and epilepsy*, eds. P.C. Jobe & H.E. Laird, pp. 191–214. Clifton, New Jersey: Humana Press.

Delgado-Escueta, A.V., Wasterlain, C.G., Treiman, D.M & Porter, R.J. (1982): In: *Status epilepticus, mechanisms of brain damage and treatment (Advances in neurology)*, Vol. 34. New York: Raven Press.

Dichter, M.A. (1989): Cellular mechanisms of epilepsy and potential new treatment strategies. *Epilepsia* **30** (Suppl. 1), S3–S12.

Dodd, P.R. & Bradford, H.F. (1976): Release of amino-acids from the maturing cobalt-induced epileptic focus. *Brain Res.* **111**, 377–388.

Dow, R.S., Fernandez-Guardiola, A. & Manni, E. (1962): The influence of the cerebellum on experimental epilepsy. *Electroencephalogr. Clin. Neurophysiol.* **14**, 383–398.

Dragunow, M. & Robertson, H.A. (1988): Localization and induction of C-fos protein-like immunoreactive material in the nuclei of adult mammalian neurons. *Brain Res.* **440**, 252–260.

Emson, P.C. (1978): Biochemical and metabolic changes in epilepsy. In: *Taurine and metabolic disorders*, eds. A. Barbeau & J.R. Huxtable, pp. 319–338. New York: Raven Press.

Faber, D.S. & Klee, M.R. (1974): Strychnine interactions with acetylcholine, dopamine and serotonin receptors in Aplysyia neurons. *Brain Res.* **65**, 109–126.

Faingold, C.L. (1987): Seizures induced by convulsant drugs. In: *Neurotransmitters and epilepsy*, eds. P.C. Jobe & H.E. Laird, pp. 215–276. Clifton, New Jersey: Humana Press.

Fariello, R.G. & Golden, G.T. (1985): Electroencephalographic models of epilepsy. In: *Epilepsy and GABA receptor agonists*, eds. G. Bartholini, L. Bossi, K.G. Lloyd & P.L. Morselli, pp. 139–148. New York: Raven Press.

Feldblum, S., Rougier, A., Loiseau, H., Cohadon, F., Morselli, P.L. & Lloyd, K.G. (1988): Quinolinic-phosphoribosyl transferase activity is decreased in epileptic human tissue. *Epilepsia* **29**, 523–529.

Fisher, R.S. & Prince, D.A. (1977): Spike-wave rhythms in cat cortex induced by parenteral penicillin. *Electroencephalogr. Clin. Neurophysiol.* **42**, 608–624.

Franceschetti, S., Bugiani, O., Panzica, F., Tagliavini, F. & Avanzini, G. (1990): Changes in excitability of CA1 pyramidal neurons in slices prepared from $AlCl_3$-treated rabbits. *Epilepsy Res.* **6**, 39–48.

Fritsch, G. & Hitzig, E. (1870): Über die elektrische Erregbarkeit des Grosshirns. *Arch. Anat. Physiol.* **37**, 300–332.

Gale, K. (1989): GABA in epilepsy: the pharmacologic basis. *Epilepsia* **30** (Suppl. 3), S1–S11.

Garant, D.S. & Gale, K. (1987): Substantia nigra-mediated anticonvulsant actions: role of nigral output pathways. *Exp. Neurol.* **97**, 143–149.

Gastaut, H., Meyer, R., Naquet, R., Cavanagh, J.B. & Beck, E. (1958): Clinical, electroencephalographic and anatomopathological study of psychomotor epilepsy induced in the cat by injection of alumina cream. In: *Temporal lobe epilepsy*, eds. M. Baldwin & P. Bayley, pp. 240–267. Springfield, Ill.: Charles C. Thomas.

Gloor, P., Quesney, L.F. & Zumstein, H. (1977): Pathophysiology of generalized penicillin epilepsy in the cat: the role of cortical and subcortical structures. *Electroencephalogr. Clin. Neurophysiol.* **43**, 79–94.

Gloor, P. & Fariello, R.G. (1988): Generalized epilepsy: some of its cellular mechanisms differ from those of focal epilepsy. *TINS* **11**, 63–68.

Gloor, P. (1989): Epilepsy: relationships between electrophysiology and intracellular mechanisms involving second messengers and gene expression. *Can. J. Neurol. Sci.* **16**, 8–21.

Goddard, G.V. (1967): Development of epileptic seizures through brain stimulation at low intensities. *Nature* **214**, 1020–1021.

Golden, G.T. & Fariello, R.G. (1984): Epileptogenic action of some direct GABA agonists: effect of manipulation of the GABA and glutamate systems. In: *Neurotransmitters, seizures and epilepsy II*, eds. R.G. Fariello, P.L. Morselli, K.G. Lloyd, L.F. Quesney & J. Engel, pp. 237–244. New York: Raven Press.

Gozzano, M. (1935): Ricerche sui fenomeni elettrici della corteccia cerebrale. *Riv. Neurol.* **8**, 216–261.

Henjyoji, E.Y. & Dow, R.S. (1965): Cobalt induced seizures in the cat. *Electroencephalogr. Clin. Neurophysiol.* **19**, 152–161.

Guerrero-Figueroa, R., Barros, A., De Balbian Vester, F. & Heath, R.G. (1963): Experimental 'petit mal' in kittens. *Arch. Neurol.* **9**, 297–306.

Hunter, J. & Jasper H.H. (1949): Effects of thalamic stimulation in unanesthetized animals. *Electroencephalogr. Clin. Neurophysiol.* **1**, 305–324.

Jasper, H.H. & Droogleever-Fortuyn, J. (1946): Experimental studies on the functional anatomy of petit mal epilepsy. *Res. Publ. Ass. Res. Nerv. Ment. Dis.* **26**, 272–298.

Jasper, H.H. (1969): Mechanisms of propagation: extracellular studies. In: *Basic mechanisms of the epilepsies*, eds. H.H. Jasper *et al.*, pp. 421–440. Boston: Little, Brown and Co.

Jennet, W.B. (1975): *Epilepsy after non-missile head injuries.* pp. 1–125. London: Heinemann.

Johnston, G.A.R. (1972): Convulsions induced in 10-day-old rats by intraperitoneal injection of monosodium glutamate and related excitant aminoacids. *Biochem. Pharmacol.* **22**, 137.

Kopeloff, L.M., Barrera, S.E. and Kopeloff, N. (1942): Recurrent convulsive seizures in animals produced by immunologic and chemical means. *Am. J. Psychiatr.* **98**, 881–902.

Kopeloff L.M. (1960): Experimental epilepsy in the mouse. *Proc. Soc. Exp. Biol.* (New York) **104**, 500–504.

Lloyd, K.G., Munari, C., Bossi, L. & Morselli, P.L. (1984): The GABA hypothesis of human epilepsy: neurochemical evidence from surgically resected identified foci. In: *Neurotransmitters, seizures and epilepsy II*, eds. R.G. Fariello, P.L. Morselli, K.G. Lloyd, L.F. Quesney & J. Engel, pp. 285–294. New York: Raven Press.

Majkowski, J. (1989): Kindling and memory. In: *The clinical relevance of kindling*, eds. T.G. Bolwig & M.R. Trimble, pp. 87–101. London: Wiley.

Marcus, E.M. & Watson, C.W. (1966): Bilateral synchronous spike wave electrographic patterns in the cat: interaction of bilateral cortical foci in the intact, the bilateral cortical callosal and adiencephalic preparation. *Arch. Neurol.* **14**, 601–610.

Marcus, E.M. (1972): Experimental models of petit mal epilepsy. A manual for the laboratory worker. In: *Experimental epilepsy*, eds. D.P. Purpura *et al.*, pp. 113–146. New York: Raven Press.

Matsumoto, H. & Ajmone-Marsan, C. (1964): Cortical cellular phenomena in experimental epilepsy: interictal manifestations. *Exp. Neurol.* **9**, 286–304.

McCulloch, W.S. (1949): Cortico-cortical connections. In: *The precentral motor cortex*, ed. P.C. Bucy, pp. 211–242. Urbana, Ill.: University of Illinois Press.

McNamara, J.O. (1986): Kindling model of epilepsy. In: *Basic mechanisms of the epilepsies. Molecular and cellular approaches (Advances in neurology)*, Vol. 44, eds. A.V. Delgado-Escueta, A.A. Ward, D.M. Woodbury & R.J. Porter, pp. 303–318. New York: Raven Press.

McNamara, J.O, Bonhaus, D.W., Crain, B.J., Geleman, R.C & Shin, C. (1987): Biochemical and pharmacologic studies of neurotransmitters in the kindling model. In: *Neurotransmitters and epilepsy*, eds. P.C. Jobe & H.E. Laird, pp. 115–160. Clifton, New Jersey: Humana Press.

McNamara, J.O. (1989): Development of new pharmacological agents for epilepsy: lessons from the kindling model. *Epilepsia* **30** (Suppl. 1), S13–S18.

Meldrum, B.S. (1983): Metabolic factors during prolonged seizures and their relation to nerve cell death. (1982): In: *Status epilepticus, mechanisms of brain damage and treatment (Advances in neurology)*, Vol. 34, eds. A.V. Delgado-Escueta, C.G. Wasterlain, D.M. Treiman & R.J. Porter. pp. 261–276. New York: Raven Press.

Meldrum, B.S. (1988): Excitatory aminoacids in neurological disease. *Curr. Opin. Neurol. Neurosurg.* **1**, 563–568.

Monaco, F., Gianelli, M., Naldi, P., Schiavella, P., Cantello, R., Torta, R., Zanalda, E., Verz, L. & Mutani R. (1991): Aminoacidi plasmatici in pazienti con epilessia generalizzata primaria e loro parenti di primo grado: studio sull'influenza dell'acido valproico. *Boll. Lega. It. Epil.* **74**, 183–187.

Morrell, F. (1961): Microelectrode studies in chronic epileptic foci. *Epilepsia* **2**, 81–88.

Morrell, F. (1979): Human secondary epileptogenic lesion. *Neurology* **19**, 558.

Moshé, L. & Ludwig, N. (1988): Kindling. In: *Recent advances in epilepsy*, eds. T. Pedley & B.S. Meldrum, pp. 21–44. Edinburgh: Curchill Livingstone.

Mutani, R. (1967a): Cobalt experimental amygdaloid epilepsy in the cat. *Epilepsia* **8**, 73–92.

Mutani, R. (1967b): Cobalt experimental hippocampal epilepsy in the cat. *Epilepsia* **8**, 223–240.

Mutani, R. (1969): L' epilessia da foci sperimentali. In: *L'epilessia*, eds. E. Lugaresi & P. Pazzaglia, pp. 29–59. Bologna: Gaggi.

Mutani, R., Bergamini, L. & Diriguzzi, T. (1969): Experimental evidence for the existence of an extrarhinencephalic control of the activity of the cobalt rhinencephalic epileptogenic focus. *Epilepsia* **10**, 351–362.

Mutani, R., Bergamini, L., Fariello, G. & Quattroccolo, G. (1973): Bilateral synchrony of epileptic discharge associated with chronic asymmetrical cortical foci. *Electroencephalogr. Clin. Neurophysiol.* **34**, 53–59.

Mutani, R. (1980): The role of corpus callosum in the interaction of multiple epileptogenic areas in neocortex. In: *Advances in epileptology*, eds. R. Canger, F. Angeleri & J.K. Penry, pp. 1–7. New York: Raven Press.

Mutani, R., Monaco, F. & Gentile, S. (1988): The experimental models of epilepsy: a critical review. In: *The rational basis of the surgical treatment of the epilepsies*, ed. G. Broggi, pp. 15–25. London: John Libbey.

Mutani, R., Cantello, R., Gianelli, M. & Bettucci, D. (1991): Rational basis for the development of new antiepileptic drugs. In: *New antiepileptic drugs. Epilepsy research 1991*, eds. F. Pisani, E. Perucca, G. Avanzini & A. Richens, (Suppl. 3): 23–28.

Mutani, R., Monaco, F., Cantello, R., Gianelli, M. & Bettucci, D. (1992): Pharmacological prophylaxis of post-traumatic epileptogenesis: an update on the experimental models. In: *Pharmacological prophylaxis of post-traumatic epilepsy*, ed. L. Murri, pp. 1–6. Ospedaletti (Italy): Pacini.

Penfield, W. (1954): Introduction. In: *The epilepsies, electro-clinical correlations*, ed. H. Gastaut, pp. 1–12. Springfield, Ill.: Charles Thomas.

Penfield, W. (1967): Epilepsy, the great teacher. The progress of one pupil. *Acta. Neurol. Scand.* **43**, 1–10.

Perry, T.L., Hansen, S., Kennedy, J., Wada, J.A. & Thompson, G.B. (1975): Aminoacids in human epileptogenic foci. *Arch. Neurol.* **32**, 752–754.

Piredda, S., Pavlick, M. & Gale, K. (1987): Anticonvulsant effects of GABA elevation in the deep prepiriform cortex. *Epilepsy Res.* **1**, 102–107.

Prince, D.A. & Farrell, D. (1969): Centrencephalic spike and wave discharges following parenteral penicillin injection in the cat. *Neurology* **19**, 309–310.

Purpura, D.P. (1953): An historical study of neurophysiologic concepts in epilepsy. *Epilepsia* **2**, 115–126.

Quesney, L.F., Gloor, P. & Zumstein, A. (1977): Pathophysiology of generalized penicillin epilepsy in the cat: the role of cortical and subcortical structures. *Electroencephalogr. Clin. Neurophysiol.* **42**, 640–655.

Quesney, L.F. & Gloor, P. (1978): Generalized penicillin epilepsy in the cat: correlation between electrophysiological data and distribution of 14–C penicillin in the brain. *Epilepsia* **19**, 35–45.

Racine, R.J. (1972a): Modification of seizure activity by electrical stimulation. I. After-discharge threshold. *Electroencephalogr. Clin. Neurophysiol.* **32**, 269–279.

Racine, R.J. (1972b): Modification of seizure activity by electrical stimulation. II. Motor seizures. *Electroencephalogr. Clin. Neurophysiol.* **32**, 281–294.

Ralston, B.L. & Ajmone-Marsan, C. (1956): Thalamic control of certain normal and abnormal cortical rhythms. *Electroencephalogr. Clin. Neurophysiol.* **8**, 559–582.

Reid, S.A. & Sypert, G.W. (1980): Acute $FeCl_3$-induced epileptogenic foci in cats: electrophysiological analyses. *Brain Res.* **188**, 531–542.

Ribak, C.E., Harris, C.B., Vaughn, J. & Roberts, E. (1989): Inhibitory GABAergic nerve terminals decrease at site of focal epilepsy. *Science* **205**, 211–214.

Ross, S.M. & Craig, C.R. (1981a): Studies on gamma-aminobutyric acid transport in cobalt experimental epilepsy in the rat. *J. Neurochem.* **36**, 1006–1011.

Ross, S.M. & Craig, C.R. (1981b): Gamma-aminobutyric acid concentration, L-glutamate, L-decarboxylase activity and properties of the gamma-aminobutyric acid post-synaptic receptor in cobalt epilepsy in the rat. *J. Neurosci.* **1**, 1388–1396.

Sherwin, A.L. & Van Gelder, N.M. (1986): Aminoacid and catecholamine markers of metabolic abnormalities in human focal epilepsy. In: *Basic mechanisms of the epilepsies. Molecular and cellular approaches (Advances in neurology)*, Vol. 44, eds. A.V. Delgado-Escueta, A.A. Ward, D.M. Woodbury & R.J. Porter, pp. 1011–1032. New York: Raven Press.

Stramka, M., Sedlak, P. & Nadvornik, P. (1977): Observation of kindling phenomenon in treatment of pain by stimulation of thalamus. In: *Neurosurgical treatment in psychiatry, pain and epilepsy*, ed. W.H. Sweet, pp. 651–654. Baltimore: University Park Press.

Sutula, T.P. (1990): Experimental models of temporal lobe epilepsy: new insights from the study of kindling and synaptic reorganization. *Epilepsia* **31** (Suppl. 3), S45–S54.

Van Gelder, N.M., Sherwin, A.L. & Rasmussen, T. (1972): Aminoacid content of epileptogenic human brain: focal versus surrounding regions. *Brain Res.* **40**, 385–393.

Van Gelder, N.M., Siatitas, I., Menini, C. & Gloor, P. (1983): Feline generalized penicillin epilepsy; changes in glutamic acid and taurine parallel the progressive increase in excitability of the cortex. *Epilepsia* **24**, 200–213.

Walker, E.A., Johnson, H.C. & Kollros, J.J. (1945): Penicillin convulsions. The convulsive effect of penicillin applied to the cortex of monkey and man. *Surg. Gynec. Obst.* **81**, 692–701.

Wasterlain, C.G. & Dwyer, B.E. (1983): Brain metabolism during prolonged seizures in neonates. In: *Status epilepticus, mechanisms of brain damage and treatment (Advances in neurology)*, Vol. 34, eds. A.V. Delgado-Escueta, C.G. Wasterlain, D.M. Treiman & R.J. Porter, pp. 241–260. New York: Raven Press.

Wasterlain, C.G, Farber, D.B. & Fairchild, M.D. (1986): Synaptic mechanisms in the kindled epileptic focus: a speculative synthesis. In: *Basic mechanisms of the epilepsies. Molecular and cellular approaches (Advances in neurology)*, Vol. 44, eds. A.V. Delgado-Escueta, A.A. Ward, D.M. Woodbury & R.J. Porter. pp. 411–433. New York: Raven Press.

Willmore, L.J. & Dubin, J.J. (1982): Formation of malonaldehyde and focal brain oedema induced by subpial injection of $FeCl_2$ into rat isocortex. *Brain Res.* **246**, 113–119.

Willmore, L.J. (1990): Posttraumatic epilepsy: cellular mechanisms and implications for treatment. *Epilepsia* **31** (Suppl.3), S67–S73.

Wong, R.K. & Prince, D.A. (1979): Dendritic mechanisms underlying penicillin-induced epileptiform activity. *Science* **204**, 1228–1231.

Woodbury, D.M. (1980): Convulsant drugs: mechanism of action. In: *Antiepileptic drugs: Mechanisms of action.* eds. G.H. Glaser, J. Kiffin Penry & D.M. Woodbury, pp. 249–304. New York: Raven Press.

Chapter 2

Basic mechanisms of focal epileptogenesis

David A. Prince

Edward F. and Irene Thiele Pimley Professor, Department of Neurology and Neurological Sciences, Stanford University School of Medicine, Stanford, CA, USA

Summary

Results of experiments in a variety of experimental models of focal epileptogenesis suggest that disturbances in regulation of intrinsic membrane excitability that lead to higher firing rates or burst generation, defects in inhibitory control mechanisms, and increased excitatory coupling in groups of neurons can all lead to development of the synchronous, excessive discharge in neuronal populations that defines focal epileptogenesis. Pathological processes may give rise to epilepsy through a variety of mechanisms focused on one or more of these regulatory processes. It is possible that novel therapeutic interventions focused on specific cellular events that are known to contribute to epileptogenesis will be effective and selective approaches to therapy in the future.

Introduction

As initially proposed by Hughlings Jackson (1890), and later confirmed in microphysiological studies, the capacity of some populations of neurons to generate excessive, high frequency, synchronous discharge underlies the development of focal cortical epileptogenesis. The electroencephalographic hallmark of this process is the interictal 'spike' of the electroencephalographer. This is a prominent field potential, associated with a large amplitude, prolonged depolarizing shift in neuronal membrane potential and bursts of action potentials in large populations of neurons (Fig. 1). The mechanisms by which these cellular events are generated are important to our understanding of the pathogenesis of clinical focal epilepsy. The results of experiments done over the past 30 years suggest that the development of focal epileptogenic discharges in a population of neurons is due to the interaction of several factors reviewed below, including (1) the existence of intrinsic membrane properties which lead to burst-generating capacities in specific subsets of neurons, (2) reduction of inhibitory control mechanisms, and (3) excitatory (predominantly synaptic) coupling among neurons of the epileptogenic region. A number of reviews of these and other aspects of the basic mechanisms of epileptogenesis are available (Prince, 1978; Delgado-Escueta *et al.*, 1986; Prince & Connors, 1986; Dichter & Ayala, 1987; Dichter, 1988). Since epilepsy is a *symptom* of disordered brain function that has many aetiologies, it is likely that different pathological processes induce seizures through different combinations of these mechanisms. The experimental findings lead to some reasonable predictions about the types of physiological alterations which might give rise to epileptogenesis in man, provide a rationale for the use of anti-convulsant drugs

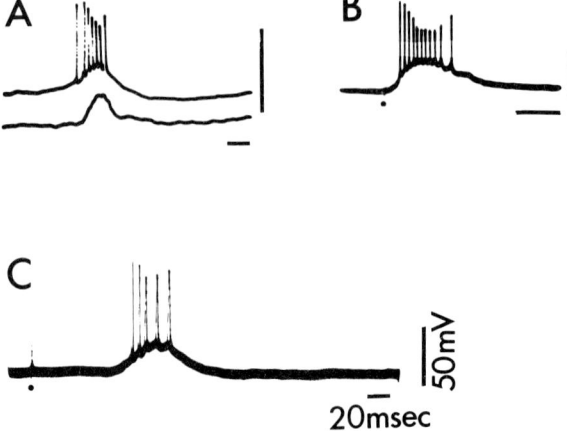

Fig. 1. Depolarization shifts (DSs) during neocortical epileptogenesis. A: Intracellular recording (upper trace) and EEG (lower trace) from alumina-cream-induced epileptogenic focus in monkey neocortex (from Prince & Futamachi, 1970, with permission); B. Intracellular recording from neuron in neocortical slice exposed to penicillin; C. Intracellular recording from neuron in human epileptogenic slice (from Prince & Wong, 1981, with permission). The event in A was spontaneous. DSs in B and C evoked by orthodromic stimulation (dots). Calibrations in A and B: 20 ms, 50 mV (from Prince et al., 1983, with permission).

that are effective in treating partial seizures and suggest interesting potential strategies for developing new therapeutic agents.

Limitations of experimental models

A large variety of preparations have been used to explore cellular mechanisms underlying interictal and ictal discharge. These extend from creation of acute and chronic epileptogenic foci *in vivo*, to induction of acute discharges in *in vitro* preparations such as brain slices and CNS cultures. It is important to emphasize that each of these models, and each method used to induce epileptogenesis, has its own peculiar advantages and limitations. For example, in the usual *in vitro* preparations, influences of subcortical structures on cortical epileptogenic foci cannot be assessed, nor can the kinds of long-term fluctuations in susceptibility to seizure discharge that are known to occur in man. More intact (*in vivo*) chronic models have advantages in this respect, but suffer from the complexities of CNS organization which often make it impossible for the investigator to obtain detailed information about the underlying pathophysiological processes. It is therefore important to carefully compare data obtained using reductionistic approaches with those from more intact animal preparations and from man. Fortunately, when this has been possible, certain basic principles of epileptogenesis have emerged.

Factors underlying the development of interictal epileptogenesis

Intrinsic burst generation in cortical neurons

Most of the features of interictal discharges seen in animals with acute foci can be replicated by exposing hippocampal or neocortical brain slices maintained *in vitro* to convulsant drugs or other agents that increase neuronal excitability (Schwartzkroin & Prince, 1978; Gutnick *et al.*, 1982; Rutecki *et al.*, 1985, 1987). In these preparations interictal discharges do not begin at random, but rather have their origin in particular subsets of nerve cells whose membrane properties endow them with the capacity to generate intrinsic burst discharges under normal conditions. In the case of the hippocampus, pyramidal cells in the CA2–CA3 area serve as pacemakers for spontaneous epileptiform events (Schwartzkroin & Prince, 1978) while in the neocortex a comparable group of bursting neurons that may initiate interictal discharges is found in layer IV–V (Connors et al., 1982; Connors, 1984; Chagnac Amitai & Connors, 1989b; Chagnac Amitai et al., 1990). The assumption that focal epileptiform discharges can be initiated by burst-generating neurons, here termed 'pacemaker cells', is supported by the demonstration that activation of a single pyramidal cell in the CA3 region of the hippocampus can lead to an interictal discharge in a cell population (Miles & Wong, 1983).

Burst generation is a mechanism for amplification of signals, since neurons which generate multiple impulses rather than a single one in response to a stimulus would tend to release more transmitter from their synaptic terminals. Under conditions where excitatory synaptic events are enhanced, or inhibitory ones depressed, synchronous burst activities in pacemaker cells can elicit intense synaptic depolarization and repetitive spiking in other ('follower') neurons and on themselves (Traub & Wong, 1982). During interictal and ictal discharges, bursts may also be initiated in axonal terminals and play an important role in amplifying and synchronizing excitatory interactions (Gutnick & Prince, 1972; Prince & Connors, 1986).

What are the cellular properties which might predispose a set of neurons to epileptogenic pacemaker activity? The behaviour of individual cells is determined in part by the balance between inward currents carried by Na and Ca and outward currents carried by K and Cl through ion channels in the cell membrane. When the slow inward currents predominate, the membrane is depolarized and a burst of spikes may result. Most cells in the hippocampus and neocortex do not generate spontaneous burst discharges, however these may result if inward currents are facilitated or outward currents are blocked. For example, drugs or transmitters such as acetylcholine, which block K channels; excessive levels of extracellular K, such as those reached during intense neural activity; or genetically-determined deficiencies in K channels may convert a non-bursting to a bursting neuron (Schwartzkroin & Prince, 1980; Benardo & Prince, 1982; Ganetsky & Wu, 1982). Excitatory amino acids may induce burst discharges by activating inward Ca currents coupled to the N-methyl-d-aspartate (NMDA) subclass of glutamate receptors (Dingledine et al., 1986).

Other data suggest that various forms of neuronal injury are accompanied by alterations in intrinsic membrane properties which alter the input-output relationships of single cells, making them intrinsically more excitable and capable of firing at higher frequencies during depolarization. For example, following axotomy there is an increase in the density of Na channels on the dendrites of mammalian motoneurons which may lead to generation of repetitive dendritic Na spikes (Sernagor et al., 1986). The relationship between depolarization and spike frequency becomes steeper in axotomized motoneurons (Heyer & Llinas, 1977), perhaps because of a decrease in a slow Ca-activated K conductance (Gustafsson, 1979). Recent studies in axotomized corticospinal neurons of rat have shown that these neurons survive in an altered state for over 1 year following such injury, and develop higher input resistances and a steeper relationship between applied current and firing frequency and decreases in slow afterhyperpolarizations which make them more excitable (Tseng & Prince, 1990).

Role of disinhibition in focal epileptogenesis

If the only requirements for development of epileptogenesis were the amplification of signals provided by subsets of neurons capable of intrinsic burst activity, and availability of appropriate excitatory connectivity to synchronize the population, seizures would be a much more common occurrence. Fortunately, post-synaptic inhibition is quite powerful and widespread in cortical circuits, and serves as a control mechanism which prevents development of synchronous epileptiform discharge. Postsynaptic inhibitory events mediated by release of the neurotransmitter γ-aminobutyric acid (GABA) serve to (1) restrict the lateral spread of epileptiform activity across the cortex ('surround inhibition'; Prince & Wilder, 1967; Dichter & Spencer, 1969), (2) decrease the spread to distant structures, (3) prevent burst generation by increasing Cl and K conductances and controlling the membrane potential (Wong & Prince, 1979), and (4) depress activity in excitatory synaptic circuits (Miles & Wong, 1987). Recently it has been shown that GABA-mediated inhibition is also important in regulating the efficacy of excitatory neurotransmission at the NMDA subclass of glutamate receptor (Staley & Mody, 1992). NMDA receptor activation contributes significantly to the development of both interictal and ictal discharges (Hoffman & Haberly, 1989; Stasheff et al., 1989). Small reductions in GABA-mediated inhibition such as are produced by some convulsant drugs (Chagnac-Amitai & Connors, 1989a) interfere with these various control mechanisms and can lead to the development of epileptogenesis. There is evidence that cortical injury may selectively affect inhibitory circuits in several models of chronic epilepsy (Riba(Riba(Riba(Ribak et al., 1982; Lancaster & Wheal, 1984; Houser et al., 1986; Sloviter 1987; Franck et al., 1988). Repetitive activation of cortical circuits causes a depression of synaptic inhibition in unlesioned tissue through decreases in the IPSP driving force due to increased $[Cl^-]_i$ and presynaptic inhibition of GABA release (McCarren & Alger, 1985; Huguenard & Alger, 1986; Deisz & Prince, 1989; Thompson & Gähwiler, 1989a). Another example of hyperexcitability secondary to decreased postsynaptic inhibition is provided by studies of immature neocortex where poorly developed inhibitory electrogenesis leads to generation of repetitive polysynaptic excitatory activity following stimulation (Luhmann & Prince, 1990).

It has become increasingly apparent that powerful presynaptic inhibitory mechanisms play an important role in controlling the level of inhibitory and excitatory electrogenesis in cortical structures. Activation of $GABA_B$ receptors by baclofen in hippocampus can have both epileptogenic effects, presumably by decreasing release of GABA (Burgard & Sarvey, 1991) and antiepileptogenic effects, perhaps via postsynaptic actions (Swartzwelder et al., 1986). Blockade of hippocampal adenosine (A-1) receptors can induce epileptiform activity (Alzheimer et al., 1989), presumably because these receptors normally control the level of excitatory transmitter release without affecting inhibitory potentials (Yoon & Rothman, 1991).

Role of excitatory postsynaptic potentials

The third vital element underlying development of epileptogenesis is the excitatory synaptic circuitry present within cortical structures. Excitatory postsynaptic potentials (EPSPs) have three important roles in this process which become apparent experimentally when inhibition is depressed. First, they serve to trigger intrinsic membrane events such as bursts in susceptible neurons (Wong & Prince, 1979). Second, propagation of impulses in excitatory synaptic circuits such as the axonal arborizations of thalamocortical neurons, or recurrent excitatory connections among pyramidal neurons in the hippocampus or neocortex, serves to synchronize the population by activation of EPSPs on groups of neurons. Finally, when the EPSPs summate through activation of recurrent and polysynaptic excitatory circuits, large postsynaptic depolarizations are evoked on groups of cells, which in turn lead to generation of repetitive high-frequency action potentials and a further cascade of excitation within the circuit (Traub et al., 1985). The summation of synaptic and intrinsic membrane currents produced by synchronous activation of large groups of cells results in an extracellular field potential characteristic of the interictal epileptiform 'spike' of the electroencephalographer. In model systems, this cascade of excitation can be initiated either by increases in the intensity of postsynaptic excitation (Rutecki et al., 1987) or small decreases in inhibitory potency (Chagnac-Amitai & Connors, 1989a).

One obvious mechanism by which cortical injury might lead to epileptogenesis through increased excitatory synaptic coupling would be development of new recurrent excitatory circuitry due to axonal sprouting. The number of recurrent excitatory connections in a population of neurons is a vital element in the development of epileptogenesis (Traub & Wong, 1982). Anatomic evidence that may indicate development of recurrent excitatory circuitry following injury has been found in the dentate gyrus of animals (Tauck & Nadler, 1985; Cronin & Dudek, 1988; Sutula et al., 1988) and has also been reported in human temporal lobes removed for epilepsy surgery (Sutula et al., 1989; Babb et al., 1991). There is also electrophysiological evidence for increased excitability with burst generation in granule cells from dentate gyri showing such recurrent mossy fibre sprouting, both in animal models (Tauck & Nadler, 1985) and in human dentate slices (Masukawa et al., 1989). Other mechanisms which might alter excitatory synaptic coupling include changes in the density and distribution of glutamate receptor subtypes on postsynaptic neurons (Hosford et al., 1991), and alterations in the NMDA subtype of glutamate receptors following repetitive seizures (Yeh et al., 1989). The importance of NMDA receptors in the development of prolonged depolarizations associated with interictal and especially ictal discharges is emphasized by experiments which show that blockade of these receptors can have potent anti-epileptic effects (Brady & Swann, 1986; Dingledine et al., 1986; Gutnick et al., 1989; Hwa & Avoli, 1991; Masukawa et al., 1991, and others).

From these data it is possible to suggest that, in the neocortex as in the hippocampus, epileptogenesis develops from interactions between populations of neurons which serve as pacemakers because of their intrinsic membrane properties and excitatory connectivity, and other groups of cells that are synchronously depolarized by the outputs of the pacemaker group. It remains to be seen whether the principles outlined above will be applicable to models of chronic epileptogenesis or to epilepsy in man. To date human epileptogenic foci studied *in vitro* using brain slice techniques have shown abnormal activities very similar to those found in both *in vivo* and *in vitro* animal models (Prince & Wong, 1981; Schwartzkroin & Knowles, 1984; Tasker & Dudek, 1991) (Fig. 1).

It is remarkable that the several classes of drugs known to be clinically effective in partial or generalized seizures have actions that relate to some of the specific mechanisms of epileptogenesis described above (Macdonald & McLean, 1986). For example, at least one effect of carbamazepine and phenytoin is to decrease the capacity of neurons to fire repetitively at high frequencies. This action, due to an influence of these agents on Na channel properties (MacDonald, 1989), would tend to limit the repetitive trains of action potentials during activation of pacemaker and follower neurons in the focus, and dampen the high frequency bursts in axonal arborizations that ultimately result in excessively large and prolonged excitatory synaptic potentials locally and in distant connected structures. Other types of anticonvulsant drugs such as phenobarbital and benzodiazepines have significant facilitatory effects on GABAergic inhibition and act, at least in part, by increasing the efficacy of released GABA (MacDonald, 1989). Other experimental drugs in this class increase GABA synthesis, or retard the reuptake of released GABA (Macdonald & Meldrum, 1989).

Mechanisms of synchronization

The intense synchronization of large groups of cells that underlies epileptiform events in the EEG is brought about by several mechanisms (Table 1). As emphasized above, activation of excitatory synaptic potentials in complex cortical circuits is a major factor in synchronization, however other mechanisms have been demonstrated *in vitro*. Large increases in extracellular K concentrations are produced by intense activity in groups of neurons (Prince et al., 1973; Moody et al., 1974), and may facilitate synaptic transmission, directly depolarize neural elements, reduce outward K-mediated currents, lead to burst discharges and thus induce interictal or ictal events in a neuronal population. Rises in $[K^+]_o$ also interfere with transport of Cl^- out of neurons and indirectly depress synaptic inhibition (Thompson et al., 1988; Thompson & Gähwiler, 1989b), Other kinds of synchronizing mechanisms include burst discharges in the axonal terminal arborizations of neurons (Gutnick & Prince, 1972), electrical interactions between groups of tightly packed cells ('ephaptic interactions'), and direct spread of current from cell to cell through non-chemical synapses ('gap junctions') (Dudek et al., 1986). All of these effects become more marked as excitation within a group of neurons increases, and such mechanisms may be important in the transition between interictal and ictal discharge, as will be discussed below.

Table 1. *Some mechanisms of synchronization in epileptogenesis*

>Activation of recurrent and polysynaptic excitatory circuits
>Increases in $[K^+]_o$
>Bursts in axonal arborizations
>Ephaptic interactions
>Electrotonic coupling via gap junctions
>Actions of neuromodulators

Interictal-ictal transitions

The reasons for transition between sporadic interictal discharge and sustained ictal episodes associated with behavioural seizures in man are unknown. From studies of conditions that give rise to experimental ictal discharge, it is possible to suggest several kinds of 'regenerative' cycles by which activity begets increasing excitation or decreased inhibition, perhaps leading to ictal events (Prince et al., 1983; Prince, 1988). Some examples of synaptic and non-synaptic factors potentially involved in the interictal-ictal transition are given in Table 2. One important mechanism may be the tendency for postsynaptic inhibition to progressively fall off in its potency as circuits are repetitively activated. This appears to be a consequence of increases in intracellular Cl concentration and decreases in GABA release, both of which make inhibition less effective (Deisz & Prince, 1989; Thompson & Gähwiler, 1989a). This, in turn, causes increased activity in excitatory circuits, activation of latent excitatory connections, increased triggering of burst discharges, etc.

Table 2. *Mechanisms of interictal-ictal transition*

Synaptic
1. Depression of GABAergic inhibition
    (a) Decreased driving force: e.g. increases in $[Cl^-]_i$ secondary to increased $[K^+]_o$ or Cl-K co-transport failure
    (b) Decreased postsynaptic Cl conductance: e.g. due to GABA-mediated pre-synaptic inhibition of GABA release, possible desensitization of receptors.
2. NMDA receptor activation; voltage-dependent EPSPs
3. Frequency potentiation of EPSPs.
4. Actions of modulators
    (a) Decreased AHPs and spike frequency accommodation: norepinephrine; ACh; serotonin
    (b) Decreased voltage-activated gKs: ACh; norepinephrine; serotonin

Nonsynaptic
1. Alterations in ionic microenvironment: e.g. increased $[K^+]_o$, decreased $[Ca^{2+}]_o$
2. Decreases in size of extracellular space
3. Failure of ion transport: Na-K pump; Cl-K co-transport
4. Presynaptic terminal bursting
5. Ephaptic interactions

Neurotransmission mediated by excitatory amino acids (glutamate, aspartate) plays a major role in development of ictal discharge. Activation of the NMDA subclass of glutamate receptor appears to be particularly important since the resulting excitatory effects are enhanced as neurons depolarize due to relief of the Mg^{2+} block of the channel (MacDonald & Nowak, 1990), potentially leading to a regenerative excitatory effect. Also, NMDA receptor activation increases the concentration of intracellular Ca through several mechanisms, and this in turn may induce long-term changes in neuronal excitability. As noted above, NMDA receptor antagonists are potent blockers of ictal discharge. In the hippocampus, such blockers prevent the evolution of the ictal discharges that develop after repetitive stimulation, but have little effect on interictal events or established ictal discharge patterns (Stasheff et al., 1989).

Another synaptic factor involved in interictal-ictal transitions might be the release of substances that

Chapter 2 BASIC MECHANISMS OF FOCAL EPILEPTOGENESIS

cause long-term increases in neuronal excitability through activation of intracellular second messenger systems coupled to changes in the conductance of membrane ion channels. Examples are the decreases in K currents produced by acetylcholine, norepinephrine and serotonin that are mediated by some classes of postsynaptic receptors. These actions make neurons more responsive to the effects of other neurotransmitters, and may result in higher firing frequencies due to depression of slow afterhyperpolarizations that normally follow repetitive discharges. Some non-synaptic mechanisms for interictal-ictal transitions including increases in $[K^+]_o$, presynaptic terminal bursting and electrical (ephaptic) interactions between neurons have been mentioned above.

How might pathological processes give rise to epileptogenesis?

From the above outline of possible pathogenic mechanisms, and from the results of a variety of other experiments, it is possible to suggest mechanisms by which disease processes might induce epilepsy (Fig. 2). It should be obvious that the list of fundamental abnormalities will turn out to be as long as the list of regulatory processes that determine the patterns of neuronal excitability and connectivity.

Evidence in some preparations suggests that inhibitory synaptic circuitry may be selectively vulnerable to injury (references above). A variety of disorders could depress functional inhibition even in the absence of such selective abnormalities of GABAergic circuits. These might include down-regulation of GABA receptors due to abnormalities in intracellular calcium concentration or state of phosphorylation (Stelzer et al., 1988), and depression in transport processes which extrude Cl

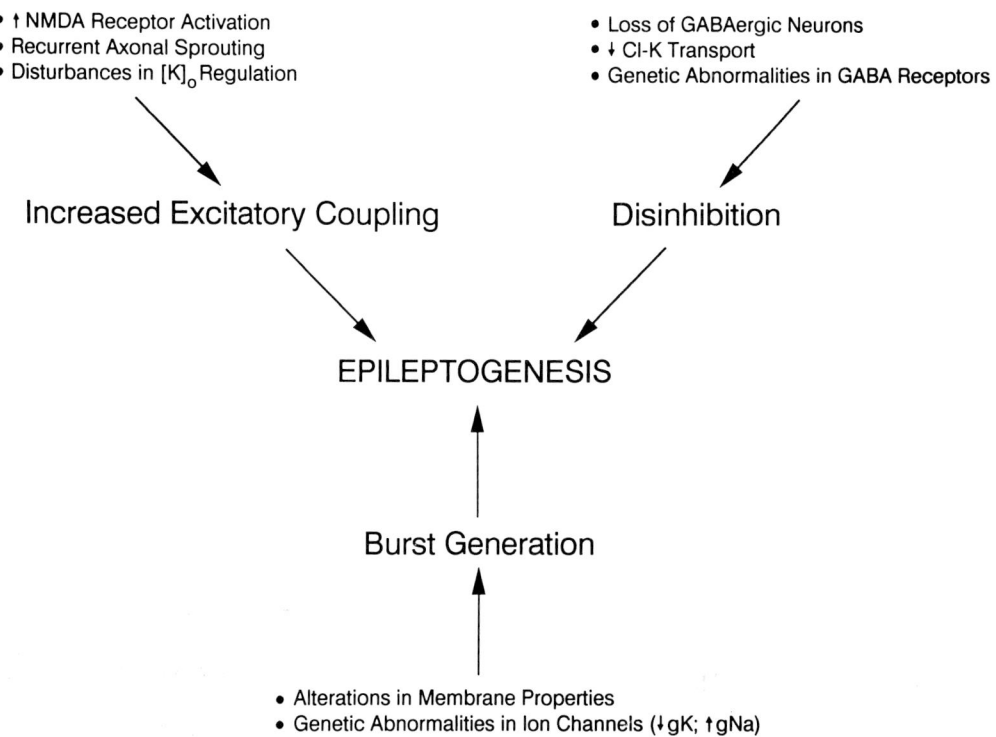

Fig. 2. Increased excitatory coupling, disinhibition and burst generation underlie epileptogenesis in cortical structures. Examples of possible contributing pathophysiological processes are shown.

from nerve cells following activation of GABA receptors (Thompson et al., 1988) such as occurs in immature neurons (Zhang et al., 1990; Luhmann & Prince, 1991). Genetic abnormalities in the GABA receptor complex have been described in animals susceptible to seizures (Olsen et al., 1985). The development of maladaptive excitatory circuitry following injury occurs in the hippocampus (references above), and such changes in connectivity may well play a role in cortical epilepsy that follows a variety of injuries. Genetic defects which affect the regulation, or even the existence of subsets of voltage-dependent ionic channels could easily give rise to burst generation and hyperexcitable states. One such mutation in *Drosophila* results in absence of a K channel and development of axonal burst discharges, excessive release of transmitter and hyperexcitability in a fly that has behavioural seizure activity (Ganetsky & Wu, 1982). Abnormalities in the uptake of the excitatory neural transmitter glutamate in injured or hypoxic cortex may well lead to excessive excitation and epileptogenesis, or even cell death through excitoxic mechanisms (Choi, 1988).

References

Alzheimer, C., Sutor, B. & ten-Bruggencate, G. (1989): Transient and selective blockade by 8-cyclopentyl-1, 3-dipropylxanthine (DPCPX) causes sustained epileptiform activity in hippocampal CA3 neurons of guinea pigs. *Neurosci. Lett.* **99**, 107–112.

Babb, T.L., Kupfer, W.R., Pretorius, J.K., Crandall, P.H. & Levesque, M.F. (1991): Synaptic reorganization by mossy fibers in human epileptic fascia dentata. *Neuroscience* **42**, 351–363.

Benardo, L.S. & Prince, D.A. (1982): Cholinergic excitation of mammalian hippocampal pyramidal cells. *Brain Res.* **249**, 315–331.

Brady, R.J. & Swann, J.W. (1986): Ketamine selectively suppresses synchronized afterdischarges in immature hippocampus. *Neurosci. Lett.* **69**, 143–149.

Burgard, E.C. & Sarvey, J.M. (1991): Long-lasting potentiation and epileptiform activity produced by $GABA_B$ receptor activation in the dentate gyrus of rat hippocampal slice. *J. Neurosci.* **11**, 1198–1209.

Chagnac-Amitai, Y. & Connors, B.W. (1989a): Horizontal spread of synchronized activity in neocortex and its control by GABA-mediated inhibition. *J. Neurophysiol.* **61**, 747–758.

Chagnac-Amitai, Y. & Connors, B.W. (1989b): Synchronized excitation and inhibition driven by intrinsically bursting neurons in cortex. *J. Neurophysiol.* **62**, 1149–1162.

Chagnac-Amitai, Y., Luhmann, H. & Prince, D.A. (1990): Burst generating and regular spiking layer 5 pyramidal neurons of rat neocortex have different morphological features. *J. Comp. Neurol.* **296**, 598–613.

Choi, D.W. (1988): Glutamate neurotoxicity and diseases of the nervous system. *Neuron.* **1(8)**, 623–634.

Connors, B.W. (1984): Initiation of synchronized neuronal bursting in neocortex. *Nature* **310**, 685–687.

Connors, B.W., Gutnick, M.J. & Prince, D.A. (1982): Electrophysiological properties of neocortical neurons *in vitro*. *J. Neurophysiol.* **48**, 1302–1320.

Cronin, J. & Dudek, F.E. (1988): Chronic seizures and collateral sprouting of dentate mossy fibers after kainic acid treatment in rats. *Brain Res.* **474**, 181–184.

Deisz, R.A. & Prince, D.A. (1989): Frequency dependent depression of inhibition in the guinea pig neocortex *in vitro* by $GABA_B$ receptor feedback on GABA release. *J. Physiol.* **412**, 513–541.

Delgado-Escueta, A., Ward, A., Woodbury, D. & Porter, R. (eds.) (1986): In: *Advances in neurology. Basic mechanisms of the epilepsies. Molecular and cellular approaches*, New York: Raven Press.

Dichter, M. (ed), (1988): In: *Mechanisms of epileptogenesis: from membranes to man.* New York: Plenum Publishing Corp.

Dichter, M.A. & Ayala, G.F. (1987): Cellular mechanisms of epilepsy: a status report. *Science* **237**, 157–164.

Dichter, M. & Spencer, W.A. (1969): Penicillin-induced interictal discharges from the cat hippocampus. II. Mechanisms underlying origin and restriction. *J. Neurophysiol.* **32**, 663–687.

Dingledine, R., Hynes, M.A. & King, G.L. (1986): Involvement of *N*-methyl-D-aspartate receptors in epileptiform bursting in the rat hippocampal slice. *J. Physiol.* **380**, 175–189.

Dudek, F.E., Snow, F.W. & Taylor, C.P. (1986): Role of electrical interactions in synchronization of epileptiform bursts: In: *Basic mechanisms of the epilepsies. Molecular and cellular approaches, (Advances in neurology)*, Vol. 44, eds. A. Delgado-Escueta, A. Ward, D. Woodbury & R. Porter, pp. 593–617. New York: Raven Press.

Franck, J.E., Kunkel, D.D., Baskin, D.G. & Schwartzkroin, P.A. (1988): Inhibition in kainate-lesioned hyperexcitable hippocampi: physiologic, autoradiographic, and immunocytochemical observations. *J. Neurosci.* **8**, 1991–2002.

Ganetsky, B. & Wu, C.F. (1982): Indirect suppression involving behavioural mutants with altered nerve excitability in *Drosophila melanogaster. Genetics* **100**, 597–614.

Gustafsson, B. (1979): Changes in motoneurons electrical properties following axotomy. *J. Physiol.* **293**, 197–215.

Gutnick, M.J., Connors, B.W. & Prince, D.A. (1982): Mechanisms of neocortical epileptogenesis *in vitro. J. Neurophysiol.* **48**, 1321–1335.

Gutnick, M.J. & Prince, D.A. (1972): Thalamocortical relay neurons: Antidromic invasion of spikes from a cortical epileptogenic focus. *Science* **176**, 424–426.

Gutnick, M.J., Wolfson, B. & Baldino, F. Jr. (1989): Synchronized neuronal activities in neocortical explant cultures. *Exp. Brain Res.* **76**, 131–140.

Heyer, C. & Llinas, R. (1977): Control of rhythmic firing in normal and axotomized cat spinal motoneurons. *J. Neurophysiol.* **40**, 480–488.

Hoffman, W.H. & Haberly, L.B. (1989): Bursting induces persistent all-or-none EPSPs by an NMDA-dependent process in piriform cortex. *J. Neurosci.* **9**, 206–215.

Hosford, D.A., Crain, B.J., Cao, Z., Bonhaus, D.W., Friedman, A.H., Okazaki, M.M., Nadler, J.V. & McNamara, J.O. (1991): Increased AMPA-sensitive quisqualate receptor binding and reduced NMDA receptor binding in epileptic human hippocampus. *J. Neurosci.* **11**, 428–434.

Houser, C.R., Harris, A.B. & Vaughn, J.E. (1986): Time course of the reduction of GABA terminals in a model of focal epilepsy; a glutamate acid decarboxylase immunocytochemical study. *Brain Res.* **383**, 129–145.

Huguenard, J.R. & Alger, B.E. (1986): Whole-cell voltage-clamp study of the fading of GABA-activated currents in acutely dissociated hippocampal neurons. *J. Neurophysiol.* **56**, 1–18.

Hwa, G.G.C. & Avoli, M. (1991): The involvement of excitatory amino acids in neocortical epileptogenesis NMDA and non-NMDA receptors. *Exp. Brain Res.* **86**, 248–256.

Jackson, J.H. (1890): The Lumleian lectures on convulsive seizures. *Br. Med. J.* **i**, 765–771.

Lancaster, B. & Wheal, H.V. (1984): Chronic failure of inhibition of the CA1 area of the hippocampus following kainic acid lesions of the CA3/4 area. *Brain Res.* **295**, 317–324.

Luhmann, H.J. & Prince, D.A. (1990): Control of NMDA receptor-mediated activity by GABAergic mechanisms in mature and developing rat neocortex. *Dev. Brain Res.* **54**, 287–290.

Luhmann, H.J. & Prince, D.A. (1991): Post-natal maturation of the GABAergic system in rat neocortex. *J. Neurophysiol.* **65**, 247–263.

Macdonald, R.L. (1989): Antiepileptic drug actions. *Epilepsia*, **30** (Suppl. 1), S19–S28.

MacDonald, J.F. & Nowak, L.M. (1990): Mechanisms of blockade of excitatory amino acid receptor channels. *TIPS* **11**, 157–171.

Macdonald, R.L. & McLean, M.J. (1986): Anticonvulsant drugs: mechanisms of action. *Adv. Neurol.* **44**, 713–736.

Macdonald, R.L. & Meldrum, B.S, (1989): Principles of antiepileptic drug action. In: *Antiepileptic Drugs*, eds. R. Levy, pp. 59–83. New York: Raven Press.

Masukawa, L.M., Higashima, M., Hart, G.J., Spencer, D.D. & O'Connor, M.J. (1991): NMDA receptor activation during epileptiform responses in the dentate gyrus of epileptic patients. *Brain Res.*, **562**, 176–180.

Masukawa, L.M., Higashima, M., Kim, J.H. & Spencer, D.D. (1989): Epileptiform discharges evoked in hippocampal brain slices from epileptic patients. *Brain Res.* **493**, 168–174.

McCarren, M. & Alger, B.E. (1985): Use-dependent depression of IPSPs in rat hippocampal pyramidal cells *in vitro. J. Neurophysiol.* **53**, 557–571.

Miles, R, Wong, R.K.S. (1983): Single neurones can initiate synchronized population discharge in the hippocampus. *Nature* **306**, 371–373.

Miles, R. & Wong, R.K.S. (1987): Inhibitory control of local excitatory circuits in guinea-pig hippocampus. *J. Physiol.* **388**, 611–629.

Moody, W.J., Futamachi, K.J. & Prince, D.A. (1974): Extracellular potassium activity during epileptogenesis. *Exp. Neurol.* **42**, 248–263.

Olsen, R.W., Wamsley, J.K., McCabe, R.T., Lee, R.J. & Lomax, P. (1985): Benzodiazepine/gamma-aminobutyric acid receptor deficit in the midbrain of the seizure-susceptible gerbil. *Proc. Natl. Acad. Sci. USA* **82**(19), 6701–6705.

Prince, D.A. (1988): Cellular mechanisms of interictal-ictal transitions. In: *Mechanisms of epileptogenesis: From membranes to man.* ed. M. Dichter, pp. 57–71. New York: Plenum Publishing Corp.

Prince, D.A. (1978): Neurophysiology of epilepsy. *Annu. Rev. Neurosci.* **1**, 395–415.

Prince, D.A. & Connors, B.W. (1986): Mechanisms of interictal epileptogenesis. *Adv. Neurol.* **44**, 275–299.

Prince, D.A., Connors, B.W. & Benardo, L.S. (1983): Mechanisms underlying interictal-ictal transitions. In: *Status Epilepticus, (Advances in Neurology),* Vol. 34, eds. A. Delgado-Escueta, C. Wasterlain, D. Treiman & R. Porter. pp. 117–118. New York: Raven Press.

Prince, D.A. & Futamachi, K.J. (1970): Intracellular recordings from chronic epileptogenic foci in the monkey. *Electroencephalogr. Clin. Neurophysiol.* **29**, 496–510.

Prince, D.A., Lux, H.D. & Neher, E, (1973): Potassium activity in rat cortex measured with ion-sensitive microelectrodes. *Brain Res.* **50**, 489–495.

Prince, D.A. & Wilder, B.J. (1967): Control mechanisms in cortical epileptogenic foci. 'Surround' inhibition. *Arch. Neurol.* **16**, 194–202.

Prince, D.A. & Wong, R.K.S. (1981): Human epileptic neurons studied *in vitro. Brain Res.* **210**, 323–333.

Ribak, C.E., Bradburne, M. & Harris, A.B. (1982): A preferential loss of GABAergic, symmetric synapses in epileptic foci: a quantitative ultrastructural analysis of monkey neocortex. *J. Neurosci.* **2**, 1725–1735.

Rutecki, P.A., Lebeda, F.J. & Johnston, D. (1985): Epileptiform activity induced by changes in extracellular potassium in hippocampus. *J. Neurophysiol.* **54**, 1363–1374.

Rutecki, P.A., Lebeda, F.J. & Johnston, D. (1987): 4-aminopyridine produces epileptiform activity in hippocampus and enhances synaptic excitation and inhibition. *J. Neurophysiol.* **57**, 1911–1924.

Schwartzkroin, P.A. & Knowles, W.D. (1984): Intracellular study of human epileptic cortex: *in vitro* maintenance of epileptic activity. *Science* **223**, 709–712.

Schwartzkroin, P.A. & Prince, D.A. (1978): Cellular and field potential properties of epileptogenic hippocampal slices. *Brain Res.* **147**, 117–130.

Schwartzkroin, P.A. & Prince, D.A. (1980): Effects of TEA on hippocampal neurons. *Brain Res.* **185**, 169–181.

Sernagor, E., Yarom, Y. & Werman, R. (1986): Sodium-dependent regenerative responses in dendrites of axotomized motoneurons in the cat. *Proc. Natl. Acad. Sci. USA* **83**, 7966–7970.

Sloviter, R.S. (1987): Decreased hippocampal inhibition and a selective loss of interneurons in experimental epilepsy. *Science* **235**, 73–76.

Staley, K.J. & Mody, I. (1992): Shunting of excitatory input to dentate gyrus granule cells by depolarizing $GABA_A$ receptor-mediated postsynaptic conductance. *J. Neurophysiol.* 1992, in press.

Stasheff, S.F., Anderson, W.W., Ciark, S. & Wilson, W.A. (1989): NMDA antagonists differentiate epileptogenesis from seizure expression in an *in vitro* model. *Science* **245**, 648–651.

Stelzer, A., Kay, A.R. & Wong, R.K. (1988): $GABA_A$-receptor function in hippocampal cells is maintained by phosphorylation factors. *Science* **241**, 339–341.

Sutula, T., Cascino, G., Cavazos, J., Parada, I. & Ramirez, L. (1989): Mossy fiber synaptic reorganization in the epileptic human temporal lobe. *Ann. Neurol.* **26**, 321–330.

Sutula, T., Xiao-Xian, H., Cavazos, J. & Scott, G. (1988): Synaptic reorganization in the hippocampus induced by abnormal functional activity. *Science* **239**, 1147–1150.

Swartzwelder, H.S., Bragdon, A.C., Sutch, C.P., Ault, B. & Wilson, W.A. (1986): Baclofen suppresses hippocampal activity at low concentrations without suppressing synaptic transmission. *J. Pharmacol. Exp. Ther.* **237**, 881–887.

Tasker, G.T. & Dudek, F.E. (1991): Electrophysiology of GABA-mediated synaptic transmission and possible roles in epilepsy. *Neurochem. Res.* **16**, 251–262.

Tauck, D.L. & Nadler, J.V. (1985): Evidence of functional mossy fiber sprouting in hippocampal formation of kainic acid treated rats. *J. Neurosci.* **5**, 1016–1022.

Thompson, S.M., Deisz, R.A. & Prince, D.A. (1988): Relative contributions of passive equilibrium and active transport to the distribution of chloride in mammalian cortical neurons. *J. Neurophysiol.* **60**, 105–124.

Thompson, S.M. & Gähwiler, B.H. (1989a): Activity-dependent disinhibition. I. Repetitive stimulation reduces IPSP driving force and conductance in the hippocampus *in vitro*. *J. Neurophysiol.* **61**, 501–511.

Thompson, S.M. & Gähwiler, B.H. (1989b): Activity-dependent disinhibition. II. Effects of extracellular potassium, furosemide, and membrane potential on ECl^- in hippocampal CA3 neurons. *J. Neurophysiol.* **61**, 512–522.

Traub, R.D. & Wong, R.K.S. (1982): Cellular mechanisms of neuronal synchronization in epilepsy. *Science* **216**, 745–747.

Traub, R.D., Wong, R.K.S., Miles, R. & Knowles, W.D. (1985): Neuronal interactions during epileptic events *in vitro*. *Fed. Proc.* **44**, 2953–2955.

Tseng, G-F. & Prince, D.A. (1990): Neuronal properties of identified corticospinal cells *in vitro* following spinal axotomy *in vivo*. *Soc. Neurosci. Abstr.* **16**, 1163.

Wong, R.K.S. & Prince, D.A. (1979): Dendritic mechanisms underlying penicillin-induced epileptiform activity. *Science* **204**, 1228–1231.

Yeh, G-C., Bonhaus, D.W., Nadler, J.V. & McNamara, J.O. (1989): *N*-methyl-D-aspartate receptor plasticity in kindling: quantitative and qualitative alterations in the *N*-methyl-D-aspartate receptor-channel complex. *Proc. Natl. Acad. Sci. USA* **86**, 8157–8160.

Yoon, K-W. & Rothman, S.M. (1991): Adenosine inhibits excitatory but not inhibitory synaptic transmission in the hippocampus. *J. Neurosci.* **11**, 1375–1380.

Zhang, L., Spigelman, I. & Carlen, P.L. (1990): Whole-cell patch study of GABAergic inhibition in CA1 neurons of immature rat hippocampal slices. *Dev. Brain Res.* **56**, 127–130.

Chapter 3

Generalized epileptogenesis

Giuliano Avanzini

Istituto Nazionale Neurologico C. Besta, Milan, Italy

Summary

Generalized epilepsies include a number of different clinical forms spanning from the most severe epileptic encephalopathies to relatively benign idiopathic epilepsies of childhood and puberty. Their pathogenetic mechanisms involve complex interactions between cortical and subcortical structures. Experimental studies dating back to the 1940s have demonstrated the special role of the thalamus in the generation of spike and wave discharges (SWD) responsible for absence seizures in petit-mal epilepsy, the prototype of the idiopathic generalized epilepsies. Further studies have led to the conclusion that SWD reflect an abnormal oscillatory pattern involving mutually interconnected cortical and thalamic neurons. Recent results obtained in a rodent genetic model highlight intrinsic thalamic rhythmogenic properties relevant to the generalized epileptogenesis. The GAERS (generalized absence epilepsy in rats from Strasbourg) model is a selected strain of Wistar rats presenting with spontaneous bilateral and synchronous 7–9 Hz. SWD are associated with behavioural arrests and facial myoclonus highly reminiscent of human petit-mal absences. In GAERS rats the role of the reticular thalamic nucleus (Rt), a GABAergic structure endowed with Ca^{2+}/K^+ dependent oscillatory properties, has been investigated by lesion experiments and pharmacological manipulation. It was concluded that Rt stands in a nodal position within a thalamo-cortico-thalamic circuit which underlies the expression of absence-like seizures in GAERS rats. The genetically-determined receptor or channel alteration, which makes this oscillatory circuit operate improperly, is now being intensively investigated. Its identification would establish a link between the electrophysiological and molecular domains, thus adding a new dimension to the approach to the generalized epileptogenesis.

The attempt to prove mutually exclusive cortical or subcortical mechanisms in primary generalized seizures should be abandoned for a more dynamic view of the interdependence between cortical and subcortical systems.
(Herbert H. Jasper, 1990)

Generalized epileptic seizures are defined as those 'in which the first clinical changes indicate initial involvement of both hemispheres ... the ictal encephalographic (EEG) patterns initially are bilateral' (ICES, 1981). Epileptic disorders with generalized seizures, identified as generalized epilepsies and generalized epileptic syndromes (ICE, 1989), include a number of different forms spanning a broad clinical spectrum. At one extreme of the range, we can put some epileptic encephalopathies of early infancy which are usually severe such as West and Lennox–Gastaut syndromes. At the other end of the spectrum are to be placed the idiopathic generalized epilepsies, in particular childhood absence epilepsy (petit mal) with school-age onset and juvenile myoclonic epilepsy (JME, Janz syndrome) with pre- to post-puberty age-related onset. By definition, patients with generalized idiopathic epilepsies have a normal interictal state, without neurological or neuroradiological signs. There is no underlying cause other than a possible hereditary predisposition suggesting a genetic aetiology. By contrast, epileptic encephalopathies are considered the consequence of known (symptomatic generalized epilepsies) or suspected (cryptogenic generalized epilepsies) disorders of the central nervous system (CNS). The prognosis is usually poor for both seizure control and psychomotor development. It is assumed that symptomatic and cryptogenic epilepsies are due to a diffuse hyperexcitable state resulting from an imbalance between excitatory and inhibitory mechanisms in cortical and subcortical structures. When symptomatic epilepsies are due to known inborn errors of metabolism the epileptogenic mechanism can be sometimes inferred from the underlying enzymatic defect. This is the case of pyridoxine-dependency leading to a defective synthesis of the inhibitory neurotransmitter γ-aminobutyric acid (GABA). In other cases the relationship between the known or suspected metabolic defect and the epileptic phenomenology is probably indirect and dependent on the non-specific damage of one or more cerebral areas including the cortex. In a large group of progressive epileptogenic encephalopathies the myoclonus either massive or segmental is the hallmark of different evolutionary clinical pictures grouped under the heading of progressive myoclonus epilepsies (PME). In spite of the efforts to define a common pathogenetic basis for myoclonus and epileptic seizures occurring in PME, the pathophysiological hypotheses are still largely speculative. The only general agreement is on the implication of subcortical (including brainstem) structures in the generation of both spontaneous and stimulus sensitive myoclonias and possibly in the pathophysiology of generalized seizures which characterize PME.

As far as the idiopathic generalized epilepsies are concerned, their genetic aetiology has been intensively investigated in recent years. The preliminary evidence of a genetic locus on the short arm of chromosome 6 for JME has been reported by two different groups (Delgado Escueta et al., 1990; Durner et al., 1991). A two-locus model of hereditary transmission where one of the loci is dominantly inherited and the other recessively inherited, has been recently suggested to account for JME and possibly for other generalized idiopathic epilepsies (Greenberg et al., 1991). At present, no information has been obtained on genetic products of the putative genes for generalized epilepsies. Therefore, the genetic approach has not contributed so far to the understanding of generalized epileptogenic mechanisms. We must turn to a more indirect approach dating back to the 1940s to find results of clinical and experimental studies aimed at investigating generalized epileptogenesis. The main object of these investigations was the petit mal (childhood absence epilepsy) which is viewed as the prototype of the generalized idiopathic epilepsies. We will summarize here the most interesting results leading to the recognition of the special role of the thalamus in the generation of spike and wave discharges (SWD) responsible for the absence seizures. A comprehensive account of this matter has been recently provided by Herbert H. Jasper to whom we owe the original development and the evolution of the concepts which we will be dealing with (Jasper, 1990).

The role of subcortical structures in animal models of petit-mal like seizures

In their paper on EEG classification of the epilepsies Jasper & Karshman (1941) first suggested that bilaterally synchronous SWD arising suddenly out of a normal EEG background must be due to a subcortical pacemaker. A few years later, in collaboration with Drooglever-Fortuyn, Jasper was able to reproduce 3/s SWD in anaesthetized cats, by 3 Hz stimulation of the intralaminar thalamus (Jasper & Drooglever-Fortuyn, 1947), the same area from which diffuse synchronous recruiting responses had been previously elicited by Morison & Dempsey (1942). The type of response (recruiting versus SWD) which can be obtained by intralaminar stimulation, depends critically on the level of arousal as was shown later by Gloor & Testa (1974). If the animal is too alert the recruiting response is observed and no SWD appear, as is known to occur in children with petit mal where the attack can be blocked by an arousing or alerting stimulus. In collaboration with Hunter, Jasper was also able to reproduce a clinical phenomenology reminiscent of the human absence by electrical stimulation of intralaminar thalamus of waking cats and monkeys (Hunter & Jasper,

1949). These absence-like seizures were characterized by staring with unresponsiveness, arrest of ongoing behaviour and even with myoclonic twitches about the face as often occurs in patients during a typical absence seizure. In the same years the concept of a centrencephalic integration system, involved in the highest level of neuronal integration underlying conscious experience, was elaborated by Penfield (1957). The term centrencephalic seizures for these generalized epileptic seizures, consisting of almost exclusively or initially a loss of consciousness, was then used by Penfield & Jasper (1954). In Penfield's view, the centrencephalic system included brainstem structures (namely the reticular formation) capable of influencing the activity of the thalamic nuclei. Monoaminergic, cholinergic and noradrenergic pathways ascending from brainstem to the thalamus and cortex were later demonstrated to modulate state-dependent reactions of the brain thus adding a new dimension to the concept of centrencephalic system.

The concept of centrencephalic seizures was challenged by experiments in animal models of generalized seizures obtained by either systemical penicillin administration (feline generalized penicillin epilepsy, FGPE) (Prince & Farrel, 1969; Gloor, 1979) or bilateral cortical application of convulsant agents to homotopic cortical areas (Marcus & Watson, 1966; Gloor, 1979). The concept of cortico-reticular seizures as opposite to that of centrencephalic seizures was put forward (Gloor, 1968; see also in Gloor & Fariello, 1988). According to this concept the cerebral cortex is primarily involved in the FGPE model with only secondary involvement of the thalamus. However, further neurophysiological studies in FGPE demonstrated that SWD reflect an abnormal oscillatory pattern of discharge involving mutually interconnected cortical and thalamic neurons (see Gloor, 1984) and that neither the cortex nor the thalamus can sustain this pattern on its own. In addition, it has been shown that the thalamocortical circuits involved in the genesis of SWD in FGPE, are the same that sustain rhythmic thalamocortical activities, which generate the EEG spindles which characterize the early stages of slow wave sleep (Gloor, 1984). Another important result of the studies on FGPE was the demonstration that the preservation of GABAergic inhibition in both cortex and thalamus is an essential factor that contributes to the synchronization of neuronal activity during SWD (Avoli et al., 1982; Kostopoulos et al., 1983; Giarretta et al., 1987) and that enhancement of GABAergic activity potentiates all experimental forms of SWD (Fariello & Ticku, 1983). It has to be noted that although the experiments carried out in FGPE have questioned the role of the thalamus as the generator of SWD, they have nevertheless stressed the essential contribution of the thalamus in sustaining their rhythmic expression. Indeed, thalamic inactivation or destruction abolishes SWD in FGPE.

This conclusion can be maintained in spite of Marcus & Watson's (1966) and Mutani's (1973) observation on the primary role of the corpus callosum in mediating bilateral synchronous discharges which, in cats with bilateral cortical foci, persist after disconnection of the cortex from its thalamic afferents. In fact, the bilateral discharges induced by homotopic cortical foci do not fit a strict definition of the petit-mal like SWD and rather reproduce some other types of human generalized seizures (see also Mutani et al., Chapter 1).

Further evidence of the role of thalamo-cortical interconnection in SWD generation comes from the genetic model GAERS (genetic absence epilepsy in rats from Strasbourg). This strain of Wistar rat, presenting with spontaneous bilateral and synchronous 7–9 Hz SWD, was selected by Vergnes et al. (1982) in the Centre de Neurochimie of Strasbourg. SWD are consistently associated with clinical manifestations (behavioural arrest and facial myoclonus) that are highly reminiscent of human absence-like seizures (see Mutani et al., Chapter 1). These absence-like seizures, lasting from 1 to 90 s, occur in all of the third generation inbred offspring after the 40th postnatal day at a mean rate of 1/min when awake. High amplitude rhythmic discharges synchronous with cortical SWD were recorded in the lateral part of the thalamus (Vergnes et al., 1987, 1990a). In addition, the same authors (Vergnes et al., 1990b) were able to suppress SWD by lesions of the lateral thalamic nuclei, thus demonstrating the role of the thalamus in SWD generation. More details on

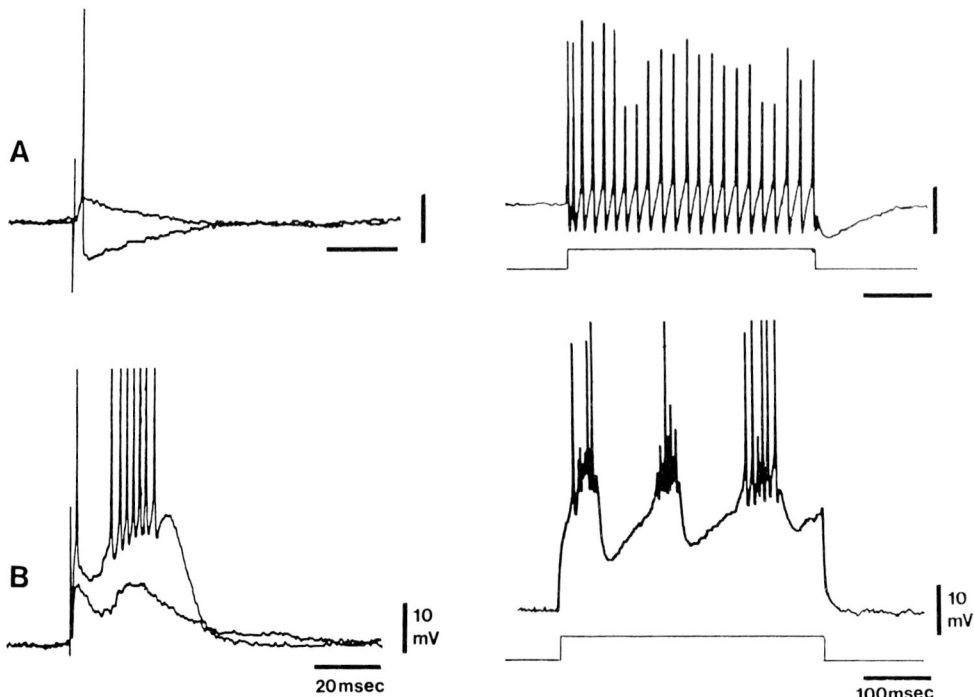

Fig. 1. *In vitro intracellular recording of an Rt neuron from a normal rat:* A, *at resting membrane potential (−58 mV);* B, *during membrane hyperpolarization (−78 mV)* **induced by steady current injection.** *Left: superimposition of postsynaptic responses evoked by* **internal capsule** *stimulations at two different intensities (infra- and supra-threshold for action potentials). Right: effect of intracellular injection of long-lasting depolarizing current pulses (from Avanzini et al., 1992b, with permission).*

the intrinsic thalamic mechanisms involved in generalized epileptogenesis in GAERS will be provided in the next section.

Rhythmogenic thalamic mechanisms and SWD

Recent observations support a central role of the thalamus in pace-setting rhythmic thalamocortical activities. From a series of experiments carried out in cats by Steriade group (Steriade & Deschenes, 1984; Steriade *et al.*, 1986, 1987; Mulle *et al.*, 1986), it became increasingly clear that the thalamic reticular nucleus (Rt) is a first-rate determinant of some rhythmic activities (namely sleep spindles).

Rt is a thin laminar nucleus which surrounds the dorsolateral and anterior portions of the dorsal thalamus. It is entirely composed of GABAergic neurons which send axons to all the other thalamic nuclei. It receives collaterals from both thalamocortical and corticothalamic systems but it does not participate directly in the thalamocortical projection.

As demonstrated for other thalamic nuclei by Deschenes *et al.* (1984) and by Jahnsen & Llinas (1984 a, b) Rt neurons can fire in two different modes, single-spike/tonic firing or bursting mode, depending on the level of membrane polarization (Kayama *et al.*, 1986; Mulle *et al.*, 1986; Avanzini *et al.*, 1989).

Intracellular recordings from *in vivo* (Mulle *et al.*, 1986) and *in vitro* (Avanzini *et al.*, 1989) Rt neurons have shown that in particular conditions bursting discharges tend to recur regularly giving

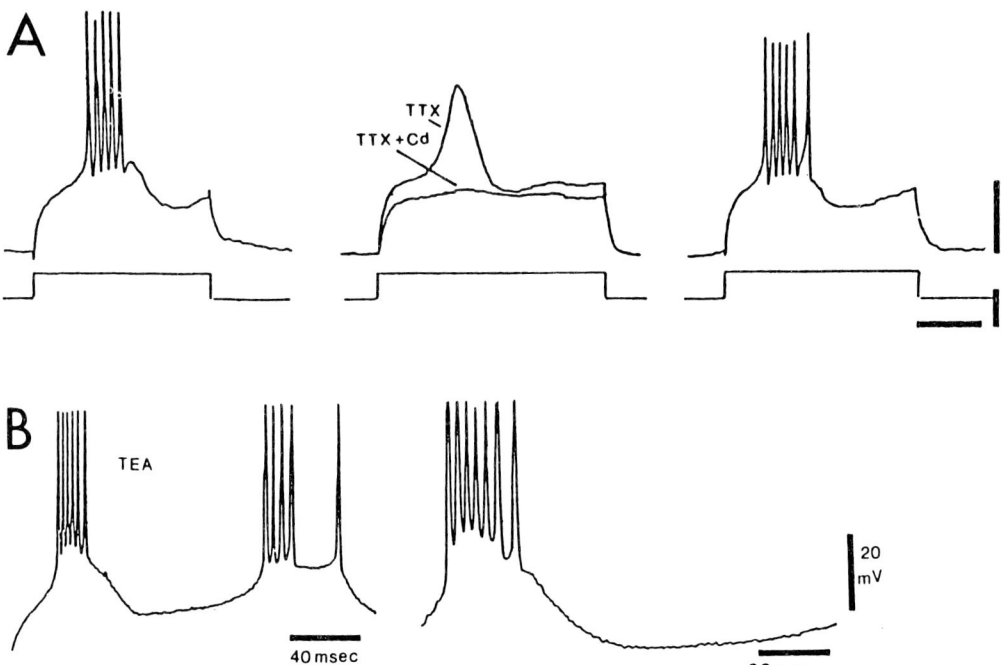

Fig. 2. A: Left: bursting response evoked by a depolarizing current pulse in a Rt neuron recorded in vitro from a normal rat. Centre: blockade of Na⁺ spikes with 1 μM TTX uncovers a Cd^{2+} (1 mM)-sensitive Ca^{2+} spike; Right: recovery of the fully developed burst after washing.
B: perfusion with TEA (20 mM) impairs the early phase of BAHP and prolongs the late slow decaying phase (from Avanzini et al., 1992a, with permission).

rise to rhythmic membrane oscillations, which are strictly correlated with EEG spindles (Mulle et al., 1986).

Intrinsic properties responsible for Rt oscillatory properties have been intensively investigated in our laboratory on *in vitro* slices prepared from Wistar rat thalamus. In addition, *in vivo* experiments aimed to investigate the implication of Rt nucleus in SWD of GAERS rats have been carried out in collaboration with the Strasbourg group. Results that may be relevant for the present discussion will be reported here in some detail.

By intracellular recording from thalamic slices burst firing was physiologically observed in Rt neurons at membrane potential values below –60 mV (Fig. 1). When Rt were stimulated directly with long lasting (600–1000 ms) and large (0.3–1 nA) depolarizing current pulses from a hyperpolarized level, repetitive 6–8 Hz bursting discharges were elicited (Fig. 1). Each burst was followed by a pronounced burst-after-hyperpolarization (BAHP) which lasted 80–120 ms (Fig. 1) resulting in a rhythmic oscillatory behaviour of the membrane potential. Perfusion with tetrodotoxin (TTX) 1 μM abolished Na⁺ spikes thus uncovering a slow all or none depolarizing potential underlying the burst, which was in turn abolished by Cd^{2+} 1 mM (Fig. 2) demonstrating its Ca^{2+} dependency.

Perfusion with tetraethylammonium (TEA) 20 mM demonstrated the bimodal nature of BAHP which consisted of a first TEA-sensitive fast phase which peaked at about 20 ms and a slower TEA-insensitive decay phase which was not reduced but rather enhanced by TEA perfusion (Fig. 2).

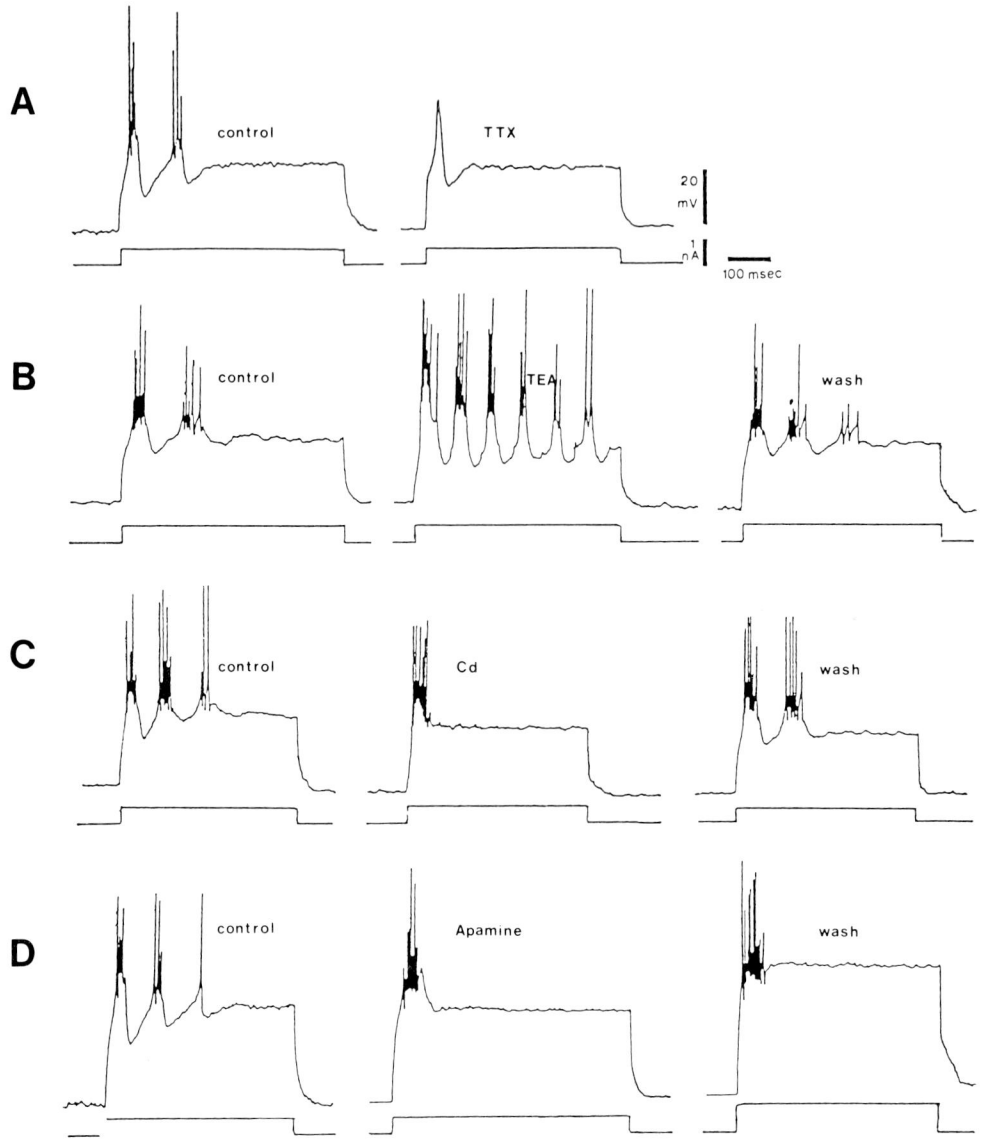

Fig. 3. Effects of TTX 1 µM (A), TEA 20 mM (B), Cd^{2+} 1 mM (C) and apamine 100 µM on rhythmic bursting behaviour of different Rt neurons recorded in vitro from normal rats (from Avanzini et al., 1989, with permission).

On the basis of these pharmacological tests the burst-BAHP sequence was attributed to a set of Ca^{2+}/K^+ membrane conductances responsible for low threshold Ca^{2+}-dependent K^+ outward currents ($K^+_{(Ca2+)}$). The apparent facilitation of the slow $K^+_{(Ca2+)}$ during TEA perfusion was explained by a TEA-induced increase in Ca^{2+} influx due to the broadening of the spike repolarization.

The existence of a well-developed biphasic BAHP was the main physiological difference between

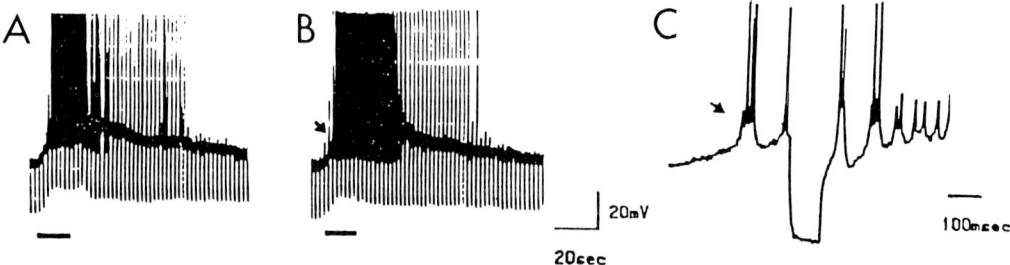

Fig. 4. Effects of 1 M glutamate (A) and 1 M aspartate (B) iontophoretic application on an Rt neuron recorded in vitro from a normal rat. The injection time is marked by a horizontal bar below the traces. C fast recording of the response depicted in B (arrow).
Membrane resistance was continuously monitored by 0.5 nA hyperpolarizing current pulses, resulting in negatively trending vertical bars in A and B. The membrane deflection induced by one such pulse is better seen in C (from Avanzini et al., 1992a, with permission).

Rt and ventralis posterior (VP) neurons. The latter consistently lacked long-lasting K^+-dependent afterhyperpolarizations and never showed a tendency to produce repetitive bursting discharges.

The effect of the following drugs was tested on oscillatory properties of Rt neurons (Fig. 3). Cadmium 1 mM, blocking $K^+_{(Ca2+)}$ conductances before a total Ca^{2+} blockade, suppressed the repetitive burst discharges. Apamine 100 mM, which blocks slow $K^+_{(Ca2+)}$ conductances did the same. On the contrary, TEA 20 mM, which suppresses the early fast $K^+_{(Ca2+)}$ current with a reciprocal enhancement of the late BAHP component, facilitated and prolonged the rhythmic discharges. The rhythmic behaviour was also abolished by TTX 1 mM in spite of a well-developed BAHP following the low-threshold Ca^{2+} spike uncovered by Na^+ blockade. This could be a consequence of the abolition of Ca^{2+} influx which occurs during Na^+ spike. Alternatively, it can be attributed to the block of a TTX-sensitive, regenerative Na^+ current activated during the burst generation.

Iontophoretic application of glutamate (0.5 and 1 M), aspartate (0.5–1 M), NMDA (20–50 mM), kainate (100 mM) and quisqualate (100 mM) induced membrane depolarization with sustained cell firing. Aspartate and NMDA were particularly effective in inducing prolonged discharges which in some neurons took the form of a burst firing associated with an apparent increase in membrane input resistance (Fig. 4). Aspartate and NMDA-induced burst firing was facilitated by slight membrane hyperpolarization.

It was therefore concluded that Rt neurons are provided with a set of Ca^{2+}/K^+ membrane conductances which enable them to produce rhythmic oscillatory activities. The putative role of Rt oscillatory properties in pacing SWD of GAERS rats was investigated by lesion experiments and by injection of Ca^{2+} blockers in Rt.

All the experiments were carried out *in vivo*. The animals were previously callosotomized to obtain an almost complete independence of SWD expression on either hemisphere (Vergnes et al., 1989). In animals with selective lesions of Rt, obtained by stereotaxic injections of ibotenic acid, SWD were completely suppressed on the ipsilateral hemisphere during the first 3 days after ibotenic acid injection. From the fourth day, low frequency (3–5 Hz) sharp waves appeared on the lesioned side and persisted throughout the observation period (up to 35 days) (Fig. 5). Their rate of expression (measured as discharge duration in seconds over 20 min of EEG) was 13.62 per cent of the corresponding SWD rate on the intact hemisphere (Avanzini et al., 1993).

In another series of experiments the local effect of Cd^{2+}, which was previously shown *in vitro* to suppress Rt oscillatory behaviour by blocking Ca^{2+} and/or $K^+_{(Ca2+)}$ membrane currents (see above),

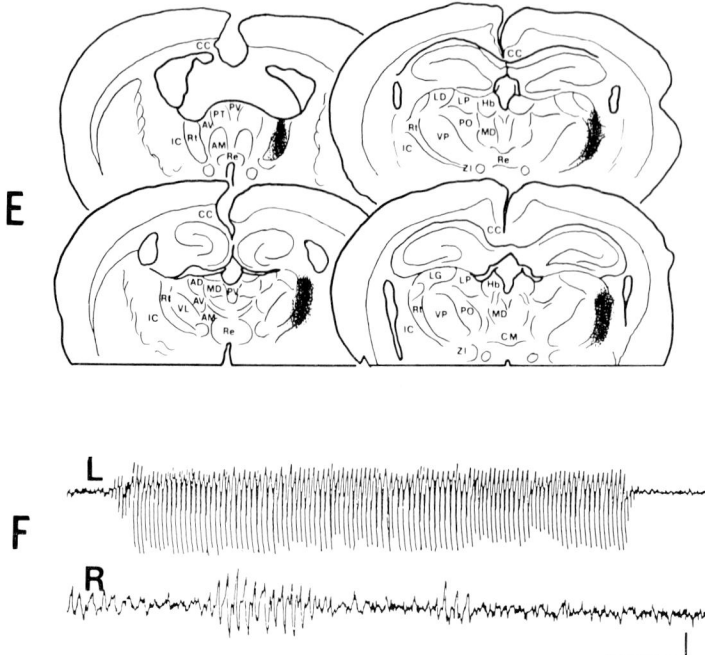

Fig. 5. Top: Schematic reconstruction of histological sections showing the extent of the lesion induced by ibotenic acid in a GAERS rat.
AD: n. anterior dorsalis; AM: n. anterior medialis; AV: n. anterior ventralis; CC: corpus callosum; CM: n. centromedianus; Hb: habenula; IC: internal capsule; LD: n. lateralis dorsalis; LG: corpus geniculatum laterale; LP: n. lateralis posterior; MD: n. medialis dorsalis; PO: posterior nuclear group; Re: n. reuniens; Rt: reticular thalamic nucleus; VL: n. ventralis lateralis; VP: n. ventralis posterior; ZI: zona incerta.
Bottom: An EEG control performed 4 days after induction of right Rt lesion in a previously callosotomized rat shows abortive low rate SWD in the right side (from Avanzini et al., 1993, with permission).

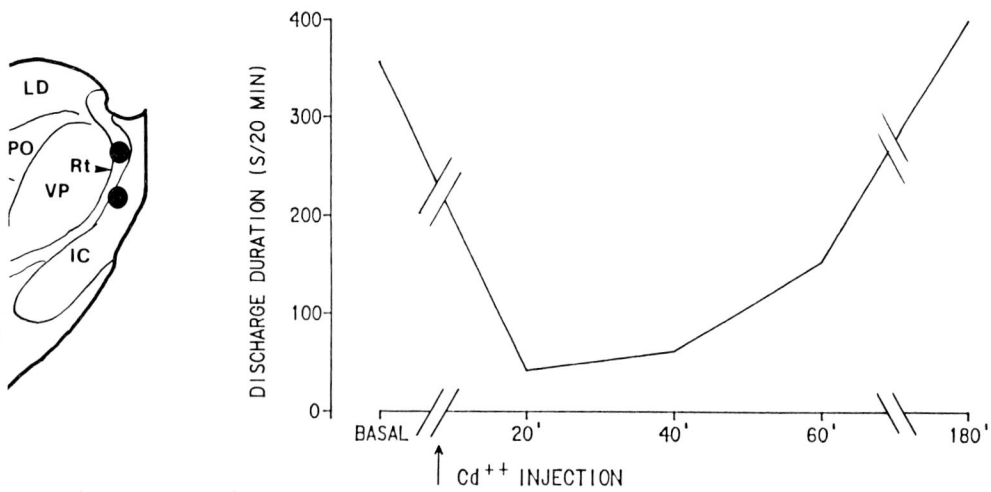

Fig. 6. Reversible antagonistic effect of unilateral Cd^{2+} injection in Rt on SWD in a callosotomized Wistar rat from the epileptic strain studied in vivo. Changes in SWD generation ipsilateral to the injection are expressed as total discharge duration (s) over 20 min (from Avanzini et al., 1993, with permission).

was tested by intrathalamic injection. Fig. 6 shows a representative example of the reversible suppressive effect of Cd^{2+} injection in the Rt on ipsilateral SWD. Significant decrements (variable in value and duration) in ipsilateral SWD activity were consistently observed in all Rt-injected animals. In contrast, rats which had received Cd^{2+} injection in the VP nucleus showed only small changes in ipsilateral SWD activity (Avanzini et al., 1993). It can be inferred that Ca^{2+}/K^+-dependent oscillatory properties of Rt play a crucial role in SWD generation.

Through its widespread efferent projections to other thalamic nuclei, Rt can impose its rhythms on thalamocortical neurons that fire in a reciprocal time relationship with the Rt, as has been demonstrated to occur in cats during spindling activity by Mulle et al. (1986). In fact, the rhythmic hyperpolarizing inhibitory postsynaptic potentials generated in thalamocortical neurons by phasic GABAergic volleys may be effective in deinactivating low threshold Ca^{2+} conductance. As a result, a generalized rhythmic bursting activity may be synchronously recruited in all of the thalamic nuclei that receive efferent fibres from the Rt. Indirect confirmation of the implication of this thalamic system in generation of SWD came from pharmacological experiments which showed that GABAergic agents facilitated SWD in GAERS (Vergnes et al., 1984) and that ethosuximide, a well-known anti-absence drug, is a potent antagonist of the Ca^{2+}-dependent T current in isolated thalamic neurons from rats (Coulter et al., 1989). Overall, these results support the idea that the Rt stands in a nodal position within the thalamocortical circuits underlying SWD in GAERS rats. This is not to say that the Rt should be necessarily viewed as the site of the primary genetically determined defect responsible for SWD. Its role in pacing rhythmic thalamocortical discharges could in fact be put into action secondarily by pathophysiological mechanisms arising elsewhere. In the *in vitro* study in normal rats, we showed that corticothalamic aspartatergic projections are particularly effective in enhancing repetitive burst firing in Rt neurons when membrane potential is set at a proper level (de Curtis et al., 1989). Thus, in GAERS an intense corticofugal output, impinging on Rt, might well set in motion the state-dependent oscillatory system, which Rt is part of, thus giving rise to 7–9 Hz SWD. According to this information, experiments are now in progress aimed to identify the basic functional defect which makes the thalamo-cortico-thalamic circuit operate improperly in GAERS. Should a specific receptor or channel alteration be recognized, this would add a new molecular dimension to the approach to the generalized epileptogenesis.

Acknowledgements

The author wishes to thank Maria Teresa Pasquali for editing assistance. The work was partially supported by the Paolo Zorzi Association for Neurosciences and by CNR-INSERM contribution N. 132.22.2 for Italian–French collaboration.

References

Avanzini, G., de Curtis, M., Marescaux, C., Panzica, F., Spreafico, R. & Vergnes, M. (1992a): Role of the thalamic reticular nucleus in the generation of rhythmic thalamo-cortical activities subserving spike and waves. *J. Neural Transm.* 35 (suppl.), 85–95.

Avanzini, G., de Curtis, M., Panzica, F. & Spreafico, R. (1989): Intrinsic properties of nucleus reticularis thalami neurones of the rat studied *in vitro*. *J. Physiol.* 416, 111–122.

Avanzini, G., de Curtis, M. & Spreafico, R. (1992b): Physiological properties of GABAergic thalamic reticular neurons studied *in vitro*: relevance to thalamocortical synchronizing mechanisms. In: *Neurotransmitters in epilepsy (Epilepsy Res. Suppl. 8)* eds. G. Avanzini, J. Engel, R. Fariello & U. Heinemann, pp. 117–124. Amsterdam: Elsevier.

Avanzini, G., Vergnes, M., Spreafico, R. & Marescaux, C. (1993): Calcium-dependent regulation of genetically determined spike and waves by the reticular thalamic nucleus of rats. *Epilepsia* 34, 1–8.

Avoli, M., Gloor, P. & Kostopoulos, G. (1982): Cortical and thalamic microphysiology of experimental spike and wave discharges. In: *Advances in epileptology XIII. Epilepsy International Symposium*, eds. H. Akimoto, H. Kasamatsuri, M. Seino & A. Ward, pp. 493–496. New York: Raven Press.

Coulter, D.A., Huguenard, J.R. & Prince, D.A. (1989): Characterization of ethosuximide reduction of low-threshold calcium current in thalamic neurons. *Ann. Neurol.* 25, 582–593.

de Curtis, M., Spreafico, R. & Avanzini, G. (1989): Excitatory amino acids mediate responses elicited *in vitro* by stimulation of cortical afferents to reticularis thalami neurons of the rat. *Neuroscience* 33, 275–283.

Delgado Escueta, A.V., Greenberg, D., Weissbecker, K., Liu, A., Treiman, L., Sparkes, R., Park, M.S., Barbetti, A. & Terasaki, P.I. (1990): Gene mapping in the idiopathic generalized epilepsy: juvenile myoclonic epilepsy, childhood absence epilepsy, epilepsy with grand mal seizures, and early childhood myoclonic epilepsy. *Epilepsia* 31 (Suppl. 3), S19–S29.

Deschenes, M., Paradis, M., Roy, J.P. & Steriade, M. (1984): Electrophysiology of neurons of lateral thalamic nuclei in cat: resting properties and burst discharges. *J. Neurophysiol.* 51, 1196–1219.

Durner, M., Sander, T., Greenberg, D.A., Johnson, K., Beck-Mannagetta, G. & Janz D. (1991): Localization of idiopathic generalized epilepsy on chromosome 6p in families of juvenile myoclonic patients. *Neurology* 41, 1651–1655.

Fariello, R.G. & Ticku, M.K.C. (1983): Minireview: the perspective of GABA replenishment treatment in the epilepsies: a critical evaluation of hopes and concerns. *Life Sci.* 33, 1629–1640.

Giarretta, D., Avoli, M. & Gloor, P. (1987): Intracellular recordings in pericruciate neurons during spike and wave discharges of feline generalized penicillin epilepsy. *Brain Res.* 405, 68–79.

Gloor, P. (1968): Generalized cortico-reticular epilepsies. Some considerations on the pathophysiology of generalized bilaterally synchronous spike and wave discharge. *Epilepsia* 9, 249–263.

Gloor, P. (1979): Generalized epilepsy with spike-and-wave discharge: a reinterpretation of its electrographic and clinical manifestations. *Epilepsia* 20, 571–588.

Gloor, P. (1984): Electrophysiology of generalized epilepsy. In: *Electrophysiology of epilepsy*, eds. P.A. Schwartzkroin & H. Wheal, pp. 107–136. London: Academic Press.

Gloor, P. & Fariello, R.G. (1988): Generalized epilepsy: some of its cellular mechanisms differ from those of focal epilepsy. *Trends Neurosci.* 11, 63–68.

Gloor, P & Testa, G. (1974): Generalized epilepsy in the cat: effects of intracarotid and intravertebral pentylenetetrazol and amobarbital injections. *Electroencephalogr. Clin. Neurophysiol.* 36, 499–515.

Greenberg, D.A., Durner, M., Delgado-Escueta, A. & Janz, D. (1991): Combined linkage analysis of juvenile myoclonic epilepsy: is there a second gene locus? *Hum. Gene Mapping* (abstract): 62–63.

Hunter, H. & Jasper, H.H. (1949): Effects of thalamic stimulation in unanaesthetized animals. *Electroencephalogr. Clin. Neurophysiol.* 1, 305–324.

ICE (1989): Proposal for revised classification of epilepsies and epileptic syndromes. Commission on classification and terminology of the International League Against Epilepsy. *Epilepsia* 30, 389–399.

ICES (1981): Proposal for revised clinical and electroencephalographic classification of epileptic seizures. Commission on classification and terminology of the International League Against Epilepsy. *Epilepsia* 22, 489–501.

Jahnsen, H. & Llinas, R. (1984a): Electrophysiological properties of guinea-pig thalamic neurones: an *in vitro* study. *J. Physiol.* 349, 205–226.

Jahnsen, H. & Llinas, R. (1984b): Ionic basis for the electroresponsiveness and oscillatory properties of guinea-pig thalamic neurones *in vitro*. *J. Physiol.* 349, 227–247.

Jasper, H.H. (1990): Historical introduction (with conclusions) In: *Generalized epilepsy. Neurobiological approaches*, eds. M. Avoli, P. Gloor, G. Kostopoulos & R. Naquet, pp. 1–15. Boston: Birkhauser.

Jasper, H.H. & Drooglever-Fortuyn, J. (1947): Experimental studies of the functional anatomy of petit mal epilepsy. *Ass. Res. Nerv. Ment. Dis. Proc.* 26, 272–298.

Jasper, H.H. & Karshman, J. (1941): Electroencephalographic classification of the epilepsies. *Arch. Neurol. Psychiatry* 45, 903–943.

Kayama, Y., Sumitomo, I. & Ogawa, T. (1986): Does the ascending cholinergic projection inhibit or excite neurons in the rat thalamic reticular nucleus? *J. Neurophysiol.* 56, 1310–1320.

Kostopoulos, G., Avoli, M. & Gloor, P. (1983): Participation of cortical recurrent inhibition in the genesis of spike and wave discharges in feline generalized penicillin epilepsy. *Brain Res.* 227, 101–112.

Marcus, E.N. & Watson, C.W. (1966): Bilateral synchronous spike and wave electrographic patterns in the cat. Interaction of bilateral cortical foci in the intact, the bilateral cortico-callosal and adiencephalic preparation. *Arch. Neurol.* 14, 601–610.

Morison, R.S. & Dempsey, E.W. (1942): A study of thalamo-cortical relations. *Am. J. Physiol.* 135, 281–292.

Mulle, C., Madariaga, A. & Deschenes, M. (1986): Morphology and electrophysiological properties of reticularis thalami neurons in cat: *in vivo* study of thalamic pacemaker. *J. Neurosci.* **6**, 2134–2145.

Mutani, R., Bergamini, L., Fariello, R.G. & Quattroccolo, G. (1973): Bilateral synchrony of epileptic discharge associated with chronic asymmetrical cortical foci. *Electroencephalogr. Clin. Neurophysiol.* **34**, 53–59.

Mutani, R., Cantello, R., Cianelli, M. & Civardi, C. (1993): Animal models of epilepsy. In: *Epileptogenic and excitotoxic mechanisms*, eds. G. Avanzini, R. Fariello, U. Heinemann & R. Mutani, pp. 5–15. London: John Libbey.

Penfield, W. (1957): Consciousness and centrencephalic organization. Proceedings of the First International Congress of Neurological Sciences. Brussels.

Penfield, W. & Jasper, H.H. (1954): *Epilepsy and functional anatomy of the human brain*. Boston: Little, Brown and Co.

Prince, D.A. & Farrel, D. (1969): Centrencephalic spike-wave discharges following parenteral penicillin injunction in the cat. *Neurology* **19**, 309–310.

Steriade, M. & Deschenes, M. (1984): The thalamus as a neuronal oscillator. *Brain Res. Rev.* **8**, 1–63.

Steriade, M., Dominich, L. & Oakson, G. (1986): Reticularis thalami neurons revisited: activity changes during shifts in states of vigilance. *J. Neurosci.* **6**, 68–81.

Steriade, M., Dominich, L., Oakson, G. & Deschenes, M. (1987): The deafferented reticular thalamic nucleus generates spindle rhythmicity. *J. Neurophysiol.* **57**, 260–273.

Vergnes, M., Marescaux, C. & Depaulis, A. (1990a): Mapping of spontaneous spike and wave discharges in Wistar rats with genetic generalized non-convulsive epilepsy. *Brain Res.* **523**, 87–91.

Vergnes, M., Marescaux, C., Depaulis, A., Micheletti, G. & Warter, J.M. (1987): Sponteneous spike and wave discharges in thalamus and cortex in a rat model of genetic petit mal-like seizures. *Exp. Neurol.* **96**, 127–136.

Vergnes, M., Marescaux, C., Depaulis, A., Micheletti, G. & Warter, J. M. (1990b): Spontaneous spike-and-wave discharges in Wistar rats: a model of genetic generalized nonconvulsive epilepsy. In: *Generalized epilepsy*, eds. M. Avoli, P. Gloor, G. Kostopoulos & R. Naquet, pp. 238–253. Boston: Birkhauser.

Vergnes, M., Marescaux, C., Lannes, B., Depaulis, A., Micheletti, G. & Warter, J.M. (1989): Interhemispheric desynchronization of spontaneous spike-wave discharges by corpus callosum transection in rats with petit mal-like epilepsy. *Epilepsy Res.* **4**, 8–13.

Vergnes, M., Marescaux, C., Micheletti, G., Depaulis, A., Rumbach, L. & Warter, J.M. (1984): Enhancement of spike and wave discharges by GABA-mimetic drugs in rats with spontaneous petit mal-like epilepsy. *Neurosci. Lett.* **44**, 91–94.

Vergnes, M., Marescaux, C., Micheletti, G., Reis, J., Depaulis, A., Rumbach, L. & Warter, J.M. (1982): Spontaneous paroxysmal electroclinical patterns in rat: a model of generalized non-convulsive epilepsy. *Neurosci. Lett.* **33**, 97–101.

Chapter 4

Mechanisms of action of antiepileptic drugs

R.G. Fariello

Department of Neurology, Thomas Jefferson University, Philadelphia, PA, USA

Summary

Insights on the mechanisms of action of antiepileptic drugs (AEDs) have been gained from the study of pathophysiological mechanisms in experimental models of fragments taken from the highly complex and non-homogeneous phenomenon called epilepsy. Other insights have been derived from the developmental process of new AEDs. Presently it is widely believed that anticonvulsant benzodiazepines and gamma-vinyl-GABA exert their antiepileptic effect by enhancing GABAergic inhibition in the brain. Several major established AEDs share the common properties of interfering with Na channels reducing the ability of neurons and axons to respectively generate and conduct high frequency discharges. Other putative mechanisms of action are even more speculative and less established. New AEDs are now synthesized to possess a specific action (for example antagonism to an excitatory receptor) and then tested experimentally and clinically. None of these designer drugs has reached widespread clinical use yet. By and large the uncertainties about the mechanisms of action of AEDs reflect poor knowledge about the fundamental steps of epileptogenesis and underscore the need for improving it. The use of more appropriate experimental models of epilepsies (rather than seizures) appears to be a suitable step toward reaching this goal.

Introduction

The discussion of the mechanisms of action of antiepileptic drugs (AEDs) is intimately intertwined with the history of how they have been developed and studied. This chapter will attempt to outline the principles that have guided such developmental processes pointing out what has been done, what has been learned, what is the present state of knowledge, but also what has not been done, what is not yet fully understood and what, perhaps, could have been done differently.

Before addressing the topic of the mechanisms of action of AEDs some preliminary concepts must be clarified. First of all, epilepsy is not a disease entity but a group of syndromic categories used for clinical operational purposes by the medical community. The unifying character of these syndromes is the repetitive occurrence of a wide variety of motor and/or behavioural abnormalities (seizures or spells) paroxysmally intruding over time into the life of the subject. Convulsions are only one type of these intrusions, consisting of sustained or rhythmic maximal contractions of striatal musculature consequent to epileptiform discharges arising in part of or in the whole cerebral grey matter. Thus, epilepsy and convulsions are not synonyms nor are AEDs and anticonvulsants the same. An AED will prevent the recurrence of seizures whether they are convulsive or not, and anticonvulsants may prevent a grand mal attack, turning it into an aura (still a type of abortive seizure) or block one convulsive episode, without being efficacious for long-term prevention of seizures. For instance, ethosuximide (ETX) is an excellent AED in petit mal, but at clinically useful doses is devoid of anticonvulsant activity; diazepam is an excellent anticonvulsant, blocking grand mal status, but a poor AED for chronic use.

Second, we must stress that today, with the notable exception of benzodiazepines (BZDs) and γ-vinylGABA (GVG), mechanism of action whose is accepted as being related to their influence on the GABA systems, the mechanism of action of all the other major clinically used AEDs still remains substantially unknown.

Third, the knowledge of the intimate mechanisms of action of AEDs is limited by the still, in a way, superficial knowledge of the mechanisms of epileptogenesis. In fact, whereas modern epileptology has made impressive advances towards the knowledge of how interictal activity (i.e. spikes) is generated within epileptic foci and, through the study of long-term potentiation and kindling, how neuronal circuits may be primed to sustain epileptiform events and spread them throughout the brain, still very little is known about the determinants of the transition from interictal activity into seizures within foci, or how seizures may abruptly originate in the entire cerebrum.

Lastly, it should be pointed out that the ideal AED ought to be exclusively acting on the epileptic activity of neurons leaving unaffected the other non-epileptic functions. This ought to be possible since epileptiform activity is hallmarked by specific electrophysiological abnormalities not otherwise found in normal neuronal aggregates, making the search for an optimal drug a reachable goal for the future.

Historical note

Seizures, having preceded the appearance of the human race on earth, have been treated through the ages with all the ingredients of magic, religion and medicine, including such ghastly methods as eating fresh gladiators' liver (Temkin, 1971).

As far as Western medicine is concerned, the first effective treatment, even though administered for the wrong premises, was bromide, introduced in England in 1857 (Locock, 1857). With the discovery of phenobarbital's antiepileptic effect in 1912 in Germany (Hauptmann, 1912), better efficacy and fewer side effects were noted. But it was only in the late 1930s that a new drug, diphenylhydantoin (phenytoin, PHT) was brought into clinical use after animal tests which still are, in their essence, the basis for AEDs screening and development today (Putnam & Merrit, 1937; Merrit & Putnam, 1938; Merrit et al., 1938). These tests consist of suppression of seizures induced first in dogs and cats and nowadays in mice and rats by administration of electrical current (maximal and minimal electroshock thresholds, EST) or chemoconvulsants, mostly pentylenetetrazol (PTZ). The initial idea that EST would provide a model of grand mal seizures and PTZ of petit mal epilepsy was soon corrected by the school of Goodman (Toman et al., 1946; Goodman et al., 1953) who pointed out the importance of the intensity of the stimulus, rather than its nature, to predict the mechanism of action and the probable clinical application of the tested compounds.

More recent studies from the same school (Piredda et al., 1985) further established the concept that minimal threshold tests, whether electrical or chemical, inducing a clonic response, identify substances that raise local stimulus threshold, whereas supramaximal tests causing tonic hind limb extension evidence the property of suppressing the spread of seizures from the site of origin. The former paradigm shows good correlation with clinical anti-petit-mal activity, the latter with anti-grand-mal. The maximal threshold test in which tonic hind leg extension is obtained with the minimally effective stimulus has no predictive value (Swinyard et al., 1989).

In spite of these firmly established facts, AEDs are still non-uniformly, on the contrary erratically, put through the series of antiseizure tests in rodents with wide variations from laboratory to laboratory both in academia and in the pharmaceutical industry. In part to obviate this confusing

Chapter 4 MECHANISMS OF ACTION OF ANTIEPILEPTIC DRUGS

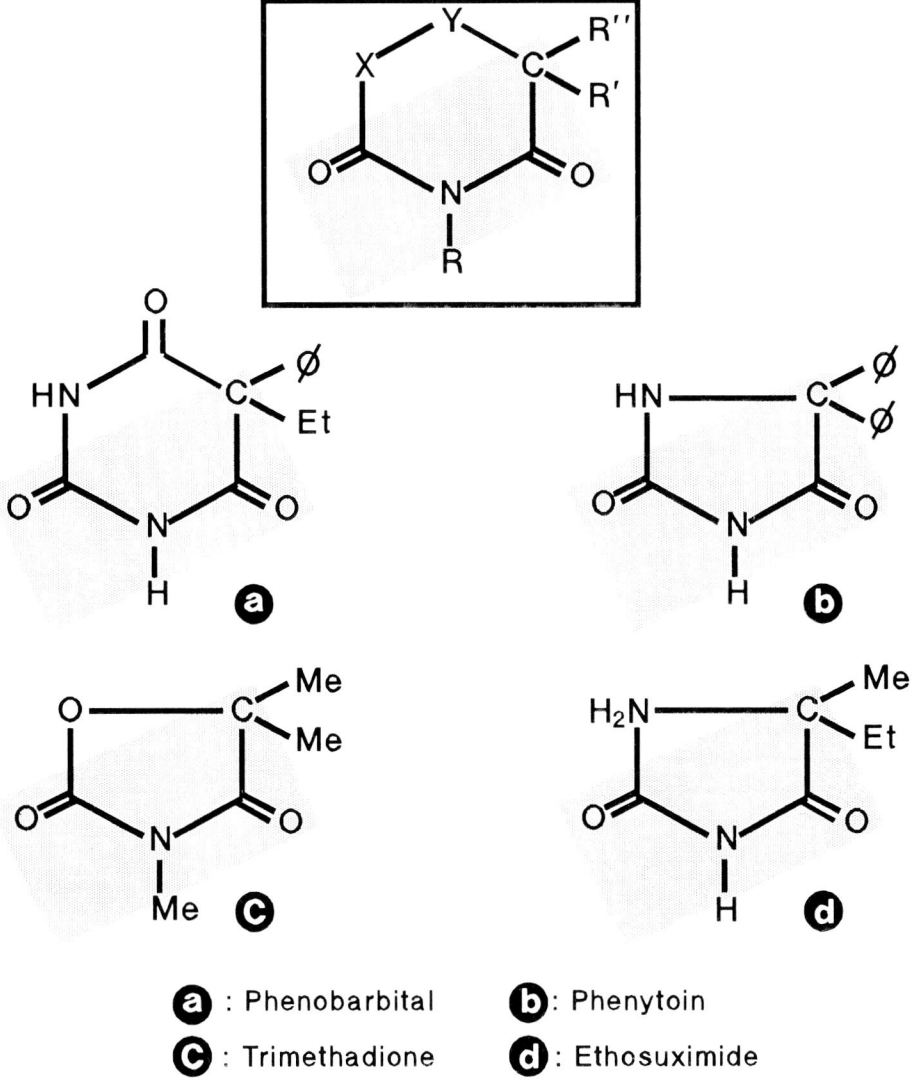

Fig. 1. Chemical skeleton of four AEDs that cover most of the spectrum of clinical efficacy. The shaded area highlights the parts in common which is also reported in the upper box.

situation the NIH has instituted a programme whereby potential AEDs are screened in a uniform way so that a reasonable comparison of efficacy and toxicity can be performed (Porter, 1986). This programme called the antiepileptic Drug Development Program, has today screened over 16,000 potential AEDs (H. Kupfenberg, personal communication).

As of the 1970s progress in the knowledge of neurobiology, especially molecular and receptorial pharmacology, prompted the elaboration of biochemical theories of epileptogenesis. A hypofunction of the GABA system was postulated as a fundamental step in experimental and, by extrapolation, clinical epileptogenesis (Fariello, 1979; Fariello *et al.*, 1991). This opened up the new era of molecular design for AEDs.

An important historical landmark was set when progabide, a GABA prodrug, was developed as an AED. Even though progabide was withdrawn from further development in the US due to a combination of limited efficacy and unacceptable risks of toxicity, nevertheless it has been the prototype of a potential AED developed on the basis of a programme of medicinal chemistry geared to design a drug to test a specific biochemical hypothesis based on solid experimental background. This event moved the field of AEDs development out of the empirical realm right into that of neurobiological science. The GABA theory of epileptogenesis contributed to the fight against epilepsy with the benzodiazepines (agents that indirectly enhance the GABA interaction with its $GABA_A$ receptor sites) and GVG, an irreversible inhibitor of GABA transaminase, a GABA catabolic enzyme. GVG is the first AED of any substance introduced into clinical use in UK and Italy since 1967, when valproic acid was first made available in France.

In the mid 1980s the emphasis of the neuroscience community shifted toward the study of the role played by excitatory neurotransmission in the pathogenesis of almost every pathological condition of the CNS with the key position assumed by the activation of the *N*-methyl-D-aspartate (NMDA) receptor. NMDA is one of the receptors for the excitatory amino acids glutamate and aspartate, believed to be important for some key physiological events, subtending learning, neuronal plasticity and memory on one hand, but on the other, leading to a cascade of excitotoxic events ensuing in neuronal damage and death when excessively or improperly used.

Similar to the GABA hypothesis mentioned before, substantial evidence links glutamate and the NMDA receptor to experimental epileptogenesis (Fariello, 1985; Dingledine *et al.*, 1990), but the clinical part of the theory is mostly, if not entirely, speculative.

Several 'designer' drugs have now been tested and are in early preclinical developmental phase to test the antiepileptic properties of competitive, non-competitive NMDA antagonists and modulators of the various allosteric sites of this complex receptor (Fisher, 1991).

The GABA and the NMDA hypothesis have introduced a new step now widely used in the screening of potential new AEDs: the receptor-binding assays. This usually extends beyond these two neurotransmitters, to involve a wide variety of other receptors which, from time to time, are believed to have relevance to epileptogenesis.

In summary, the history of AEDs began in the realm of magic, moved into the area of empirical observation, and then through medicinal chemistry principles of the modification of existing drugs, ended in the very recent era in which drugs are first designed to possess a specific pharmacological action, desired according to the present knowledge of the epileptogenesis. A screening procedure is then initiated to test on one hand how successfully the intended goal has been reached (i.e. a glutamate antagonist will be assayed for its affinity to the various receptor subtypes, its specificity and its full or partial activity in *in vitro* and *in vivo*) and on the other hand to establish efficacy through the battery of the seizure models induced by chemoconvulsants and electrical currents. In parallel, neurotoxicity is tested in rodents assessing coordination impairment in a series of motor performances, in order to establish the therapeutic index (TI). TI is defined as the numerical expression of efficacy versus toxicity:

$$TI = ED_{50}/TD_{50}.$$

Obviously the developmental process outlined above has great intrinsic limitations. First, several of the used testing paradygms are by themselves afflicted by lack of knowledge of their mechanisms of action. Thus, it is unreasonable to expect that they provide clues as to the mechanisms of action of the tested compounds. For instance it remains to be established why the electrical current produces a jump at minimal threshold and a full blown tonic hindlimb extension followed by massive repetitive myoclonic jumps at supramaximal intensity. As a consequence, the suppression of these phenomena by any drug cannot provide insights into its mechanism of action other than the empirical observation that blockade of the minimal EST relates to a locally raised threshold response, whereas the suppression of the supramaximal response indicates reduction of the spread of the epileptic response throughout the brain.

Second, several of the tests were originally biased and able to screen drugs with one predominant mechanism of action without giving indication about possible others. To illustrate this point let us consider the bicuculline-induced convulsion test.

Bicuculline produces convulsions by blocking $GABA_A$ receptors throughout the brain. Thus this test will screen, as excellent AEDs, drugs acting as GABA agonists (BZDs for instance) providing no more than an *in vivo* confirmation of their demonstrated *in vitro* agonistic activity on the GABA system. For other compounds such as PHT the test may at the most suggest some activity on the GABA system or on other systems that secondarily may influence GABAergic tone.

Third, it must be pointed out that no one of the developmental steps presently used really tests an antiepileptic effect as compared to a simple antiseizure effect (see Introduction). Models of epilepsy do exist naturally in the animal kingdom (see Fisher, 1989; Löscher & Schmidt, 1988, for review) but for mostly practical and economical reasons these have been constantly overlooked by both the academic and industrial scientific community in the development of AEDs.

Some of these naturally occurring epilepsies, such as the ones seen in beagles, poodles, cats and cynomolgus baboons, bear important resemblances to human epileptic syndromes. Other naturally occurring neurological syndromes may be models of very rare human conditions (as appears to be the case for photosensitive myoclonic seizures in *Papio papio* baboons, Naquet & Meldrum, 1972), or even uncertainly related to the human epilepsies, as the sound-induced running fits in mice (Swinyard *et al.*, 1963) and other rodents (Jobe *et al.*, 1984).

The need for new AEDs greatly rests on the unmet goal of a satisfactory state of the art for the treatment of partial complex seizures. In the development of new AEDs, none of the presently utilized tests reliably predict efficacy against partial complex seizures nor can these tests be considered a satisfactory model of this condition (Fariello & Golden, 1985). It is auspicious that some of the naturally occurring epileptic syndromes in animals characterized by partial seizures with or without generalization can be introduced in the screening and developmental process of new AEDs.

In essence, since the introduction of DPH, for over 30 years AEDs have been sought by applying principles of medicinal chemistry to known molecules in the attempt to improve efficacy and tolerability. In the more recent past, drugs are designed to accomplish a specific biochemical test (i.e. receptor ligation, uptake or enzyme inhibition, etc.) and then put through the developmental phases in the laboratory. Still, a substantial number of compounds reach clinical testing after having been serendipitously found effective in the battery of electrically and chemically induced convulsions described above. Eventually, when a drug is established as a potential AED, studies are designed to discover its intimate mechanism of action on normal and epileptiform neuronal activity. Even in the case of 'designer' drugs, targeted for a specific mechanism of action, the relevance of the mechanism to the anticonvulsant and antiepileptic effect is rarely established with certainty, even after years of approved, widespread clinical use.

Mechanisms of action shared by different AEDs

The great majority of clinically established AEDs derive from a limited number of chemical compounds. Some major anti-grand-mal and petit-mal drugs belong to ever more restricted chemical series sharing major structural analogies (Porter, 1986). As illustrated in Fig. 1 barbiturates, hydantoines, succinamides and trimethadione share striking structural similarities in spite of their diversified clinical spectrum of efficacy. Therefore, it appears logical to ask whether a common mechanism of action is shared by all these chemically related molecules. In general, the evidence supporting the action of various AEDs on a common 'pharmacophore' is tenuous, but an effect on the Na channel in the neuronal membrane appears to be the best hypothetical candidate. However, as pointed out by Macdonald & McLean (1986) in a series of *in vitro* studies, such an effect is not always evident at therapeutic drug concentrations. When only toxic levels exert a given action, then this is unlikely to contribute to the clinically observed antiepileptic action. As far as the Na channel is concerned, whereas phenobarbital (PB), PHT, primidone (PM), carbamazepine (CBZ), sodium valproate (VPA) and potent anticonvulsant BZPs all show effects, only PHT, CBZ and VPA can modify Na channel permeability at therapeutic levels. Na channels in neuronal membranes are key regulators of cellular excitability as they exist in a resting, open or inactive state. The equilibrium among these states is dependent on voltage, time and frequency of use. Sustained (high frequency) repetitive firing (SRF) is an intrinsic property of some neurons which bears important resemblances with epileptic discharges and is mainly regulated by Na channels. AEDs (and local anaesthetics as well) although leaving unaffected the initial action potential (AP) will limit the capability of generating the train of APs that follow and eventually block SRF, probably by binding to the Na channel in their inactive state (see Macdonald & Meldrum, 1989, for review).

Another mechanism of action, shared by various classes of AEDs, is the functional enhancement of the GABAergic tone achieved through either direct action on the receptor or intervention on the metabolic pathways. The $GABA_A$ receptor is a tetrameric complex of α and β subunits, the latter containing binding sites for two GABA molecules. Within the several crossings of the neuronal membrane made by the receptor protein, there is a Cl^- channel whose opening generates, in most conditions, hyperpolarizing currents. Anticonvulsant BZPs bind to an allosteric modulatory site that enhances the binding of GABA to the receptor (Skerrit *et al.*, 1982; Bormann, 1988) and increases the channel's currents by increasing the frequency of the opening events. Anticonvulsant barbiturates bind to another regulatory allosteric site (sensitive also to convulsant barbiturates and picrotoxin) and prolong the duration of the currents (Twyman *et al.*, 1989).

GABA metabolism *in vitro* and in animal experiments is altered by VPA which both inhibits two GABA-degrading enzymes (GABA transaminase (GABA-T) and succinic-semialdehyde-dehydrogenase, Harvey *et al.*, 1975) and increases the GABA synthesizing enzyme, glutamic acid decarboxylase (GAD) (Löscher, 1981). Whether this mechanism plays any role in the clinical setting is still a matter of debate. By and large, the data supporting increased availability of the neurotransmitter fraction of the GABA pool in the VPA-treated epileptic population are scanty and far from definitive (Fariello & Smith, 1989).

GVG (Vigabatrin®) is a designer drug that irreversibly inhibits GABA-T with a mechanism called suicidal, as it becomes itself a substrate for the enzyme (Lippert *et al.*, 1977). GVG is now an established AED in several European countries: its clinical efficacy is associated with elevated GABA levels in the CSF (Pitkaanen *et al.*, 1988).

PHT too has been shown in a molluscan preparation to possess GABAmimetic properties (Ayala *et al.*, 1977), diminishing the rate of closing of the Cl^- channel. Doubts exist regarding the clinical relevance of this experimental data (De Lorenzo, 1989).

Whereas other mechanisms of action are theoretically possible or even have been demonstrated in experimental settings, they remain nevertheless speculative at this time in regard to their clinical relevance. These postulated mechanisms include action on the excitatory transmission (Macdonald & Meldrum, 1989) and on the purinergic system (Dragunow, 1988). Lamotrigine, a potential AED in an advanced phase of clinical development, appears to be the first compound that will have, as its putative mechanism of action, a reduction of glutamate release at synaptic terminals (Leach *et al.*, 1986).

Anatomical substrate of antiepileptic action

The epilepsies represent an ensemble of events exquisitively dynamic in their essence from both the temporal and spatial point of view. Of all the known substrates of partial seizures, the most stable appears to be the epileptic focus, even though the idea of a changing, migrating or shifting focus has been proposed several times in the history of epileptology. The presence of focal epileptiform activity modifies the excitability of the entire brain (Chrigel & Dimov, 1967) and may show tendency to disseminate spatially (Udvarhely & Walker, 1965). Complex circuits become established, the activity of which may propagate, sustain, activate or inhibit epileptiform events both in their interictal and ictal states. AEDs may exert a stabilizing action at the level of the focus itself, on normal pathways at rest or when used for transmission of epileptic signals, or on newly created epileptic circuitries. Nuclei that, once involved in the epileptogenic process, possess the property of rapidly diffusing or modulating it are thought to be important not only for the generalization of focal activity but perhaps also for triggering or suppressing at the onset ictal events in distant regions (Fariello, 1976). For instance, the pivotal role of the substantia nigra in controlling generalized seizures has been recognized long ago (Fariello & Hornykiewicz, 1979). Microinjection of GVG and direct GABA agonists in the pars compacta of the substantia nigra prevents some generalized seizures (Gale, 1985). Discrete lesions or pharmacological manipulations of several other cerebral structures may suppress various types of seizures, including models of generalized petit mal discharges (Miller & Ferrendelli, 1988; Buzsaki *et al.*, 1988). Thus, AEDs may show preferential or selective action at one or more of these regulator loci, in addition to the effect at the focus. The study of this potential regional pharmacology of drugs is an open field that may yield promising results, which in turn may help the understanding of the highly complex interplay between intrafocal, perifocal and distant circuits in the regulation of cerebral excitability.

Conclusions

In conclusion, the comprehension of the mechanisms of action of AEDs is limited primarily as a consequence of our limited knowledge of the mechanisms of epileptogenesis. The fact that an AED may counteract some elementary phenomena of the interictal spike generating process will not help clarifying the antiepileptic property of that drug until we know the exact place of the interictal spike in epileptogenesis (Fariello & Garant, 1992). If we do not study real models of epilepsy (as opposed to fragmental models of seizures) it is unlikely that we can reach the necessary understanding to properly target pharmacological research. Several effective AEDs show common mechanisms of action. Particularly in the ability to act on Na channels, limiting the SRF of neurons offers an acceptable logical explanation of how high frequency use of neuronal pathways may be selectively dampened by these drugs. Whether this research path has been throughly explored having already provided the best results, or still has potential versus more innovative research avenues, is one of the major unsolved debates regarding the present attempts to improve the pharmacological armamentarium of physicians in their millenial fight against the epilepsies.

References

Ayala, G.F., Lin, S. & Johnston D. (1977): The mechanism of action of diphenylhydantion on invertebrate neurons. I. Effects on basic membrane properties. *Brain Res.* **121**, 245–258.

Bormann J. (1988): Electrophysiology of GABA A and GABA B receptor subtypes. *TINS* **11**, 112–116.

Buzsaki, G., Bickford, R.G., Ponomareff, G., Thall, J., Mandel, R. & Gage, F.H. (1988): Nucleus basalis and thalamic control of neocortical activity in the freely moving rat. *J. Neurosci.* **8**, 4007–4026.

Chrigel, E. & Dimov, S. (1967): Excitability changes throughout the neocortex induced by a localized spiking focus. *Epilepsia* **8**, 137–151.

De Lorenzo, R.J. (1989): Phenytoin. Mechanisms of action. In: *Antiepileptic drugs*, eds. R. Levy, R. Mattson, B. Meldrum, J.K. Penry & F.E. Dreyfuss, (3rd edn), pp. 143–158. New York: Raven Press.

Dingledine, R., McBain, C.J. & McNamara J.D. (1990): Excitatory amino acid receptor in epilepsy. *TINS* **11**, 334–338.

Dragunow, M. (1988): Purinergic mechanisms in epilepsy. *Prog. Neurobiol.* **31**, 85–108.

Fariello, R.G. (1976): Forebrain influences an amygdaloid acute focus in the cat. *Exp. Neurol.* **51**, 515–528.

Fariello, R.G. (1979): The role of GABAergic mechanisms in the epilepsies. In: *Advances in epileptology*, Vol. 15. pp. 17–24. New York: Raven Press.

Fariello, R.G. (1985): Biochemical approaches to seizure mechanisms: the GABA and glutamate systems. In: *The epilepsies*, eds. R.J. Porter & P.L. Morselli, pp. 1–19. London: Butterworths.

Fariello, R.G. & Hornykiewycz, O. (1979): Substantia nigra and metrazol threshold in rats. Correlation with striatal dopamine metabolism. *Exp. Neurol.* **65**, 202–208.

Fariello, R.G. & Golden, G.T. (1985): In: *Electroencephalographic models of epilepsy*, Vol. 3. eds. G. Bartholini, P.L. Morselli & K.G. Lloyd, pp. 139–147. New York: Raven Press.

Fariello, R.G. & Smith M. (1989): Valproate: mechanism of action. In: *Antiepileptic drugs*, eds. R. Levy, R. Mattson, B. Meldrum, J.K. Penry & F.E. Dreifuss 3rd edn), pp. 567–575. New York: Raven Press.

Fariello, R.G. & Garant, D.S. (1992): Neurotransmitter pharmacology of the epilepsies: discrepancies between animal model and human conditions. *Epi. Res. Suppl.* **8**, 21–27.

Fariello, R.G., Forchetti, C.M. & Fisher, R.S. (1991): GABAergic function in relation to seizure phenomena In: *Neurotransmitters and epilepsy*, eds. R.S. Fisher & J.T. Coyle, pp. 77–94. New York: Wiley-Liss.

Fisher, R.S. (1989): Animal models of the epilepsies. *Brain Res. Rev.* **14**, 245–278.

Fisher, R.S. (1991): In: *Glutamate and epilepsy*, eds. R.S. Fisher & J.T. Coyle, pp. 131–145. New York: Wiley-Liss.

Gale, K. (1985): Mechanisms of seizure control mediated by γ-aminobutyric acid: Role of the substantia nigra. *Fed. Proc.* **44**, 2414–2424.

Goodman, L.S., Grewal, M.S., Brown, W.C. & Swinyard, E.A. (1953): Comparison of maximal seizures evoked by pentylenetetrazol (Metrazol) and electroshock in mice, and their modification by anticonvulsants. *J. Pharmacol. Exp. Ther.* **108**, 168–176.

Harvey, P.K.B., Bradford, H.F. & Davisson, A.N. (1975): The inhibition effect of sodium *n*-dipropylacetate on the degradative enzymes of the GABA shunt. *FEBS Lett.* **52F**, 251–254.

Hauptmann, A. (1912): Luminal bei Epilepsie. *Muncher Med. Wochenschr.* **59**, 1907–1909.

Jobe, P.C., Ko, K.T. & Daily J.W. (1984): Abnormalities in norepinephrine turnover rate in the central nervous system of the genetically epilepsy-prone rat. *Brain Res.* **290**, 357–360.

Leach, M., Harden, C.M. & Miller, A.A. (1986): Pharmacological studies of lamotrigine, a novel potential antiepileptic drug. II Neurochemical studies of the mechanisms of action. *Epilepsia* **27**, 490–497.

Lippert, B., Metcalf, B.W., Jung, M.J. & Casara, P. (1977): 4-Amino-hex-5-enoic acid a selective catalytic inhibitor of 4 aminobutyric acid aminotransferase in mammalian brain. *Eur. J. Biochem.* **4**, 441–445.

Locock, C. (1857): Discussion of a paper by E.H. Sieveking. Analysis of 52 cases of epilepsy observed by the author. *Lancet* **i**, 527.

Löscher, W. (1981): Valproate induced changes in GABA metabolism at the subcellular level. *Biochem. Pharmacol.* **30**, 1364–1366.

Löscher, W.L. & Schmidt, D. (1988): Which animal models should be used in the search for new antiepileptic drugs? A proposal based on experimental and clinical considerations. *Epilepsy Res.* **2**, 145–181.

Macdonald, R.L. & McLean, M.J. (1986): Anticonvulsant drugs: mechanisms of actions. In: *Basic mechanisms of the epilepsies. Molecular and cellular approaches. (Advances in neurology)*, Vol. 44, eds. A.V. Delgado-Escueta, A.A. Ward, D.M. Woodbury & R.J. Porter, pp. 713–736. Raven Press: New York.

Macdonald, R.L. & Meldrum, B.S. (1989): Principles of antiepileptic drug action. In: *Antiepileptic drugs*, eds. R. Levy, T. Mattson, B. Meldrum, J.K. Penry & F.E. Dreyfuss (3rd edn), pp. 59–83. New York: Raven Press.

Merritt, H.H. & Putnam, T.J. (1938): Sodium diphenyl-hydantoinate in the treatment of convulsive disorders. *JAMA* **111**, 1068–1073.

Merritt, H.H., Putnam, T.J. & Schwab, D.M. (1938): A new series of anticonvulsant drugs tested by experiments on animals. *Arch. Neurol. Psychiatry* **39** 1003–1015.

Miller, J.W. & Ferrendelli, J.A. (1988): Brain stem and diencephalic structures regulating experimental generalized (pentylentetratol) seizures in rodents. In: *Anatomy of epileptogenesis*, eds. B.S. Meldrum, J.A. Ferrendelli & H.G. Wiese, pp. 57–69. London: John Libbey.

Naquet, R. & Meldrum, B.S. (1972): Photogenic seizures in baboons In: *Experimental models of epilepsy. A manual for the laboratory worker*, eds. D. Purpura, J.K. Penry, D.M. Woodbury, D.B. Tower & R.D. Walter, pp. 373–406. Raven Press: New York.

Piredda, S.G., Woodhead, J.H. & Swinyard, E.A. (1985): Effects of stimulus intensity on the profile of anticonvulsant activity of phenytoin ethosuximide and valproate. *J. Pharmacol. Exp. Ther.* **222**, 741–745.

Pitkaanen, A., Matilainen, R., Ruutiainen & Riekkinen, P. (1988): Levels of total γ-aminobutyric acid (GABA), free GABA and homocarnosine in cerebrospinal fluid of epileptic patients before and during vinylGABA treatment. *J. Neurol. Sci.* **88**, 83–93.

Porter, R.J. (1986): Antiepileptic drug: efficacy and inadequacy: In: *New anticonvulsant drugs*, eds. B.S. Meldrum & R.G. Porter, pp. 3–15. London: John Libbey.

Putnam, T.J. & Merritt H.H. (1937): Experimental determination of the anticonvulsant properties of some phenyl derivatives. *Science* **85**, 525–526.

Skerrit, J.H., Willow, M. & Johnson, G.A. (1982): Diazepam enhancement of low affinity GABA binding to rat brain membranes. *Neurosci. Lett.* **29**, 63–66.

Swinyard, E.A., Castellion, A.W., Fink, G.B. & Goodman L.S. (1963): Some neurophysiological and neuropharmacological characteristics of audiogenic seizure susceptible mice. *J. Pharmacol. Exp. Ther.* **140**, 375–384.

Swinyard, E.A., Woodhead, J.H., White, H.S. & Franklin, M.R. (1989): General principles. Experimental selection, quantification and evaluation of anticonvulsants. In: *Antiepileptic drugs*, eds. R.H. Levy, F.E. Dreifuss, R.H. Mattson, B.S. Meldrum & J.K. Penry (3rd edn), pp. 85–102. New York: Raven Press.

Temkin, O. (1971): *The falling sickness*, (2nd edn), pp. 323. Baltimore, London: Johns Hopkins Press.

Toman, J.E.P., Swinyard, E.A. & Goodman L.S. (1946): Properties of maximal seizures and their alteration by anticonvulsant drugs and other agents. *J. Neurophysiol.* **9**, 231–240.

Twyman, R.E., Rogers, C.J. & Macdonald, R.L. (1989): Differential regulation of GABA A receptor channels by diazepam and phenobarbital. *Ann. Neurol.* **25**, 213–220.

Udvarhely, G.B. & Walker, A.E. (1965): Dissemination of acute focal seizures in the monkey. I From cortical foci. *Arch. Neurol.* **12**, 333–356.

Chapter 5

GABA-mediated potentials and epileptogenesis

Massimo Avoli and Granger G.C. Hwa

Montreal Neurological Institute and Department of Neurology and Neurosurgery, McGill University, Montreal, QC, Canada H3A 2B4

Summary

This paper reviews the involvement of GABA-mediated potentials in epileptogenesis by taking into consideration data obtained in models of epilepsy as well as findings observed in human cortex removed from epileptic patients.

Introduction

Following the discovery of large amounts of gamma-aminobutyric acid (GABA) in the brain more than 40 years ago (Roberts & Frankel, 1950; Awapara *et al.*, 1950), a large body of evidence has accumulated indicating that this monocarboxylic amino acid is the main transmitter at inhibitory synapses in the mammalian cortex (for review see Avoli, 1988; Krnjevic, 1991). Furthermore, based on the fact that normal brain function depends upon the balance between excitatory and inhibitory processes in neuronal circuits, it has been proposed that a decreased efficacy or loss of GABA function might be responsible for the appearance of seizure activity and even constitute a hallmark of epileptic syndromes (Avoli, 1988).

The main aim of this paper is to review evidence on the involvement of GABA-mediated potentials in the genesis of epileptiform discharges recorded in different models of epilepsy. In addition, we shall also report some findings regarding GABA-mediated mechanisms in human cortical samples removed from epileptic patients. In doing so we shall summarize the physiological and pharmacological characteristics of the actions exerted by synaptically released GABA upon hippocampal and neocortical neurons.

Cortical GABA-mediated mechanisms

GABA exerts pre- and postsynaptic actions in mammalian cortical structures. The presynaptic mechanism operates by reducing the release of transmitter (from both excitatory and inhibitory synapses) via the activation of $GABA_A$ and $GABA_B$ receptor subtypes (see below). The postsynaptic mechanism is usually associated with a hyperpolarizing action that brings the postsynaptic membrane to potentials that are near or more negative than rest. By doing so, the inhibitory postsynaptic effect opposes depolarizing influences (e.g. those caused by excitatory postsynaptic potentials, EPSPs) and thus reduces the tendency to fire action potentials.

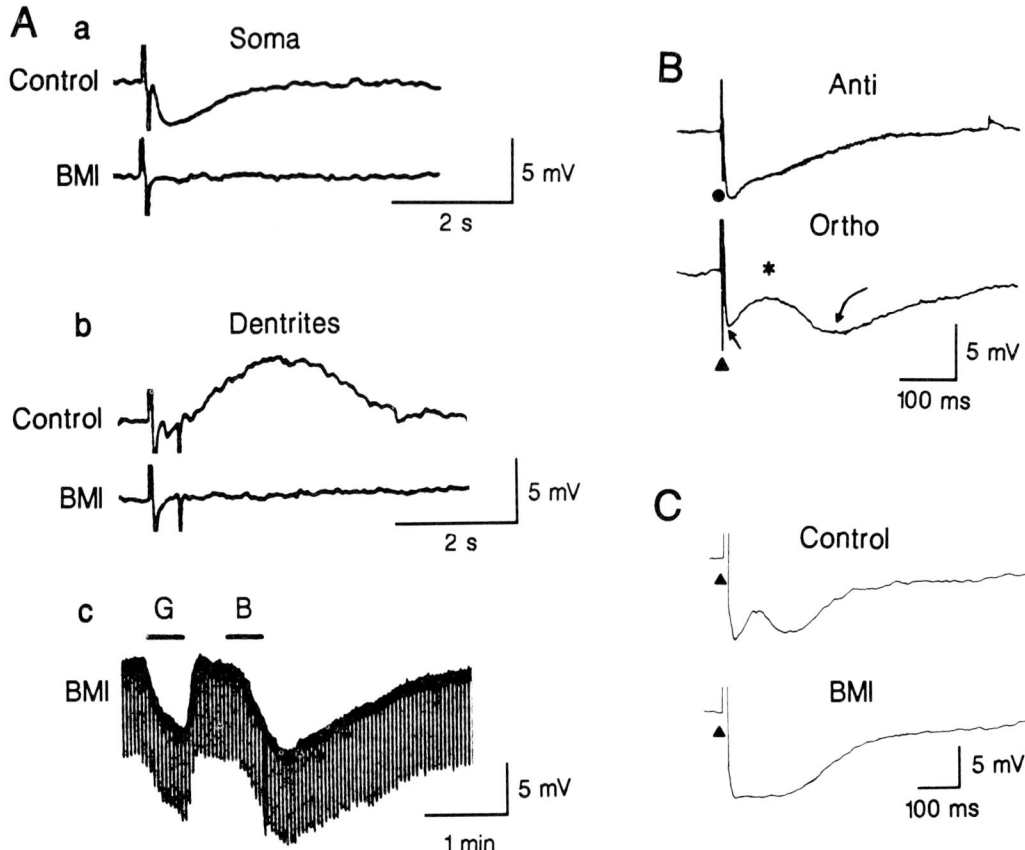

Fig. 1. (A). Effects of GABA ionophoresis on CA1 hippocampal neurons. (a) GABA application onto the soma induces a hyperpolarizing potential (control) that is sensitive to the GABA$_A$ antagonist bicuculline methiodide (BMI). (b) In contrast, when GABA is applied onto the dendrites, a BMI-sensitive depolarization potential can be observed. (c) In the presence of BMI, application of either GABA (G) or baclofen (B) onto the soma is sufficient to hyperpolarize the membrane. B: GABA receptor-mediated inhibitory postsynaptic potential (IPSP) evoked by antidromic stimulation of the alveus (anti) or orthodromic stimulation of the stratum radiatum (ortho). Note that the orthodromic response is compromised by an early hyperpolarizing component (straight arrow), followed by a depolarizing component (asterisk), then a late hyperpolarizing component (curved arrow). (C) The depolarizing component is sensitive to the dendritic application of BMI. Aa and Ab from Alger and Nicoll (1982); Ac from Dutar and Nicoll (1988); B and C from Avoli (1992).

The presynaptic action in cortical structures can only be analysed indirectly by recording the postsynaptic cells. Hence the understanding of this function is limited, as it derives from extrapolations of data observed in the postsynaptic cell. By contrast, much evidence has been accumulated for the postsynaptic effects of GABA. As illustrated in Fig. 1, three main effects can be attributed to the action of this inhibitory transmitter on hippocampal and neocortical cells. First, focal application of GABA to the somatic region of pyramidal cells causes a hyperpolarization due to an increased membrane conductance to Cl$^-$ (Alger & Nicoll, 1982; Connors et al., 1988) (Fig. 1Aa). Such a mechanism also underlies the early hyperpolarizing inhibitory post-synaptic potentials (IPSP) recorded in pyramidal cells, is blocked by bicuculline and thus is caused by the activation of GABA$_A$ receptor subtypes (Figs. 1Aa, 2A). This IPSP is mainly caused by the activation of recurrent inhibitory circuits, and in the hippocampus is mediated by basket cells terminating on or

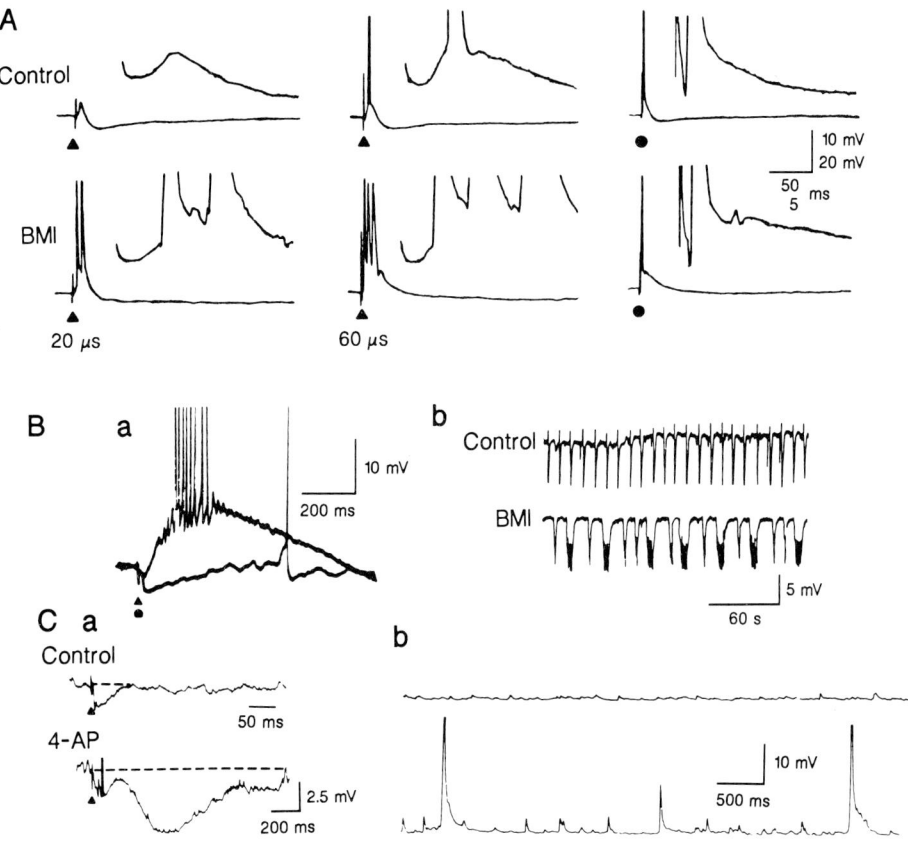

Fig. 2. (A) The blockade of $GABA_A$ receptor-mediated IPSP with BMI readily induces the appearance of epileptiform activity in CA1 hippocampal neurons (BMI, 20 & 60 µs). Orthodromic stimulation is illustrated by a triangle, and antidromic stimulation by a circle. B: Under the perfusion of low-$[Mg^{2+}]_o$ medium, an alvear stimulus (circle) elicits an IPSP at a time when orthodromic stimulation (triangle) induces an epileptiform discharge (a). The presence of synaptic inhibition in low-$[Mg^{2+}]_o$ epileptogenesis can also be revealed by the application of BMI (b). C: In the presence of 4-aminopyridine (4AP), epileptiform activities occur spontaneously in CA3 hippocampal neurons (b) while their inhibitory mechanism is potentiated (a). A from Tancredi and Avoli (1987); B from Tancredi et al. (1990); C from Perreault & Avoli (1991).

near the soma of pyramidal cells. Second, GABA application on dendrites evokes a hyperpolarization that is resistant to bicuculline, is associated with opening K$^+$ channels and is due to the activation of $GABA_B$ receptor subtypes, so termed after the agonist baclofen (Blaxter & Carlen, 1985; Newberry & Nicoll, 1984, 1985) (Fig. 1Ac). This response is similar to the late hyperpolarization that is observed following orthodromic activation of hippocampal and neocortical pyramidal cells (curved arrow in Fig. 2B, Ortho) (Blaxter & Carlen, 1980; Newberry & Nicoll, 1985; Connors et al., 1988). Finally, GABA application to the dendrites of cortical pyramidal cells can elicit a depolarizing response that is blocked by bicuculline (Fig. 1Ab). The ionic mechanism responsible for this depolarizing response is not well understood. On the one hand it has been proposed that it might be caused by an outward movement of Cl$^-$ which would require a different Cl$^-$ gradient in the dendrites and soma of pyramidal cells (Misgeld et al., 1986; Müller et al., 1989). On the other hand, the $GABA_A$-mediated depolarization might be due to an inward movement of some cations such as Na^+ and Ca^{2+} (Alger & Nicoll, 1982). It should also be mentioned that GABA-mediated depolarizations might be due to an increase in permeability to HCO_3 (see Krnjevic, 1991). A synaptic counterpart of the depolarizing effect induced by GABA has recently been characterized in CA1 pyramidal cells (Avoli, 1992), where it is seen following orthodromic activation and appears as a transient depolarization situated between the early and late IPSP (Fig. 1C). This depolarizing component is selectively blocked by local application of $GABA_A$ antagonists on the apical dendrites of pyramidal cells (Fig. 1C, BMI).

Postsynaptic $GABA_A$ and $GABA_B$ receptor subtypes are also very different in their molecular nature since the former type is directly linked with the opening of Cl^- channels (and therefore qualify as an ionotropic receptor), while the latter opens K^+ channels through the activation of a pertuxis toxin-sensitive G-protein (hence it represents a metabotropic receptor) (Andrade et al., 1986; Dutar & Nicoll, 1988; Thalmann, 1988).

GABA-mediated potentials and cortical epileptogenesis

There is no doubt that a decrease or loss of inhibition mediated through GABA receptors is paralleled by the appearance of epileptiform activity and eventually seizures. Accordingly, substances that are capable of interfering with GABA synthesis, release or postsynaptic effects possess potent convulsive effects (see for review, Avoli, 1988). At a more basic level, several *in vitro* studies have demonstrated that convulsants such as bicuculline, picrotoxin or penicillin induce stimulus-induced or spontaneously occurring epileptiform discharges while blocking the $GABA_A$ receptor-mediated hyperpolarizing IPSP (Dingledine & Gjerstad, 1980; Schwartzkroin & Prince, 1980; Tancredi & Avoli, 1987) (Fig. 2A). These epileptiform discharges when recorded with an extracellular electrode resemble the interictal focal spikes or sharp waves that are seen during EEG studies performed in epileptic patients (so-called interictal epileptiform activity). However, more recent studies in which different experimental manipulations were employed to induce epileptiform activity have shown that $GABA_A$-mediated potentials can be recorded at a time when epileptiform interictal discharges are seen (Fig. 2B, C). These procedures include perfusion of the brain slices with medium containing low Mg^{2+} (Tancredi et al., 1990) or the K^+-channel blocker tetraethylammonium or 4-aminopyridine (4AP) (Rutecki et al., 1987, 1990; Perreault & Avoli, 1991). Interestingly, it has been demonstrated that 4AP-induced epileptiform interictal activity in the CA3 subfield of adult rat hippocampus is recorded at a time when the recurrent IPSP is increased in amplitude and duration (Fig. 2C). Therefore, although a decrease in the efficacy leads to the appearance of epileptiform activity, this mechanism does not represent a *sine qua non* condition for the generation of interictal epileptiform discharges.

Experiments performed with 4AP have also demonstrated that hippocampal cells generate a synchronous GABA-mediated potential that corresponds at the intracellular level to a depolarization due to the activation of $GABA_A$ receptors located on the dendrites of pyramidal cells (Fig. 3A) (Perreault & Avoli, 1989, 1991, 1992; see also Michelson & Wong, 1991). This GABA-mediated, synchronous potential can be observed at the same time in the three main areas of the hippocampus even following blockade of receptors for the excitatory amino acid transmitter (Fig. 3B) (Perreault & Avoli, 1992). A similar phenomenon has been reported in the guinea-pig neocortex (Aram et al., 1991). It is of interest that in the immature hippocampus the synchronous GABA-mediated potential precedes and thus appears to initiate ictal-like discharges (Fig. 3C) (Avoli, 1990). Therefore, $GABA_A$-mediated mechanisms are not only operant during interictal and ictal discharges, but they can even participate in the process of initiation of ictal activity.

GABAergic inhibition in the human neocortex

The unequivocal role of GABA in the genesis of seizures has been demonstrated in humans as well. Thus, convulsions were reported to occur in infants who were fed milk formula that had accident-

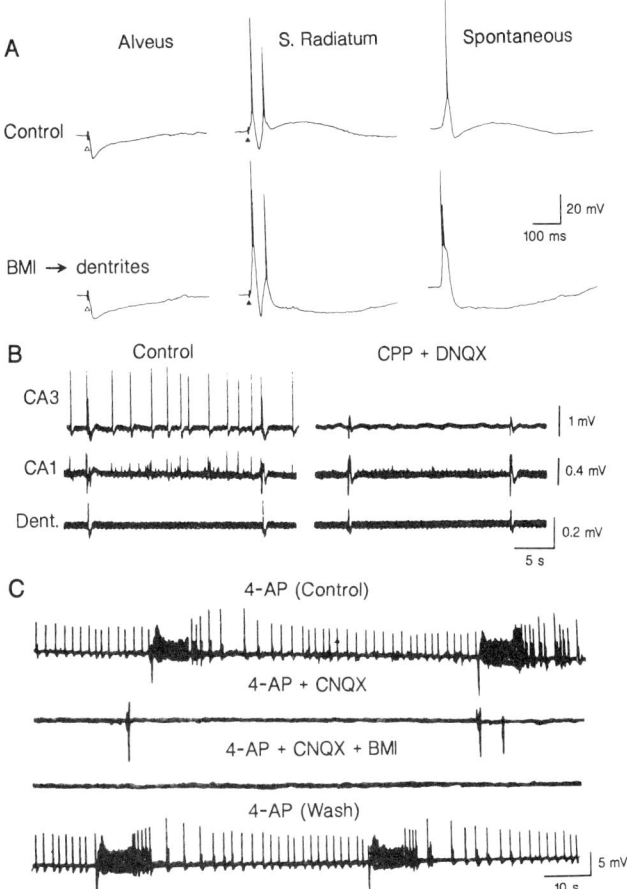

Fig. 3. Synchronous GABA-mediated potentials recorded from 4AP-treated hippocampal slices of adult (A,B) and immature (C) rats. A: Intracellular recording from a CA1 neuron indicates that the stimulus-induced or spontaneously occurring GABA-mediated potential can be blocked by the application of BMI onto the dendrites. B: Simultaneous extracellular recordings from the CA1, CA3 and dentate regions show that only the epileptiform discharge and not the synchronous GABA-mediated potential is sensitive to excitatory amino acid antagonists CPP and DNQX. C: Extracellular recordings from the CA3 region show that the synchronous GABA-mediated potential (4AP+CNQX) is sensitive to BMI (4AP+CNQX+BMI). A from Perreault & Avoli (1989); B from Perreault & Avoli (1992); C from Avoli (1990).

ally been made deficient in pyridoxine (also termed vitamin B_6) (Malony & Parmalee, 1954; Hunt et al., 1954; Coursin, 1954). Pyridoxine is the coenzyme for the formation of GABA from glutamic acid by means of glutamic acid decarboxylase (GAD).

However, a decreased efficacy of GABA-mediated mechanisms, GABA content and/or related enzymatic activity remains to be demonstrated as yet in the brain tissue obtained from epileptic patients. Thus, biochemical studies have failed in revealing any difference between cortical areas found to be spiking and non-spiking during electrocorticography (for review see Sherwin & van Gelder, 1986), while Tursky et al. (1976) did not find any difference in the GAD activity of hippocampi removed from epileptic patients as compared to analogous tissue obtained from non-epileptic patients.

During the last decade, several investigators have used the *in vitro* slice preparation to characterize,

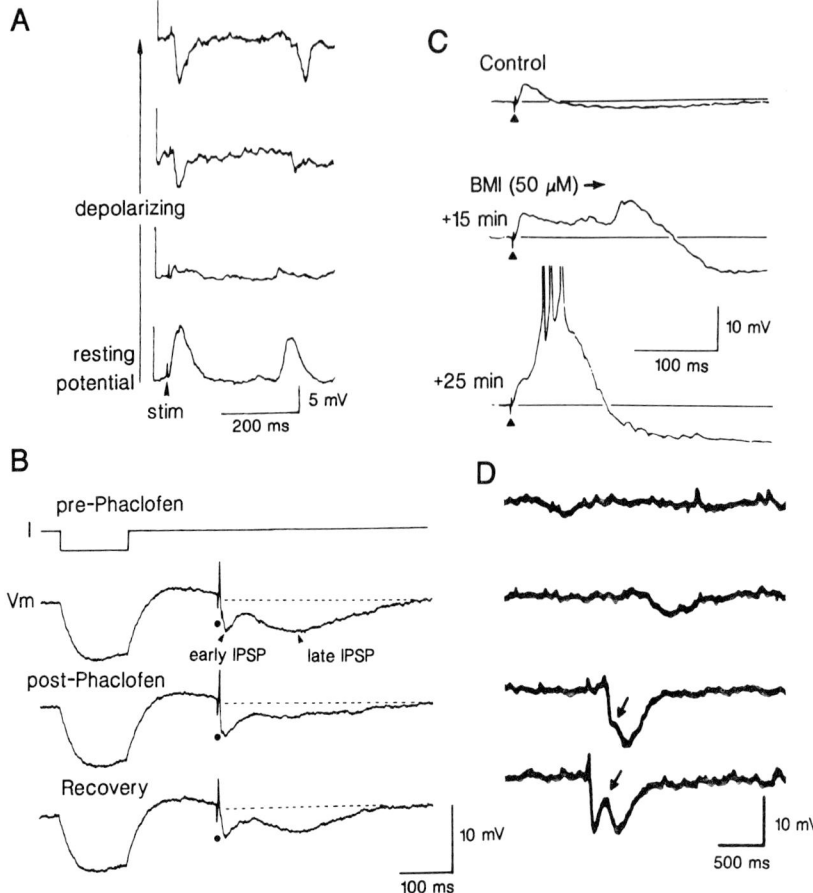

Fig. 4. GABA-mediated potentials recorded from epileptic human neocortical slices. A: Depolarization of the membrane from resting level reveals a stimulus-induced or spontaneously occurring IPSP. B: Both early and late IPSPs are discernible following extracellular stimulation. The late IPSP is sensitive to the GABA$_B$ antagonist phaclofen. C: In contrast, the early IPSP is sensitive to the GABA$_A$ antagonist BMI. Note that BMI readily induces the appearance of epileptiform discharge. D: Progressive development of spontaneously occurring GABA-mediated potentials following the application of 4-aminopyridine. A from Schwartzkroin & Haglund (1986); B from McCormick (1989); C from Hwa et al. (1991); D from Avoli et al. (1988).

at the pharmacological and electrophysiological levels, the inhibitory potentials generated by human neurons located in epileptogenic cortical areas. Although an initial report by Schwartzkroin et al. (1983) indicated that neurons in slices obtained from 'active' epileptogenic areas have less effective hyperpolarizing IPSPs than cells in slices taken from nearby tissue, successive studies have failed to confirm this finding. For instance, a more recent paper from the same laboratory has demonstrated the presence of spontaneous GABA-mediated potentials in human, presumably hippocampal, cells (Schwartzkroin & Haglund, 1986) (Fig. 4A). As illustrated in Fig. 4B, studies of the human neocortex removed from epileptic patients in McCormick's laboratory (1989) have revealed that the GABA-mediated potentials seen in normal cortical neurons of lower mammalian species (see section above, and compare with Fig. 1C) can be induced by focal stimuli. Similar conclusions have been made in our laboratory by analysing stimulus-induced synaptic responses in cells located in slices of human epileptogenic neocortex (Avoli & Olivier, 1989; Hwa et al., 1991)

(Fig. 4B). It should also be mentioned that in the presence of 4AP hippocampal and neocortical cells recorded in slices obtained from epileptic patients generate synchronous, depolarizing potentials that are blocked by bicuculline (Fig. 4D).

Although these electrophysiological studies do not allow us to conclude whether GABA-mediated potentials in the human epileptogenic cortex are unchanged as compared to normal tissue, they indicate that inhibitory mechanisms are present and from a qualitative point of view display remarkable similarities with the GABA-mediated events described in normal animals.

Conclusions

The findings reviewed above indicate that the inhibitory transmitter GABA induces three distinct postsynaptic responses in the mammalian cortex. We have also presented evidence indicating that epileptiform activity and seizures do appear following a decreased efficacy of GABA. In line with this view, some antiepileptic drugs can exert their action by potentiating GABA potentials (see Fariello, Chapter 4). However, depending upon the experimental procedures used, epileptiform discharges can also be seen at a time when GABA is preserved or even enhanced. Finally, inhibitory potentials generated by cortical cells in human epileptogenic tissue display features that are remarkably similar to those seen in analogous structures of normal animals.

Acknowledgement

This work was supported by MRC of Canada (grant MA-8109), by the FRSQ and by the Savoy Foundation.

References

Alger, B.E. & Nicoll, R.A. (1982): Pharmacological evidence for two kinds of GABA receptor on rat hippocampal pyramidal cells studied *in vitro*. *J. Physiol.* **328**, 125–141.

Andrade, R., Malenka, R.C. & Nicoll, R.A. (1986): A G-protein couples serotonin and $GABA_B$ receptors to the same channels in hippocampus. *Science* **234**, 1261–1265.

Aram, J.A., Michelson, H.B. & Wong, R.K.S. (1991): Synchronized GABAergic IPSPs recorded in the neocortex after blockade of synaptic transmission mediated by excitatory amino acids. *J. Neurophysiol.* **65**, 1034–1041.

Avoli, M. (1988): GABAergic mechanisms and epileptic discharges. In: *Neurotransmitters and cortical function*, eds. M. Avoli, *et al.*, pp. 187–205. New York: Plenum Press.

Avoli, M. (1990): Epileptiform discharges and a synchronous GABAergic potential induced by 4-aminopyridine in the rat immature hippocampus. *Neurosci. Lett.* **117**, 93–98.

Avoli, M. (1992): Synaptic activation of $GABA_A$ receptors causes a depolarizing potential under physiological conditions in rat hippocampal pyramidal cells. *Eur. J. Neurosci.* **4**, 16–26.

Avoli, M. & Olivier, A. (1989): Electrophysiological properties and synaptic responses in the deep layers of the human epileptogenic neocortex *in vitro*. *J. Neurophysiol.* **61**, 589–606.

Avoli, M., Perreault, P., Olivier, A. & Villemure, J-G. (1988): 4-Aminopyridine induces a long-lasting depolarizing GABA-ergic potential in human neocortical and hippocampal neurons maintained *in vitro*. *Neurosci. Lett.* **94**, 327–332.

Awapara, J., Landua, A.J., Fuerst, R. & Seale, B. (1950): Free γ-aminobutyric acid in brain. *J. Biol. Chem.* **187**, 35–39.

Blaxter, T.J. & Carlen, P.L. (1985): Pre-and postsynaptic effects of baclofen in the rat hippocampal slice. *Brain Res.* **341**, 195–199.

Connors, B.W., Malenka, R.C. & Silva, L.R. (1988): Two inhibitory postsynaptic potentials and $GABA_A$ and $GABA_B$ receptor-mediated responses in neocortex of rat and cat. *J. Physiol.* **406**, 443–468.

Coursin, D.B. (1954): Convulsive seizures in infants with pyridoxine-deficient diet. *JAMA* **154** 406.

Dingledine, R. & Gjerstad, L. (1980): Reduced inhibition during epileptiform activity in the *in vitro* hippocampal slice. *J. Physiol.* **305**, 297–313.

Dutar, P. & Nicoll, R. (1988): Pre- and postsynaptic $GABA_B$ receptors in the hippocampus have different pharmacological properties. *Neuron* **1**, 585–591.

Hunt, A.D., Stokes, J., McCrory, W.W. & Stroud, H.H. (1954): Pyridoxine dependency: report of a case of intractable convulsions in an infant controlled by pyridoxine. *Pediatrics* **13**, 140.

Hwa, G.G.C., Avoli, M., Olivier, A. & Villermure, J.G. (1991): Bicuculline-induced epileptogenesis in the human neocortex maintained *in vitro*. *Exp. Brain Res.* **83**, 329–339.

Krnjevic, K. (1991): Significance of GABA in brain function. In: *GABA mechanisms in epilepsy*, eds. G. Tunnicliff and B.U. Raess, pp. 47–87. New York: Wiley-Liss, Inc.

Malony, C.J. & Parmalee, A.H. (1954): Convulsions in young infants as a result of pyridoxine (vitamin B_6) deficiency. *JAMA* **154**, 405.

McCormick, D.A. (1989): GABA as an inhibitory neurotransmitter in human cerebral cortex. *J. Neurophysiol.* **62**, 1018–1027.

Michelson, H.B. & Wong, R.K.S. (1991): Excitatory synaptic responses mediated by $GABA_A$ receptors in the hippocampus. *Science* **253**, 1420–1423.

Misgeld, U., Deisz, R.A., Dodt, H.U. & Lux, H.D. (1986): The role of chloride transport in post-synaptic inhibition of hippocampal neurons. *Science* **232**, 1413–1415.

Müller, W., Misgeld, U. & Lux, H.D. (1989): γ-Aminobutyric acid-induced ion movements in the guinea pig hippocampal slice. *Brain Res.* **484**, 184–191.

Newberry, N.R. & Nicoll, R.A. (1984): Direct hyperpolarizing action of baclofen on hippocampal pyramidal cells. *Nature* **308**, 450–452.

Newberry, N.R. & Nicoll, R.A. (1985): Comparison of the action of baclofen with γ-aminobutyric acid on rat hippocampal pyramidal cells *in vitro*. *J. Physiol.* **360**, 161–185.

Perreault, P. & Avoli, M. (1989): Effects of low concentrations of 4-aminopyridine on CA1 pyramidal cells of the hippocampus. *J. Neurophysiol.* **61**, 953–970.

Perreault, P. & Avoli, M. (1991): Physiology and pharmacology of epileptiform activity induced by 4-aminopyridine in rat hippocampal slices. *J. Neurophysiol.* **65**, 771–785.

Perreault, P. & Avoli, M. (1992): 4-Aminopyridine-induced epileptiform activity and a GABA-mediated long-lasting depolarization in the rat hippocampus. *J. Neurosci.* **12**, 104–115.

Roberts, E. & Frankel, S. (1950): γ-Aminobutyric acid in brain: its formation from glutamic acid. *J. Biol. Chem.* **187**, 55–63.

Rutecki, P.A., Lebeda, F.J. & Johnston, D. (1987): 4-Aminopyridine produces epileptiform activity in hippocampus and enhances synaptic excitation and inhibition. *J. Neurophysiol.* **57**, 1911–1924.

Rutecki, P.A., Lebeda, F.J. & Johnston, D. (1990): Epileptiform activity in the hippocampus produced by tetraethylammonium. *J. Neurophysiol.* **64**, 1077–1088.

Schwartzkroin, P.A. & Haglund, M.M. (1986): Spontaneous rhythmic synchronous activity in epileptic human and normal monkey temporal lobe. *Epilepsia* **27**, 523–533.

Schwartzkroin, P.A. & Prince, D.A. (1980); Changes in excitatory and inhibitory synaptic potentials leading to epileptogenic activity. *Brain Res.* **183**, 61–76.

Schwartzkroin, P.A., Turner, D.A., Knowles, W.D. & Wyler, A.R. (1983): Studies of human and monkey 'epileptic' neocortex in the *in vitro* slice preparation. *Ann. Neurol.* **13**, 249–257.

Sherwin, A.L. & van Gelder, N. (1986): Amino acid and catecholamine markers of metabolic abnormalities in human focal epilepsy. *Adv. Neurol.* **44**, 1011–1032.

Tancredi, V. & Avoli, M. (1987): Control of spontaneous epileptiform discharges by extracellular potassium: an *'in vitro'* study in the CA1 subfield of the hippocampal slice. *Exp. Brain Res.* **67**, 363–372.

Tancredi, V., Hwa, G.G.C., Zona, C., Brancati, A. & Avoli, M. (1990): Low magnesium epileptogenesis in the rat hippocampal slice: electrophysiological and pharmacological features. *Brain Res.* **511**, 280–290.

Thalmann, R.H. (1988): Evidence that guanosine triphosphate (GTP)-binding proteins control a synaptic response in brain: effect of pertussis toxin and GTP S on the late inhibitory postsynaptic potential of hippocampal CA3 neurons. *J. Neurosci.* **8**, 4589–4602.

Tursky, T., Lassanova, M., Sramka, M. & Nadvornik, P. (1976): Formation of glutamate and GABA in epileptogenic tissue from human hippocampus *in vitro*. *Acta. Neurochir. Suppl.* **23**, 111–118.

Chapter 6

Morphological aspects of neocortical maturation

Roberto Spreafico and Carolina Frassoni

Istituto Nazionale Neurologico C. Besta, Milan, Italy

Summary

During cortical ontogenesis, the formation of transient structures is observed before the establishment of the final laminate cortex present in adult animals. Although the intimate mechanisms subserving the processes of cortical genesis are not known, both genetic and environmental factors play a role in determining the ultimate fate of cortical neurons. Proliferation, migration, differentiation, maturation and programmed cell death are the major steps involved during cortical maturation. These mechanisms involve both projecting and non-projecting neurons. Although the term 'differentiation' is mainly applied to the morphological aspect of neurons, its significance must be also expanded to indicate the maturation of functional characteristics of cell lineage. Thus, in addition to the morphological variations observed during development, the maturation of neurochemical systems (e.g. neurotransmitters and receptors) must be considered. These two aspects are mutually integrated since maturation of biochemical processes may influence the morphogenetic aspects of developing cortex.

Introduction

The cerebral vesicles are recognized, during human embryonic development, around the 40th postovulatory day. At the beginning of neocortical development, a homogeneus population of undifferentiated cells is present. These matrix cells, organized as a pseudostratified columnar epithelium, will generate the neuronal and glial elements of the neocortex. The final laminated cortex of the adult mammals is therefore generated, through the formation of transient structures, by means of different basic mechanisms. Both intrinsic and environmental mechanisms have been suggested to be important during development (McConnell, 1988). Despite the large number of experimental works, the intimate mechanisms leading the processes of cortical genesis are not yet completely understood, but environment seems to play a major role in determining the ultimate fate of cortical cells. From an undifferentiated cell population, the neocortex is generated through successive and apparently irreversible steps each of which implies, for a single cell, decisions that progressively restrict its choices (McConnell, 1992). Thus, during cortical ontogenesis, a cascade of self-restricting events are observed (Fig. 1). Proliferation is the first step in development but further and successive mechanisms such as migration, differentiation, maturation and programmed cell death have to be regarded as fundamental events for the formation of the mature cortex (Fig. 2).

After the appearance of the ventricular zone (VZ), formed by the undifferentiated cells (Fig. 3A), a new area is recognized below the pial surface and named the marginal zone (MZ, Fig. 3B).

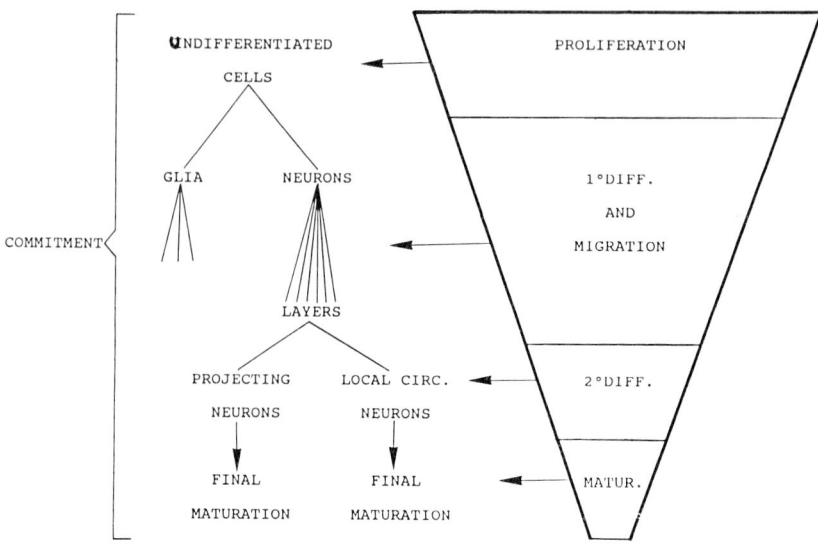

Fig. 1. Progressive steps during cortical ontogenesis. From undifferentiated cells a cascade of self-restricting events (triangle on the right) are observed during the development of neocortex.

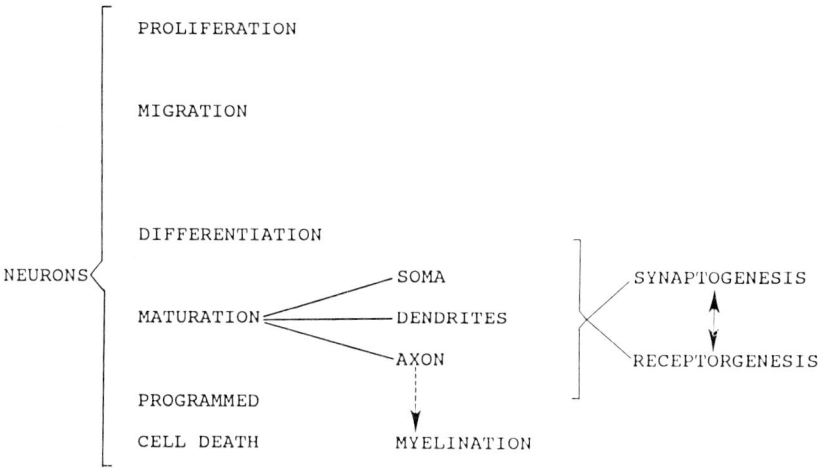

Fig. 2. Events observed during the different steps of the evolution of the cortical maturation.

Following the proposal of the Boulder Committee (1970) this area is classified as a neuronal free region since it would be deprived of neurons in the early developmental stages. Although this hypothesis is still supported (Rakic, 1982), a new interpretation on the formation of this area has been proposed (Marin Padilla, 1988). The data, obtained mainly from Golgi material, suggest that the formation of early synapses in the MZ determined by the first cortical afferences, originating presumably from the brainstem, would promote the maturation of the neurons scattered in the subpial region. This primitive neurofibrillary organization, named primordial plexiform layer

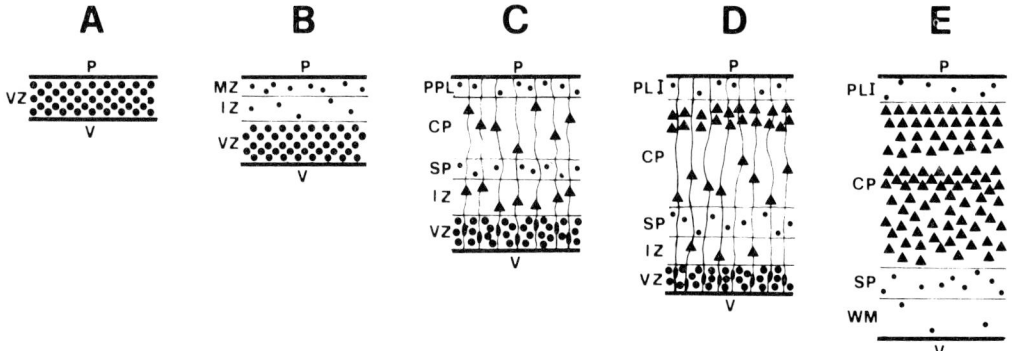

Fig. 3. Schematic drawing showing different stages of the neocortical development. Triangles indicate migrating neurons climbing on the fibres of the radial glial cells. P: pial surface; V: ventricular surface; VZ: ventricular zone; MZ: marginal zone; IZ: intermediate zone; PPL: primordial plexiform layer; CP: cortical plate; SP: subplate; PLI: perspective layer I; WM: white matter.

(PPL), marks the beginning of cortical neurogenesis and precedes the formation of all the other cortical layers (Fig. 3C). Thus the PPL contains the first differentiating neuronal elements in the embryonic cortex and, during the early phases of the ontogenesis, the PPL and its derivatives (see later) will be the only 'functional' regions of the developing cortex (Marin Padilla, 1984). These events can be dated in human embryos around the 6–8th gestational week. Subsequently, after the last mitotic cycle, the neuroblasts from the ventricular zone migrate upword, presumably attracted by the functioning PPL (Marin Padilla, 1984). The arrival of the first migratory neurons splits the PPL in two regions. The upper portion, close to the pial surface, will become the future layer I and thus is defined as perspective layer I (PLI, Fig. 3D). The second one, below the newly arrived neurons that are forming the cortical plate (CP), is named subplate (SP, Fig. 3C–E). Below the SP a further region mainly formed by embryonic white matter is recognized: the intermediate zone (IZ). This area separates the SP from the VZ (Fig. 3C and D).

During further developmental stages, the CP is expanding and the three regions (SP, IZ and VC) progressively reduce their size. From the CP, layers II–VI will originate, while the three zones will disappear giving way to the white matter (Fig. 3E). It must be noticed that during the development the SP has an important role as the waiting compartment of afferent fibres growing from subcortical structures particularly from the thalamus (Shatz, 1992). The incoming fibres penetrate into the SP and contact the cells of this region until the migrating neuroblasts, forming the CP, reach their maturation and appropriate location. Later on, the majority of SP neurons die by a mechanism of programmed cell death and the fibres are free to reach their appropriate final target. The few remaining neurons will be incorporated in the white matter and will survive also in the adult cortex. As mentioned above, the enlargement of CP is determined by subsequent waves of migrating neuroblasts following an inside–outside sequence (Rakic, 1972). This term has been introduced to indicate the pattern of generation and displacement of neurons in different cortical layers. After the last mitotic division, the early generated neuroblasts migrate guided by the fibres of radial glial cells spanning from the pial surface to the VZ where cell bodies reside (Rakic, 1971, Fig. 3B, C, D). Migrating neurons move toward the pial surface and form the superficial border of CP below the PLI, (Fig. 3B, C, D). A subsequent wave of migrating neurons passes through the early migrated cells reaching the superficial position displacing the early migrated cells downward. Following this sequence, the CP is expanded and the last generated neurons will reside in the most superficial layer below the PLI. After the completion of cortical migration, the radial glial fibres disappear (Schmechel & Rakic, 1979). This inside–outside sequence explains why early generated and mi-

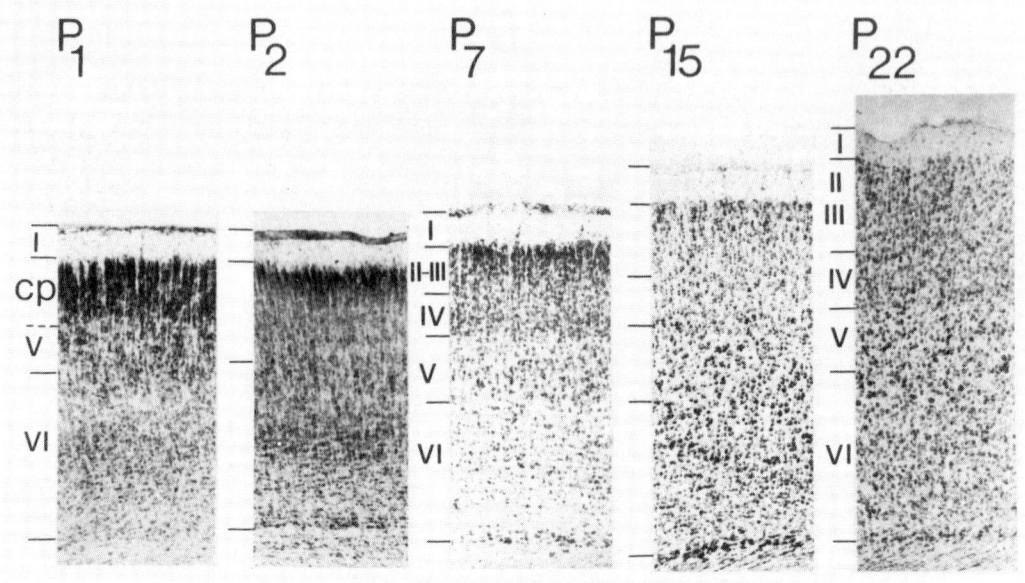

Fig. 4. Low-power photomicrographs showing the postnatal differentiation of the cortex in the rat. Note that in this animal not all the cortical layers are differentiated during the first postnatal week.

grated neurons will form the deep layer of the neocortex, displaced downward by the cells generated later forming the most superficial layer. Only layer I is not included in this mechanism.

In humans the migratory events have been divided into five stages spanning from the 8th to approximately the 16th gestational week. At the 5th month of gestation, only a few proliferative cells are evident in the VZ mainly generating glial cells since, by this time, all the neurons of the human cortex have been generated. Recent studies directed the attention to the presence of some molecules that seem to play an important role, during the migration, in the recognition of the final target of cells and their neurites (Easter et al., 1985). It is therefore clear that pathological events, during this period of gestation, can disrupt the normal sequential event, generating inappropriate locations and connections of neurons such as the neuronal migration disorders now detectable *in vivo* by NMR.

During the migratory events, and particularly at the last stages, the cellular differentiation also takes place. Only few studies have been performed on human brain on this topic (Marin Padilla, 1984, 1988), and most of our knowledge derives from experimental animals and particularly from the rat. In this animal the embryonic period (E) is 21 days and part of the developmental events continue also during the postnatal (P) period (Fig. 4). The neuronal differentiation of perikaryon (including the cytoplasmatic rearrangement), the expansion of neuronal processes with the formation of synapses and the neurochemical differentiation with the appearance of neurotransmitters and receptors, are the main events observed.

The term 'differentiation' is not restricted to the maturation of neuronal morphology but also implies the maturation of its functional characteristics. This phenomenon includes signals for cell recognition, the production of specific receptors and the expression of neurotransmitter phenotype. Most of these processes of differentiation can continue for a long time after the basic plan of the cortex is laid down and neurons have been formed.

In the past the neuronal specificity was postulated and explained on the basis of nerve cell recog-

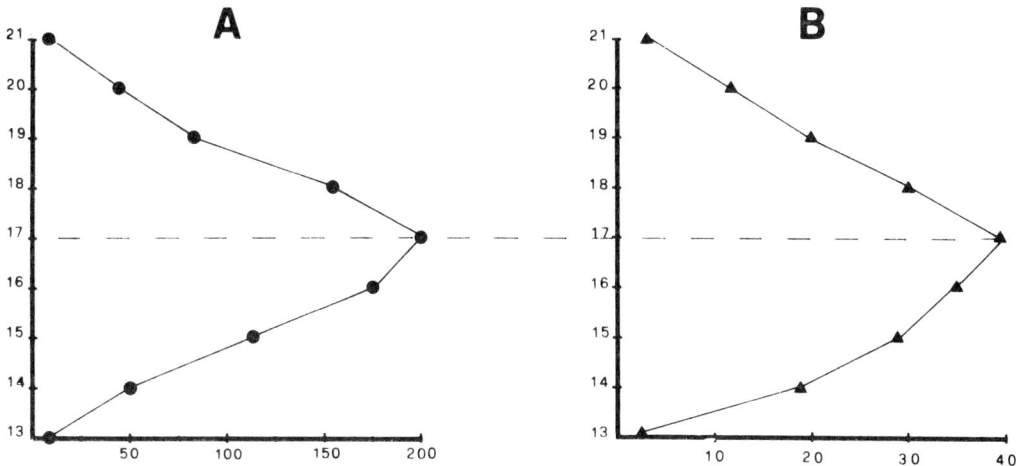

Fig. 5. Histogram showing the generation of cortical projecting neurons (A) and of GABAergic interneurons (B) in the rat. The neurons are generated through the period of cortical neurogenesis, but peak, in both cases, at E_{17}. X axis: number of neurons; Y axis: time of origin (gestational day) (modified from Miller, 1988).

nition. The pioneering work of Sperry and his coworkers postulated the theory of chemo-affinity suggesting that, during axogenesis and synaptogenesis, specific membrane labels are present to allow mutual recognition between pre- and postsynaptic elements. More recently, experiments indicate that the cell recognition is only part of a more complex mechanism for the establishment of appropriate connectivity. The importance of competitive interaction in the formation of connections in vertebrates' central nervous systems has become increasingly evident. It has been suggested that the great ability of the central nervous system to adapt to an ever-changing external evironment is due to the long-lasting synaptic malleability promoted by the long-term competitive interaction (Easter et al., 1985). Two main mechanisms contribute to the definitive formation of brain network: selection and exuberance. During differentiation the neurite outgrowth is guided to select the correct target and the appropriate location to form synapses. But axons grows exuberantly in the sense that they are forming transient synapses during the development that do not persist in adulthood. During later stages of development, the exuberant connection will be eliminated by programmed cell death, reorganization of axonal and dendritic arborization and retraction of axon collaterals. Two types of neurons are present in the adult cortex: the projecting neurons (PN), termed also as Golgi type I or extrinsic neurons, and local circuit neurons (LCN) defined also as Golgi type II, intrinsic neurons or interneurons. Although for many years, projecting neurons have been thought to be generated before the local circuit neurons, recent data demonstrated that generation, migration and differentiation of both types of cells occur concurrently (Miller, 1985; Fig. 5).

In the rat, the morphological differentiation of projecting neurons occurs in the postnatal period, and it is only at the end of the 4th postnatal week that perikaryons of pyramidal neurons reach their adult configuration. During the same period, most of the intracellular changes also take place particularly in the rough endoplasmic reticulum. Nevertheless, because of the time of birth and of migration schedules, the differentiation of these cells is not synchronous through all the layers (Miller, 1981).

Within the first week, somatic spines appear as a transient feature being almost absent in mature cells. During these phases of development, axosomatic synapses appear and the presynaptic elements presumably derive from axons of local circuit neurons. The large increase of the neuropil observed during the first postnatal weeks, is due to the growth and expansion of dendritic tree with the production of dendritic spines. At the distal end of the expanding dendrite, the dendritic growth cone is observed as an irregularly shaped swelling, frequently contacted by immature type I synapses. Dendritic growth is maximum between P_3 and P_9, and will be completed by the 3rd postnatal week with the concomitant disappearance of the growth cone. Dendritic spines appear around the middle of the first postnatal week and their density progressively increases until the 4th week. With the appearance of spines, the formation of dendritic synapses also start.

Although, axons elongation begins before neurons complete their migration, they do not seem to form synapses before the migration is completed. The first axonal synapses (asymmetric or Grey type I) appear at P_0 presumably originating from axon collaterals of pyramidal neurons or from corticocortical projections. Contribution to these synapses from thalamic axons seems to be in the minority. Thalamocortical fibres, in fact, lying in the waiting compartment of the SP, are distributed in different cortical layers of the rat by P_2–P_3 coinciding with the appearance of the first recorded evoked potential. By this period, the first corticothalamic fibres are already distributed within the thalamic nuclei (Wise & Jones, 1977). The generation time of LCN has been made possible by means of two combined methods: autoradiography, using tritiated thymidine and immunocytochemistry, using an antibody against GABA. GABA positive neurons are found to be generated between E_{13} and E_{21}, following an orderly inside–outside sequence (Miller, 1986a, b). The LCN, like the projecting neurons, begin their morphogenesis at the end of migration. Differences of the morphological aspect of the variety of LCN can be appreciated during the first postnatal week and the final morphology is completed by the 3rd postnatal week. Therefore, no significant changes in the complexity of dendritric tree can be appreciated after P_{20}.

The axons of LCN grow very little during the first postnatal week and a rapid increase is observed during the 2nd and 3rd postnatal week. The type II synapses appear around P_3 (Miller, 1986a) and progressively increase from the soma, to proximal and distal dendrites.

It can be argued, therefore, that the most important difference in the maturation and development of the two types of cortical cells is referred to the growth of axons. In fact, the growing axons of projecting neurons are forming synapses, about 1 week before those of LCN (Miller, 1988). This could explain the physiological results (Kriegstein et al., 1987) showing that excitatory postsynaptic potentials can be elicited at P_1, in contrast to the inhibitory postsynaptic potentials that are absent through all the 1st postnatal week. Therefore differences in the synaptogenesis between projecting neurons and LCN have been regarded as morphological bases for seizure susceptibility in infants (Vernadakis & Woodbury, 1969; Miller, 1986a,b).

In addition to the morphogenetic aspect of differentiation, the maturation of systems responsible for the uptake, synthesis, release, reception and degradation of neuroactive compounds are observed during development. In the last decade biochemical, physiological and immunocytochemical studies contributed to the identification of neurotransmitter pathways and receptor-second messenger systems involved during maturation events. Differences in maturation of several neurotransmitter systems, according to distinct ontogenetic patterns, have been postulated (Johnston & Coyle, 1981; Johnston, 1988).

The efficiency of a certain neurotransmitter system is dependent on the differential maturation of uptake, synthetic and degradative systems and on receptor-second messenger systems. It is known that cortical neurotransmitters are activated very early during the ontogenesis and in some instances postsynaptic compounds may develop independently of their respective presynaptic elements.

The excitatory and inhibitory neurotransmitters and their receptors are the most important neurochemical systems in the cortex. Glutamate and aspartate are considered the main candidates for excitatory neurotransmission in the cortex. In particular glutamate has been studied during development and it is suggested to be a major excitatory neurotransmitter in the visual cortex (Kvale et al., 1983; Tsumoto et al., 1987). The postsynaptic effect of the excitatory neurotransmitters is mediated by the activation of NMDA and non-NMDA receptor channels. Recent experimental evidence suggests that NMDA are linked to plasticity in the developing neurons system and that NMDA channels are initially expressed in cortical neurons before extensive elaboration of dendrites and the formation of synapses (Lo Turco *et al.*, 1991).

Similar experiments demonstrate that migrating neurons, still in the ventricular zone, express GABA-activated channels (Lo Turco *et al.*, 1990). These data are in agreement with the morphological experiments demonstrating the presence of GABA and $GABA_A$ receptors very early during the cortical embryogenesis (Cobas *et al.*, 1991). These experimental data support the idea that the neurochemical systems, and particularly the neurotransmitter–receptor complex, develop heterogeneously during the ontogenesis. Furthermore, as stated by Johnston (1988) 'these systems may have dual roles in the developing nervous system, serving to transfer messages or to provide trophic signals to adjacent neurons. Maturational differences in biochemical processes involved in neurotransmission may determine the relative influence of these systems in developing brain.'

Acknowledgements

The authors wish to thank Marina De Negri and Maria Teresa Pasquali for editing assistance. The work was partially supported by the Paolo Zorzi Association for Neurosciences.

References

Boulder Committee (1970): Embryonic vertebrate central nervous system: revised terminology. *Anat. Rec.* **166**, 257–262.

Cobas, A., Fairen, A., Alvarez-Bolado, G. & Sanchez, M. P. (1991): Prenatal development of the intrinsic neurons of the rat neocortex: a comparative study of the distribution of GABA-immunoreactive cells and $GABA_A$ receptor. *Neurosciences* **40**, 375–397.

Easter, Jr. S.S., Purves, D., Rakic, P. & Spitzer, N. C. (1985): The changing view of neural specificity. *Science* **230**, 507–511.

Johnston, M. V. (1988): Biochemistry of neurotransmitters in cortical development. In: *Cerebral cortex*, Vol. 7, eds. A. Peters & E.G. Jones. pp. 211–236. New York, London: Plenum Press.

Johnston, M. V. & Coyle, J. T. (1981): Development of central neurotransmitters systems. *Ciba Found. Symp.* **86**, 251–270.

Kriegstein, A. R., Suppes, T. & Prince, D. A. (1987): Cellular and synaptic physiology and epileptogenesis of developing rat neocortical neurons 'in vitro'. *Dev. Brain Res.* **34**, 161–171.

Kvale, I., Fosse, V. M. & Fonnum, F. (1983): Development of neurotransmitters parameters in the lateral geniculate body, superior colliculus and visual cortex of the albino rat. *Dev. Brain Res.* **7**, 137–145.

Lo Turco, J.J., Blanton, M. G. & Kriegstein, A.R. (1990): Appearance of functional voltage and aminoacid gated channels on embryonic neocortical neurons. *Soc. Neurosci. Abstr.* **16**, 797.

Lo Turco, J. J., Blanton, M. G. & Kriegstein, A. R. (1991): Initial expression of endogenous activation of NMDA channels in early neocortical development. *J. Neurosci.* **11**, 792–799.

Marin Padilla, M. (1984): Neurons of layer I. A developmental analysis. In: *Cerebral cortex*, Vol. 1, eds. A. Peters & E. G. Jones. pp. 447–478. New York, London: Plenum Press.

Marin Padilla, M. (1988): Early ontogenesis of the human cerebral cortex . In: *Cerebral cortex*, Vol. 7, eds. A. Peters & E.G. Jones, pp. 1–34. New York, London: Plenum Press.

McConnell, S. (1988): Development and decision-making in the mammalian cerebral cortex. *Brain Res. Rev.* **13**, 1–23.

McConnell, S. (1992): The control of neuronal identity in the developing cerebral cortex. *Curr. Opin. in Neurobiol.* **2**, 23–27.

Miller, M. W. (1981): Maturation of rat visual cortex I. A quantitative study of Golgi impregnated pyramidal neurons. *J. Neurocytol.* **10**, 859–878.

Miller, M.W. (1985): Co-generation of retrogradely labelled cortico-cortical projection and GABA-immunorective local circuit neurons in neocortex. *Dev. Brain Res.* **23**, 187–192.

Miller, M.W. (1986a): Maturation of rat visual cortex III. Postnatal morphogenesis and synaptogenesis of local circuit neurons. *Dev. Brain Res.* **25**, 163–178.

Miller, M.W. (1986b): The migration and neurochemical differentiation of gamma-aminobutyric acid (GABA)-immunoreactive neurons in the rat visual cortex as demonstrated by immunocytochemical-autoradiographic technique. *Dev. Brain Res.* **25**, 271–285.

Miller, M.W. (1988): Development of projection and local circuit neurons in neocortex. In: *Cerebral cortex*, Vol. 7, eds. A. Peters & E.G. Jones, pp. 133–175. New York, London: Plenum Press.

Rakic P. (1971): Guidance of neurons migrating to the fetal monkey neocortex. *Brain Res.* **33**, 471–476.

Rakic, P. (1972): Mode of cell migration to the superficial layers of fetal monkey neocortex. *J. Comp. Neurol.* **145**, 61–84.

Rakic, P. (1982): Early developmental events: cell lineage, acquisition of neuronal position and areal and laminar developments. In: *Developmental and modifiability of cerebral cortex*, eds. P. Rakic & P.S. Goldman-Rakic, pp. 439–451. Cambridge MA: MIT Press.

Schmechel, D.E. & Rakic, P. (1979): A Golgi study of radial glial cells in developing monkey telencephalon: morphogenesis and transformation into astrocytes. *Anat. Embryol.* **156**, 115–152.

Shatz C.J. (1992): How are specific connections formed between thalamus and cortex? *Curr. Opin. Neurobiol.* **2**, 78–82.

Tsumoto, T., Hagihera K., Sato, H. & Hata, Y. (1987): NMDA receptors in the visual cortex of young kittens are more effective than these in adult cats. *Nature* **327**, 513–514.

Vernadakis, A. & Woodboury, D.M. (1969): The developing animal as a model. *Epilepsia* **10**, 163–178.

Wise, S.P. & Jones, E.G. (1977): Cells of origin and terminal distribution of descending projections of the rat somatic sensory cortex. *J. Comp. Neurol.* **175**, 129–158.

Chapter 7

Noradrenergic and peptidergic neurotransmission in hippocampal kindling

A. Vezzani, A. Monno, M. Rizzi, A. Galli, C. Bendotti and R. Samanin

Mario Negri Institute for Pharmacological Research, Laboratory of Neuropharmacology, Milan, Italy

Summary

In this study we investigated the role of hippocampal noradrenergic and peptidergic neurotransmission in kindling epileptogenesis using biochemical indices. Biochemical measurements were done at stage 2 (pre-convulsive stage) and stage 5 (tonic-clonic seizures) in rats electrically kindled in the dorsal hippocampus.

Presynaptic noradrenergic function was assessed by measuring norepinephrine (NE) release from kindled and contralateral hippocampi (CA1–CA3 or dentate gyrus (DG) slices). Two min electrical stimulation induced a frequency-dependent NE release (two-, four- and eightfold above spontaneous release measured respectively at 2, 5 and 10 Hz) which did not significantly differ from that observed in shams (implanted with electrodes but not stimulated). Spontaneous release of NE from kindled and control hippocampi did not differ as well. Isoproterenol-mediated cAMP accumulation and NE-stimulated phosphatidylinositol turnover (PI) were studied as postsynaptic markers of the functional status of α_1- and β_1-adrenoceptors respectively. Isoproterenol induced a dose-dependent increase above basal values in cAMP accumulation (from 40 per cent at 0.01 µM to 180 per cent at 10 µM ($P < 0.01$)) which did not differ between stages 2 and 5 and shams. NE (1–1000 µM) induced a dose-dependent, prazosin-sensitive increase in inositol phosphate (^{3}H-IP) accumulation in the presence of LiCl in hippocampal slices. A significantly higher increase was found at stages 2 ($P < 0.05$) and 5 ($P < 0.05$ and $P < 0.01$) compared to controls at all doses studied. No differences were observed in the basal cAMP or ^{3}H-IP concentrations in kindled versus controls. In another series of experiments we investigated whether the synthesis of somatostatin (SOM) or its release were modified during hippocampal kindling. Northern blot analysis showed that preprosomatostatin (ppSOM) mRNA levels were significantly elevated ($P < 0.05$) in the dorsal hippocampus bilaterally at stage 5 while they were unchanged in the cortex and striatum. The spontaneous and KCl-stimulated release of SOM from hippocampal slices was significantly enhanced in kindled rats ($P < 0.01$) compared to shams. The infusion of 7 pmol/h SOM at the site of hippocampal stimulation 4 days before and 7 days after the beginning of kindling significantly increased the cumulative afterdischarge (AD) and the number of stimulations necessary to reach stage 5 by 80 per cent ($P < 0.05$) and 62 per cent ($P < 0.05$) respectively.

These results show that modifications in noradrenergic and peptidergic neurotransmission occur in kindling and suggest that these neuronal systems have a role in the development of kindling epileptogenesis.

Kindling is a phenomenon of epileptogenesis and synaptic plasticity which develops over time in response to repeated electrical or chemical stimulation of various brain areas. The biochemical and molecular mechanisms involved in the establishment and maintenance of this phenomenon are not clear.

Recent reports indicate that activation of *N*-methyl-*d*-aspartate (NMDA) receptors significantly contribute to the induction of kindling as shown by the ability of selective antagonists of these receptors to delay its development (Peterson et al., 1984; Cain et al., 1988; Croucher et al., 1988; Vezzani et al., 1988). Moreover, NMDA-type receptors become involved in synaptic transmission after kindling of the amygdala or hippocampus and an increased postsynaptic sensitivity to NMDA has been seen after kindling of the stratum radiatum *in vitro* (Mody & Heinemann, 1987; Stelzer et al., 1987). These modifications do not appear to be consequent to changes in receptor density or affinity (Okazaki et al., 1989; Yeh et al., 1989 Vezzani et al., 1990).

A failure of GABA mediated paired-pulse depression in CA1 (Michelson et al., 1989) and an enhanced glutamate release in CA3 (Jarvie et al., 1990) are long lasting effects which may contribute to the hyperexcitability of the kindled tissue but do not appear to be closely involved in NMDA receptor activation.

Noradrenergic and peptidergic (SOM-containing) neurons have been shown to modulate in a complex manner the excitability of the pyramidal and granule cells in the hippocampus (Mancillas et al., 1986; Nicoll et al., 1987). These neuronal systems have also been shown to have a role in convulsive phenomena (Mason & Corcoran, 1979; Higuchi et al., 1983; Kato et al., 1983; Wu et al., 1987; Marksteiner & Sperk, 1988; Sloviter, 1988; Marksteiner et al., 1990; Vezzani et al., 1991b) and in the expression of long-term plasticity in the CNS involving the NMDA receptors (Stanton & Sarvey, 1987; Burgard et al., 1989; Matsuoka et al., 1991).

We studied whether repetitive electrical kindling stimulation caused alterations in hippocampal noradrenergic neurotransmission at pre- and postsynaptic levels using various biochemical indices. In addition, Northern blot analysis of preprosomatostatin (ppSOM) mRNA as well as the release of SOM in the hippocampus were investigated as a measure of the functional status of these peptidergic neurons.

Material and methods

Sprague–Dawley male rats (240–260 g, Charles River, Italy) were housed at constant temperature (23 °C) and relative humidity (60 per cent) with a fixed 12 h light–dark cycle and free access to food and water.

Kindling procedure

The animals underwent kindling by electrical stimulation of the dorsal hippocampus (upper blade of dentate gyrus (DG)) as previously described (Vezzani et al., 1988). Constant current stimuli were delivered to the left hippocampus through a bipolar electrode (recording electrode) twice daily for 5 days and once daily for 2 days (weekend), at intervals of at least 6 h. The parameters of stimulation were 50 Hz, 2 ms monophasic rectangular wave pulses for 1 s, the current intensity ranging between 60 and 200 µA. Animals were stimulated until stage 2 (stereotypies and occasional retraction of a forelimb) (12 ± 1 stimuli) (mean ± SEM) or three consecutive stage 5 (tonic-clonic seizures with rearing and falling) (24 ± 2 stimuli) were reached according to Racine's classification (Racine, 1972). Behaviour was observed and afterdischarge (AD) duration was measured in the kindled hippocampus after each stimulation. Control rats were implanted with electrodes and handled in the same way as the experimental rats but were not electrically stimulated.

Light microscopic analysis of Nissl-stained 40 µm cryostat sections was made (Vezzani et al., 1986) on completion of kindling to verify the electrode placement in the granule cells of the DG.

Biochemical assays

For biochemical determinations, rats kindled at stages 2 and 5, and their controls, were killed, respectively, 48 h and 1 week after the last stimulation.

l-[^{3}H]NE release

Experimental conditions for the uptake and release of L-[^{3}H]NE release from hippocampal slices were done as previously described (Vezzani et al., 1991b).

Fractional release was calculated as ^{3}H released into the medium during each 5 min fraction as a percentage of the ^{3}H content of the slice during that interval. The effect of stimulation was calculated as the fractional release during electrical stimulation (S2) divided by the baseline spontaneous release (S1), the latter being the average of three samples before electrical stimulation. Stimulated release was assessed as the average of the sample collected during stimulation and the one after.

Somatostatin release

Coronal slices of dorsal hippocampi 250 µm, were prepared using, a McIllwain chopper and placed in oxygenated Krebs–Ringer solution (Vezzani et al., 1991b) (KRB) at 37 °C for 30 min. Then the slices were placed in basket-shaped sieves (four slices/sieve) in a series of wells (48-well tissue culture clusters) containing 500 µl oxygenated KRB at 37 °C and they were transferred every 5 min through the wells. After a 40 min wash-out to achieve a steady spontaneous efflux, a 20 min baseline was collected followed by 10 min stimulation in oxygenated KRB containing elevated KCl concentration (50 mM) and proportionally lowered NaCl. The medium was collected and assayed with a sensitive RIA and a specific antibody as described by Lindefors et al. (1987). The antibody was generated in white rabbits as described by Eféndic et al. (1978) and generously supplied by Dr E. Brodin (Dept. of Pharmacology, Karolinska Institute, Stockholm).

The spontaneous efflux and the effect of elevated KCl on basal release are expressed as fmol of SOM measured in the medium in 10-min fractions. The spontaneous efflux was reckoned by considering the two samples immediately preceding KCl stimulation.

cAMP accumulation

cAMP accumulation was measured by the method of Magistretti & Schorderet (1984) as previously described (Vezzani et al., 1991b). Proteins were measured in the pellets by the method of Lowry et al. (1951).

Phosphatidylinositol (PI) turnover

PI hydrolysis was measured by the method of Brown et al. (1984) and the various inositol phosphates were eluted together in a pooled fraction by the method of Berridge et al. (1982) as previously described (Vezzani et al., 199b1).

Northern blot

Total mRNA was isolated from brain tissue with guanidine isothiocyanate as described by Chirgwin et al. (1979). Northern blot analysis was performed as previously described (Bendotti et al., 1991). Each RNA sample was run twice on Northern blots and the mean of two experiments was used for statistical analysis.

Osmotic minipumps

Osmotic minipumps (14 days, Alzet Model 2002, Alza Corp., Palo Alto, CA) were prepared as previously described (Vezzani et al., 1991a). Minipumps were implanted at the back of the neck and connected by a short length of tubing to an injection needle fitting into a guide cannula and protruding 3.0 mm in order to reach the upper blade of the DG (site of electrical stimulation). A 10 mm stainless steel tube was used as a guide cannula, implanted unilaterally on top of the dura as previously described (Vezzani et al., 1991). Continuous infusions were done at a constant speed (0.5 µl/h) for 11 days (4 days before and 7 days after the beginning of kindling). At the end of the infusion period the animals (experimental and control) were lightly anaesthetized to remove the minipumps at least 5 h before the electrical stimulation. Kindling was continued until stage 5 seizures were observed. Experimental animals were implanted with minipumps filled with 5 µg/218 µl SOM-14 (Sigma Chemical Co., St Louis, MO) in 0.1 M phosphate buffered saline (pH 7.4) (PBS) containing 0.2 per cent BSA (Sigma Chemical Co., St Louis, MO). Controls were implanted with minipumps containing 0.2 per cent BSA in PBS. Naive rats (implanted with electrodes but without minipumps) were also used as controls.

Statistical analysis

One-way ANOVA followed by Tukey's test and Dunnett's or Duncan's test (two-tailed comparisons) were used for, respectively, single and multiple comparisons between the experimental groups and their controls.

Results

Electrical stimulation of the dorsal hippocampus initially triggered a high-frequency, high-amplitude AD. The length of the AD significantly increased at stage 5 compared to the beginning of kindling (Fig. 1).

To study whether modifications occurred in noradrenergic neurotransmission, we assessed field electrical-stimulated NE release from hippocampal slices as presynaptic marker of noradrenergic activity, NE-stimulated PI turnover and isoproterenol-induced cAMP accumulation were studied as postsynaptic markers of the functional status of α_1- and β_1-adrenoceptors.

Figure 2 shows the effect of electrical stimulation at various frequencies (2, 5 and 10 Hz) on the

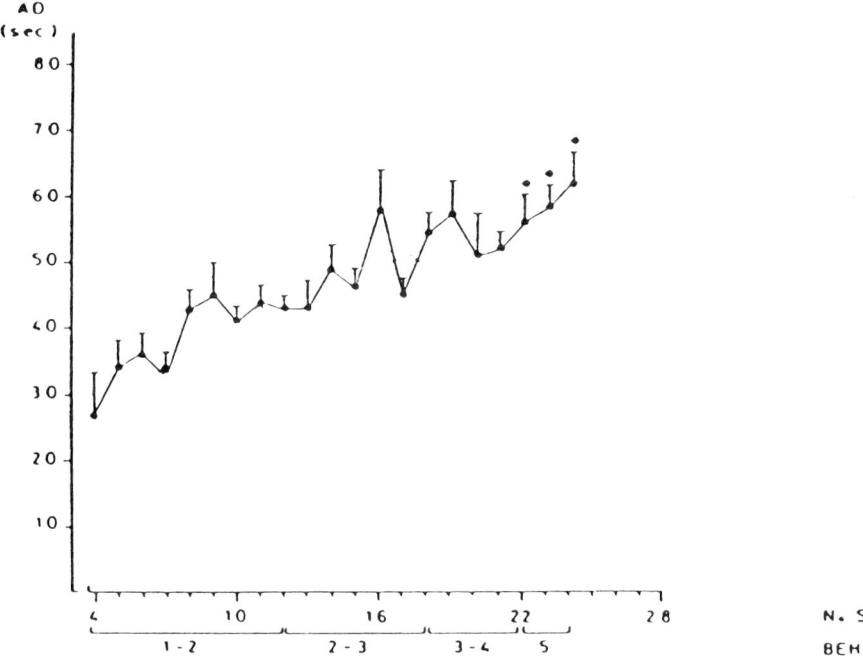

Fig. 1. Focal afterdischarge (AD) duration and behavioural seizures during the development of hippocampal kindling.
Each point represents the average AD duration (s) (mean ± SE) in the kindled hippocampus after each stimulation (n = 5). Bottom line represents the behavioural stages occurring during kindling with the increasing number of stimulations. Asterisks indicate the occurrence of stage 5 behavioural seizures.

fractional release of NE from stratum pyramidale CA1–CA3 and DG slices at stage 2 (left panel) and 5 (right panel) of hippocampal kindling. Ca^{2+}-dependent NE release (80 per cent of the electrically stimulated release as measured by omitting Ca^{2+} and adding 1 mM EGTA to the perfusing solution) was directly related to the frequency of stimulation, as shown by about two-, four- and eightfold increases above spontaneous release at 2, 5, and 10 Hz respectively. No significant differences were observed in the release of NE from CA1–CA3 and DG slices from the stimulated and contralateral hippocampus at stages 2 and 5 of kindling as compared to controls.

Figure 3 shows the isoproterenol-stimulated cAMP accumulation in hippocampi at stages 2 and 5 of kindling and in sham-treated animals. A dose-related increase above basal value in cAMP accumulation was seen in controls, ranging from about 40 per cent at 0.01 μM to 180 per cent at 10 μM ($P < 0.01$, Dunnett's test). No significant differences were observed in the basal cAMP concentration or in the effect of NE (0.001–10 μM) on cAMP accumulation in hippocampi of kindled rats compared to shams (Tukey's test).

Figure 4 shows the effect of various concentrations of NE (1–1000 μM) on PI turnover in hippo-

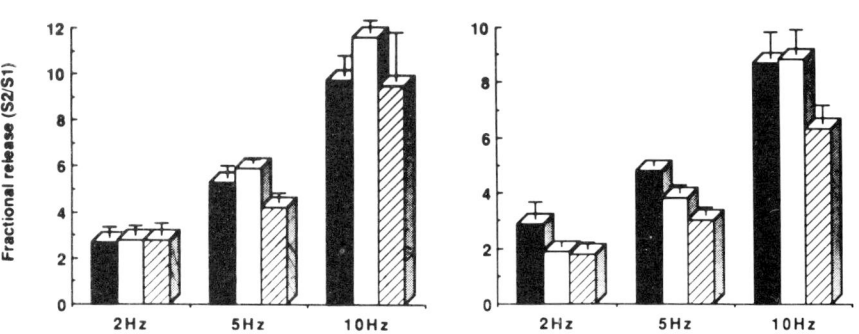

Fig. 2. L-[^{3}H]NE release from stratum pyramidale CA1–CA3 and dentate gyrus slices of stage 2- (left side) and stage 5- (right side) kindled rats. Data are mean ± SEM values, in fractional release during stimulation (S2) divided by the baseline of spontaneous release (S1) from three experiments (n = 3 rats/group/experiment). Sham represents rats implanted with electrodes but not stimulated. Kindled ipsi and contra refer respectively to the stimulated and contralateral hippocampus. Slices were stimulated at the indicated frequencies for 2 min; samples were collected every 5 min. The speed of perfusion was 0.5 ml/min. Rats were killed 48 h after the last stimulation (stage 2) or 1 week after the last seizure (stage 5).

campi of kindled rats as compared to shams. NE induced a dose-dependent increase in PI turnover as measured by [^{3}H]IP accumulation in the slices in the presence of LiCl. The maximal stimulation, about 350 per cent above basal values, was reached at 100 µM ($P < 0.01$; Dunnett's test). The effect of NE on PI turnover was mediated by stimulation of α_1-adrenoceptors as demonstrated by the fact that 1 µM prazosin abolished the effect of 10 and 100 µM NE in slices taken from naive rats (data not shown). A significantly larger increase in ^{3}H-IP accumulation was seen in stage 2 ($P < 0.05$, Tukey's test) and stage 5 ($P < 0.05$ and $P < 0.01$, Tukey's test) compared to shams at the same doses (Fig. 4 A,B). No significant differences were found in the basal concentrations of IP between rats kindled at stages 2 and 5 and their respective shams (data not shown). The enhanced accumulation of ^{3}H-IP in kindled rats was maintained one month after stage 5 acquisition (per cent of basal: NE 100 µM, control 446 ± 17; kindling 511 ± 21 (n = 5), $P < 0.01$, Tukey's test). ^{3}H-IP accumulation induced by carbachol (10–1000 µM) was not modified by kindling (data not shown).

In another series of experiments we investigated whether the synthesis of SOM or its release was modified during hippocampal kindling.

At stage 2 ppSOM mRNA contents was increased by about 35 per cent compared to controls in the dorsal hippocampus ipsilateral and contralateral to the site of stimulation (Fig. 5). Further enhancement of ppSOM mRNA, 88 per cent above controls ($P < 0.05$, Duncan's test), was observed at stage 5 in the stimulated hippocampus while a 20 per cent increase was observed in the contralateral one. No changes in mRNA were observed in striatum and cerebral cortex at stages 2 and 5.

Preliminary experiments on naive animals had shown a concentration-dependent increase in the spontaneous efflux of SOM in response to 25–100 mM KCl. The 50 mM KCl-stimulated release was submaximal (about 16-fold above spontaneous efflux) and completely suppressed in the virtual absence of Ca^{2+} (Vezzani et al., 1992).

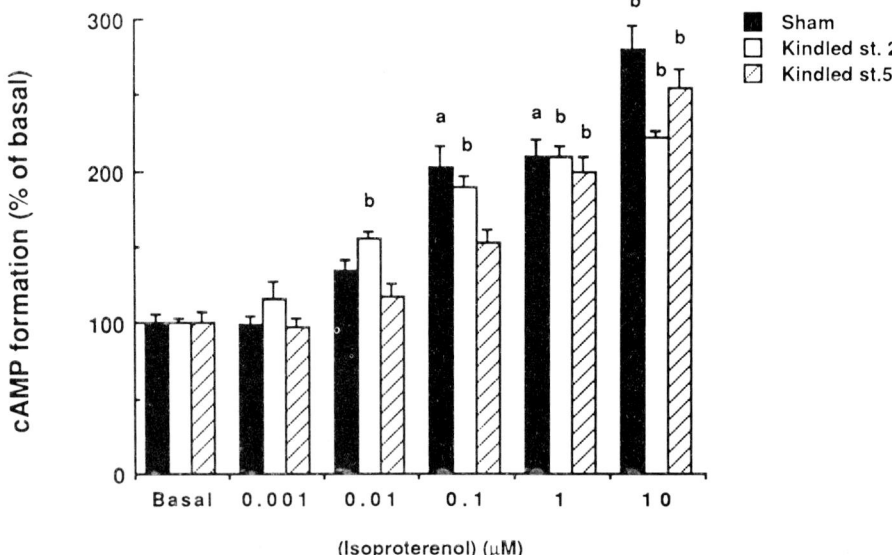

Fig. 3. Isoproterenol-induced cAMP accumulation in hippocampi of stage 2- and stage 5-kindled rats. Data are means ± SEM (n = 10 rats/group) expressed as per cent increase above basal values ((pmol/mg prot.); sham, 5.03 ± 0.3; stage 2, 4.74 ± 0.15; stage 5, 5.3 ± 0.4). Rats were killed 48 h after the last stimulation (stage 2) or 1 week after the last seizure (stage 5). Statistical analysis of data was done on absolute values. a, $P < 0.05$; b, $P < 0.01$ vs respective basal (Dunnett's test).

The 50 mM KCl-induced SOM release from hippocampal slices of kindled rats was enhanced by 66 per cent and 95 per cent ($P < 0.01$, Tukey's test) at stage 2 and by 51 per cent and 96 per cent at stage 5 ($P < 0.01$, Tukey's test) in the stimulated and contralateral hippocampus respectively as compared to shams (Fig. 5).

The spontaneous efflux of SOM was enhanced by 160 per cent and by 95 per cent at stage 5 in the stimulated and contralateral hippocampus respectively compared to shams ($P < 0.01$, Tukey's test) (Table 1) (Vezzani et al., 1992).

In a final experiment we studied the effect of 11-day intrahippocampal infusion of 7 pmol/h SOM on the rate of kindling development.

As shown in Table 2, in the post-infusion period the peptide increased the cumulative AD and the

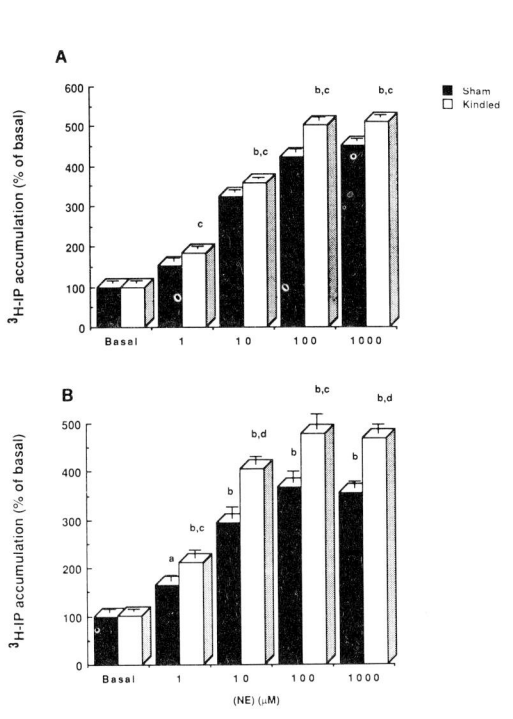
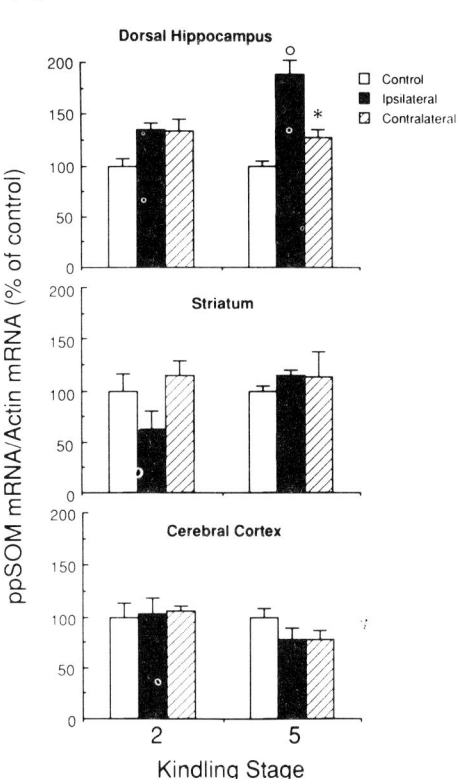

Fig. 4. Norepinephrine (NE)-stimulated PI turnover in hippocampi of stage 2-(A) and stage 5-(B) kindled rats. Data are means± SEM of three experiments (n = 6 rats/group/experiment). [³H]IP accumulation was expressed as per cent increase above basal values. Rats were killed 48 h after the last stimulation (stage 2) or 1 week after the last seizure (stage 5). Statistical analysis of data was done on absolute values.
a, $P < 0.05$; b, $P < 0.01$ vs respective basal (Dunnett's test); c, $P < 0.05$; d, $P < 0.01$ vs sham at the same dose (Tukey's test).

Fig. 5. Depolarization (50 mM KCl)-induced somatostatin release from hippocampi of stage 2- and stage 5-kindled rats.
Data are means ± SEM of two experiments (n = 5 rats/group/experiment). Somatostatin release (fmol/ml) is expressed as percentage increase above baseline (the spontaneous efflux in the two samples immediately preceding the depolarization). Baseline values are reported in Table 1.
**$P < 0.01$ vs respective sham by Tukey's test.

number of stimulations to stage 5 by 80 per cent ($P < 0.05$, Student's t-test) and by 50 per cent ($P < 0.05$, Student's t-test) respectively compared to controls.

Table 1. *Somatostatin release from hippocampal slices of stage 2-kindled rats (fmol/ml)*

Sham		19.7 ± 1.5	
	Stage 2		*Stage 5*
Kindled ipsi	24.3 ± 2.1		51.1 ± 7*
Kindled contra	19.8 ± 1.7		39.5 ± 2.4*

Data are means ± SE (n = 10). *$P < 0.01$ *vs* sham by Tukey's test.
Kindled ipsi and contra refer to simulated and contralateral hippocampus respectively.

Table 2. *Effect of somatostatin infusion in the hippocampus on the rate of acquisition of stage 5 seizures*

	No. of stimulations		Cumulative AD (s)	
	Infusion	Post-infusion	Infusion	Post-infusion
Control (0.2% BSA)	12	14 ± 3	366 ± 18	432 ± 89 (7)
Som-14 (7 pmol/h)	12	21 ± 3*	358 ± 26	778 ± 100* (8)

Data are means ± SE. Number of animals in parentheses.
Somatostatin (Som-14) (5 μg/minipump/218 μl) was continuously infused (0.5 μl/h) for 11 days (4 before and 7 after the beginning of kindling) at the site of electrical stimulation (upper blade of dentate gyrus). The animals were stimulated until they reached three consecutive stage 5 seizures.
*$P < 0.05$, Student's t-test.

Discussion

Our study has shown that significant changes in noradrenergic and peptidergic neurotransmission occur in the hippocampus during kindling epileptogenesis.

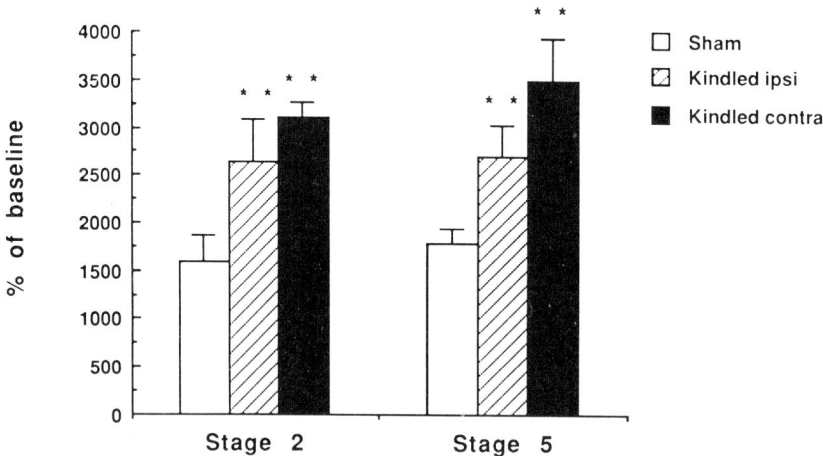

Fig. 6. *PreproSOM mRNA levels in rat hippocampus at different stages of hippocampal kindling. The ppSOM mRNA levels are shown relative to the contents of β-actin mRNA and are expressed as a percentage of controls.*
Each column represents the mean ± SE (vertical bar) of at least three separate samples.
*°$P < 0.05$ vs control; *$P < 0.05$ vs ipsilateral (Duncan's test).*

Selective and long-lasting modifications in the functional status of α_1-adrenoceptors occur during kindling in the absence of changes in NE release from presynaptic nerve terminals under basal and stimulated conditions (Vezzani et al., 1991b).

β_1-Adrenoceptor-mediated cAMP accumulation was not altered in kindling (Vezzani et al., 1991b) while stimulation of PI turnover by NE was enhanced at the early preconvulsive stage (stage 2) and remained higher than controls for at least 1 month after the last stage 5 seizure. The persistence of this effect makes it unlikely that it was a mere consequence of seizure activity. The lack of changes in carbachol-stimulated PI hydrolysis at stage 5 suggests that the enhanced response induced by NE was not due to a non-specific increase in the activity of phospholipase C.

The enhanced effect of NE on PI turnover was not due to an increase in the density and/or affinity of α_1-binding sites (unpublished). An enhanced coupling of the receptors with phospholipase C as well as transynaptic mechanisms may be involved. Phospholipase C activation induced by NE in hippocampus has been shown to be potentiated by GABA-receptor stimulation (Ruggiero et al., 1987) and GABA release is enhanced in CA1 following kindling (Kamphuis et al., 1990). Glutamate has been reported to inhibit NE-stimulated PI turnover in naive rats (Nicoletti et al., 1986). A failure of this heteroreceptor regulation in kindling may lead to the enhancement of the α_1-adrenoceptor response.

The effect on NE-induced PI turnover is similar to that observed for ibotenate-dependent stimulation although it lasted longer (Iadarola et al., 1986). This suggests that IP hydrolysis and the associated intracellular events are part of the mechanisms that accompany permanent changes in the excitability of the hippocampus following kindling or, more in general, phenomena of synaptic plasticity. This is supported by a recent finding of a selective increase in excitatory amino acid and NE-induced PI turnover associated with the late (maintenance) phase of LTP (Aronica et al., 1991).

α_1-Adrenoceptors appear to mediate the inhibitory effects of endogenous NE released by locus ceruleus stimulation on hippocampal pyramidal neurons (Curet & de Montigny, 1988). Suppressant effects of NE through α_1-adrenoceptors on Ca^{2+}-dependent regenerative potentials in DG (Stanton et al., 1989) and on NMDA-induced responses in cortical neurons (Lehmenkuhler et al., 1991) have been reported. In accordance with this evidence, we have shown an inhibitory effect of NE through α_1-adrenoceptors on seizure activity induced in the hippocampus by NMDA-receptor stimulation (Wu et al., 1987). Amplification of the α_1-adrenoceptor-linked second messanger system may, therefore, be aimed at blunting the enhanced neuronal excitation of the kindled hippocampus. On the other hand, hyperactivity of metabotropic receptors as a result of an initial activation of NMDA-receptor, may lead to enhanced intracellular Ca^{2+} mobilization and activate a cascade of intracellular events which may ultimately lead to structural synaptic changes (Cavazos & Sutula, 1990; Geinisman et al., 1990) and/or modulation of gene expression. Further studies are needed to clarify the mechanisms and functional significance of this phenomenon.

We have found an increased synthesis of SOM in the hippocampus at stage 5 (Bendotti et al., 1991). This finding together with the higher extracellular concentration of SOM under resting and depolarizing conditions in the hippocampus of kindled rats, indicates an enhanced activity of these peptidergic neurons in kindling.

We have found that continuous infusion of pmol amounts of SOM on granule cells of the DG at the site of stimulation retards the development of kindling. Thus, the increased availability of SOM in the extracellular compartment may represent a local endogenous mechanisms to counteract kindling epileptogenesis. In accordance, we have recently shown that SOM has an inhibitory effect on limbic seizures induced by kainic acid and quinolinic acid in the hippocampus (Vezzani et al., 1991c). This suggests this peptide may be one factor controlling the excessive excitation caused by glutamate during kindling. Our results support and extend previous evidence of a role of brain SOM in convulsive phenomena (Higuchi et al., 1983; Kato et al., 1983; Marksteiner & Sperk, 1988; Sloviter, 1988; Marksteiner et al., 1990; Vezzani et al., 1991c). In view of the loss of SOM in the hippocampus of temporal lobe epilepsy patients (de Lanerolle *et al.*, 1989), it is worth considering the possibility that this neuropeptide has a role in the pathophysiology of this human disorder.

In summary, our study emphasizes the importance of a modulatory role of hippocampal noradrenergic and peptidergic neurons on kindling epileptogenesis. Our data together with electrophysiological and functional studies suggest that NE- and SOM-containing neurons in the hippocampus act in concert to antagonize the epileptic discharge and/or its generalization.

Abbreviations: AD, afterdischarge; DG, dentate gyrus; EEG, electroencephalography; IP, inositol phosphates; NE, norepinephrine; NMDA, N-methyl-D-aspartic acid; PI, phosphatidyl inositol.

References

Aronica, E., Frey, U., Wagner, M., Schroeder, H., Krug, M., Ruthrich, H., Catania, M.V., Nicoletti, F. & Reymann, K.G. (1991): Enhanced sensitivity of 'metabotropic' glutamate receptors after induction of long-term potentiation in rat hippocampus. *J. Neurochem.* **57**, 376–383.

Bendotti, C., Vezzani, A., Serafini, R., Servadio, A., Rivolta, R. & Samanin, R. (1991): Increased preproneuropeptide Y mRNA in the rat hippocampus during the development of hippocampal kindling: comparison with the expression of preprosomatostatin mRNA. *Neurosci. Lett.* **132**, 175–178.

Berridge, M.J., Downes, C.P. & Hanley, M.R. (1982): Lithium amplifies agonist-dependent phosphotidylinositol responses in brain and salivary glands. *Biochem. J.* **206**, 587–595.

Brown, E., Kendall, D.A. & Nahorski, S.R. (1984): Inositol phospholipid hydrolisis in rat cerebral cortical slices. I. Receptor characterization. *J. Neurochem.* **42**, 1379–1387.

Burgard, E.C., Decker, G. & Sarvey, J.M. (1989): NMDA receptor antagonists block norepinephrine-induced long-lasting potentiation and long-term potentiation in rat dentate gyrus. *Brain Res.* **482**, 351–355.

Cain, D.P., Desborough, K.A. & McKitrick, D.J. (1988): Retardation of amygdala kindling by antagonism of NMD-aspartate and muscarinic cholinergic receptors: evidence for the summation of excitatory mechanisms in kindling. *Exp. Neurol.* **100**, 179–187.

Cavazos, J. E. & Sutula, T. P. (1990): Progressive neuronal loss induced by kindling: a possible mechanism for mossy fiber reorganization and hippocampal sclerosis. *Brain Res.* **527**, 1–6.

Chirgwin, M. E., Przybyla, A.E., MacDonald, R. J. & Rutter, W.J. (1979): Isolation of biologically active ribonucleic acid from sources enriched in ribonucleases. *Biochemistry* **18**, 5294–5299.

Croucher, M.J., Bradford, H.F., Sunter, D.C. & Watkins, J.C. (1988): Inhibition of the development of electrical kindling of the prepyriform cortex by daily focal injections of excitatory amino acid antagonists. *Eur. J. Pharmacol.* **152**, 29–38.

Curet, O. & de Montigny, C. (1988): Electrophysiolocal characterization of adrenoceptors in the rat dorsal hippocampus. II. Receptors mediating the effect of synaptically released norepinephrine. *Brain Res.* **475**, 47–57.

de Lanerolle, N.C., Kim, J.H., Robbins, R.J. & Spencer, D.D. (1989): Hippocampal interneuron loss and plasticity in human temporal lobe epilepsy. *Brain Res.* **495**, 387–395.

Eféndic, S., Nylen, A., Roovete, A. & Uvnas-Wallensten, K. (1978): Effect of glucose and arginine on the release of immunoreactive somatostatin from the isolated rat pancreas. *FEBS. Lett.* **22**, 33–35.

Geinisman, Y., de Toledo-Morrell, L. & Morrell, F. (1990): The brain's record of experience: kindling-induced enlargement of the active zone in hippocampal perforated synapses. *Brain Res.* **513**, 175–179.

Higuchi, T., Sikand, G.S., Kato, N., Wada, J.A. & Friesen, H.G. (1983): Profound suppression of kindled seizures by cysteamine: possible role of somatostatin to kindled seizures. *Brain Res.* **288**, 359–362.

Iadarola, M.J., Nicoletti, F., Naranjo, J.R., Putnam, F. & Costa, E. (1986): Kindling enhances the stimulation of inositol phospholipid hydrolysis elicited by ibotenic acid in rat hippocampal slices. *Brain Res.* **374**, 174–178.

Jarvie, P.A., Logan, T.C., Geula, C. & Slevin J.T. (1990): Entorhinal kindling permanently enhances Ca^{2+}-dependent L-glutamate release in regio inferior of rat hippocampus. *Brain Res.* **508**, 188–193.

Kamphuis, W., Huisman, E., Dreijer, A.M.C., Ghijsen, W.E.J.M., Verhage, M. & Lopes da Silva, F.H.. (1990): Kindling increases the K^+-evoked Ca^{2+}-dependent release of endogenous GABA in area CA1 of rat hippocampus. *Brain Res.* **511**, 63–70.

Kato, N., Higuchi, T., Friesen, H.G. & Wada, J.A. (1983): Changes in immunoreactive somatostatin and β-endorphine content in rat brain after amygdaloid kindling. *Life Sci.* **32**, 2415–2422.

Lehmenkuhler, C., Walden, J. & Speckmann, E.-J. (1991): Decrease of N-methyl-D-aspartate responses by noradrenaline in the rat motorcortex in vivo. *Neurosci. Lett.* **121**, 5–8.

Lindefors, N., Brodin, E. & Ungerstedt, U. (1987): Microdialysis combined with a sensitive radioimmunoassay. *J. Pharmacol. Methods* **17**, 305–312.

Lowry, O. H., Rosebrough, N.J., Farr, A.L. & Randall, R.J. (1951): Protein measurement with the Folin phenol reagent. *J. Biol. Chem.* **193**, 265–275.

Magistretti, P.J. & Schorderet, M. (1984): VIP and noradrenaline act synergistically to increase cyclic AMP in cerebral cortex. *Nature* **308**, 280–282.

Mancillas, J.R., Siggins, G.R. & Bloom, F.E. (1986): Somatostatin selectively enhances acetylcholine-induced excitations in rat hippocampus and cortex. *Proc. Natl. Acad. Sci. USA* **83**, 7518–7521.

Marksteiner, J., Lassman, H., Saria, A., Humpel, C., Meyer, D.K. & Sperk, G. (1990): Neuropeptide levels after pentylenetetrazol kindling in the rat. *Eur. J. Neurosci.* **2**, 98–103.

Marksteiner, J. & Sperk, G. (1988): Concomitant increase of somatostatin, neuropeptide Y and glutamate decarboxylase in the frontal cortex of rats with decreased seizure threshold. *Neuroscience* **26**, 379–385.

Mason, S.T. & Corcoran, M.E. (1979): Catecholamines and convulsions. *Brain Res.* **170**, 497–507.

Matsuoka, N., Kaneko, S. & Satoh, M. (1991): Somatostatin augments long-term potentiation of the mossy fiber-CA3 system in guinea-pig hippocampal slices. *Brain Res.* **553**, 188–194.

Michelson, H.B., Kapur, J. & Lothman, E.W. (1989): Reduction of paired pulse inhibition in the CA1 region of the hippocampus by pilocarpine in naive and in amygdala-kindled rats. *Exp. Neurol.* **104**, 264–271.

Mody, I. & Heinemann, U. (1987): NMDA receptors of dentate gyrus granule cells participate in synaptic transmission following kindling. *Nature* **326**, 701–704.

Nicoletti, F., Iadarola, M. J., Wroblenski, J.T. & Costa, E. (1986): Excitatory amino acid recognition sites coupled with inositol phospholipid metabolism: developmental changes and interaction with α_1-adrenoceptors. *Proc. Natl. Acad. Sci. USA* **83**, 1931–1935.

Nicoll, R.A., Madison, D.V. & Lancaster, B. (1987): Noradrenergic modulation of neuronal excitability in mammalian hippocampus. In: *Psychopharmacology, The third generation of progress*, ed. H.Y. Meltzer, pp. 105–112. New York: Raven Press.

Okazaki, M.M., McNamara, J.O. & Nadler, J.V. (1989): N-Methyl-D-aspartate receptor autoradiography in rat brain after angular bundle kindling. *Brain Res.* **482**, 359–364.

Peterson, D.W., Collins, J.F. & Bradford, H.F. (1984): Anticonvulsant action of amino acid antagonist against kindled hippocampal seizures. *Brain Res.* **311**, 176–180.

Racine, R.J. (1972): Modification of seizure activity by electrical stimulation, II. Motor seizure. *Electroencephalogr. Clin. Neurophysiol.* **32**, 281–294.

Ruggiero, M., Corradetti, R., Chiarugi, V. & Pepeu, G. (1987): Phospholipase C activation induced by noradrenaline in rat hippocampal slices is potentiated by GABA-receptor stimulation. *EMBO J.* **6**, 1595–1598.

Sloviter, R.S. (1988): Decreased hippocampal inhibition and a selective loss of interneurons in experimental epilepsy. *Science* **235**, 73–76.

Stanton, P.K., Mody, I. & Heinemann, U. (1989): Down-regulation of norepinephrine sensitivity after induction of long-term neuronal plasticity (kindling) in the rat dentate gyrus. *Brain Res.* **476**, 367–372.

Stanton, P.K. & Sarvey, J.M. (1987): Norepinephrine regulates long-term potentiation of both the population spike and dendritic EPSP in hippocampal dentate gyrus. *Brain Res. Bull.* **18**, 115–119.

Stelzer, A., Slater, N.T. & Bruggencate, G. (1987): Activation of NMDA receptors blocks GABAergic inhibition in an *in vitro* model of epilepsy. *Nature* **326**, 698–701.

Vezzani, A., Forloni, G.L., Serafini, R. & Samanin, R. (1991a): Neurodegenerative effects induced by chronic infusion of quinolinic acid in rat striatum and hippocampus. *Eur. J. Neurosci.* **3**, 40–46.

Vezzani, A., Monno, A., Razzi, M., Galli, A., Barrios, M. & Samanin, R. (1992): Somatostatin release is enhanced in the hippocampus of partially and fully kindled rats. *Neuroscience* **51**, 41–46.

Vezzani, A., Rizzi, M., Serafini, R., Vigano', G. & Samanin, R. (1991b): Changes in pre- and postsynaptic components of noradrenergic transmission in hippocampal kindling in rats. *Brain Res.* **557**, 210–216.

Vezzani, A., Serafini, R., Samanin, R. & Foster, A. (1990): Autoradiographical analysis of excitatory amino acid binding sites in rat hippocampus during the development of hippocampal kindling. *Brain Res.* **526**, 113–121.

Vezzani, A., Serafini, R., Stasi, M.A., Vigano', G., Rizzi, M. & Samanin, R. (1991c): A peptidase-resistant cyclic octapeptide analog of somatostatin (SMS 201–995) modulates seizures induced by quinolinic acid and kainic acid differently in the rat hippocampus. *Neuropharmacology* **30**, 345–352.

Vezzani, A., Wu, H.Q., Moneta, E. & Samanin, R. (1988): Role of the N-methyl-D-aspartate receptors in the development and maintenance of hippocampal kindling in rats. *Neurosci. Lett.* **87**, 63–68.

Vezzani, A., Wu, H.Q., Tullii, M. & Samanin, R. (1986): Anticonvulsant drugs effective against human temporal lobe epilepsy prevent seizures but not neurotoxicity induced in rats by quinolinic acid: electroencephalographic, behavioural and histological assessments. *J. Pharmacol. Exp. Ther.* **239**, 256–262.

Wu, H. Q., Tullii, M., Samanin, R. & Vezzani, A. (1987): Norepinephrine modulates seizures induced by quinolinic acid in rats: selective and distinct roles of α-adrenoceptor subtypes. *Eur. J. Pharmacol.* **138**, 309–318.

Yeh, G.C., Bonhaus, D.W., Nadler, J.V. & McNamara, J.O. (1989): N-methyl-D-aspartate receptor plasticity in kindling: quantitative and qualitative alterations in the N-methyl-D-aspartate receptor-complex. *Proc. Natl. Acad. Sci. USA* **86**, 8157–8160.

Chapter 8

Epileptogenesis in the hippocampus of the isolated guinea-pig brain maintained *in vitro*: a model for limbic seizures

Marco de Curtis*, Denis Paré and Rodolfo R. Llinas

*Department of Physiology and Biophysics, New York University, New York, NY 10016, USA and *Dipartimento di Neurofisiologia, Istituto Nazionale Neurologico C. Besta, 20133 Milan, Italy*

Summary

The limbic system has a particularly low threshold for the generation of epileptic activity. The structural and functional characteristics of the hippocampal formation play a significant role in this propensity of the limbic lobe to hypersynchronization. The isolated guinea-pig brain preparation maintained *in vitro* by arterial perfusion was utilized to study with electrophysiological techniques the epileptiform activity induced in the hippocampus by repetitive high frequency stimulation of the entorhinal cortex (EC). Two stages in the epileptiform discharges are described here. In stage 1, isolated population spikes (occurring at 1–3 Hz) originated from pyramidal neurons in the Cornu Ammonis area 3 (CA3) and spread to all level of the entorhinal cortex-hippocampal loop, except in the dentate gyrus (DG). The epileptiform activity evolved to stage 2 only when a large population spike was recruited in the dentate gyrus. In this phase rhythmic re-entrant activation of the entorinal-hippocampal-entorhinal loop was observed with simultaneous extra- and intracellular recordings from EC, DG, CA3 and CA1 hippocampal subfields. The pattern of epileptiform activity recalls the early electroencephalographic events observed during the onset of hippocampal seizures recorded with depth electrodes in epileptic patients affected by temporal lobe epilepsy.

Introduction

The hippocampus is regarded as one of the cortical structures having the lowest threshold for generation of epileptiform activity (Liberson *et al.*, 1951). The abnormal firing of hippocampal cortical neurons during partial complex seizures in humans shows peculiar characteristics of onset that have been described in epileptic patients investigated with stereo-electro-encephalographic procedures for surgical removal of the epileptogenic focus (Walsh & Delgado-Escueta, 1984). In this population of patients, selected on the basis of rigorous electroclinical criteria (refractoriness to pharmacological treatment, monofocal origin of the seizures, etc.), depth electrodes were implanted in the temporal lobe to locate the epileptogenic area (Fig. 1). In most of these cases, the ictal discharge at the onset of the electroclinical seizure was characterized by fast 15–25 Hz rhythmic spikes that progressively increased in amplitude and recruited surrounding brain areas, thus causing diffusion of the epileptiform activity and occasionally leading to secondary generalization. The hippocampal mechanisms involved in this pattern of electrical onset and its spread to nearby structures are not completely understood yet.

Many factors are known to be determinant in the hyperexcitability leading to generation of epileptic activity in the hippocampus. The most relevant for the discussion of this paper are:

(1) *The unidirectional loop organization of intrinsic hippocampal connectivity.* Anatomical (Amaral & Witter, 1989) and physiological (Andersen, 1975) studies have revealed that the main subfields of the hippocampal formation, namely the dentate gyrus (DG), the areas CA3 and CA1, the subiculum and the entorhinal cortex (EC) constitute a largely unidirectional multisynaptic loop. As a result, impulses arising in the EC (the main source of cortical afferents to the hippocampus) can be channelled back to the EC through the sequential activation of dentate granule cells, pyramidal cells of CA3 and CA1 as well as those of the subiculum. Such a strongly wired closed circuit arrangement might enhance the hippocampal excitability via the possible resonant reactivation of the loop (de Curtis *et al.*, 1991; Buzsaki *et al.*, 1991).

(2) *Intrinsic membrane properties and microcircuit.* The pyramidal neurons of the CA3 subfield area display peculiar intrinsic electrophysiological membrane properties and contribute to a prominent system of associative connections, which have been studied extensively on slices *in vitro* and by computational modelling (see Traub & Miles, 1991, for review). In particular CA3 neurons can generate high threshold calcium spikes subtending bursting discharges in response to synaptic inputs (Schwartzkroin & Prince, 1978; Wong & Traub, 1983). This bursting propensity could constitute a loop gain system that would reinforce the tendency of the entorhinal-hippocampal loop to resonate. In addition, the system of excitatory recurrent synapses and the existence of electrotonic coupling between CA3 pyramidal neurons (McVicar & Dudek, 1981) provide structural and functional substrates for the genesis of synchronized events by this hippocampal region and explain the tendency of CA3 pyramids to generate epileptiform activity in disinhibited conditions (Wong & Traub, 1983).

(3) *Morphological abnormalities associated with epilepsy.* Among the neuropathological findings in hippocampi of patients with temporal lobe epilepsy, abnormal synaptic transformations occurring in the DG have been given major attention in recent years in an attempt to explain epileptogenic hyperexcitability. Sutula *et al.* (1989) and Babb *et al.* (1991) demonstrated the presence of neuronal loss and mild sclerosis in the DG and hilus of epileptic patients affected by focal hippocampal

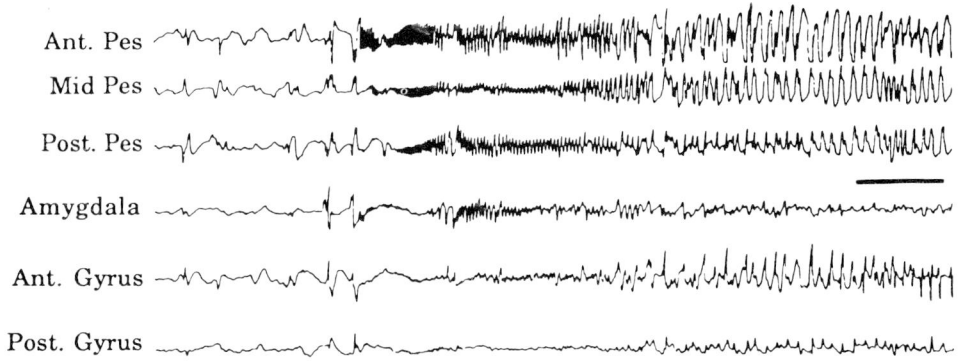

Fig. 1. Typical recording of an epileptic focus in the hippocampus of a patient with complex partial seizures originating from the temporal lobe. The patient was studied with depth electrodes positioned in the limbic lobe (anterior, medium and posterior pes of the hippocampus, amygdala, anterior and posterior parahippocampal gyri) for surgical treatment of the epilepsy (modified with permission from Walsh & Delgado-Escueta, 1984).

epilepsy. This neuronal damage was associated to a remodelling of the intrinsic DG synaptic network. With a Timm staining for zinc that selectively labels mossy fibres (because of their high content of zinc) these authors demonstrated the appearance of newly formed granule cell axon collaterals sprouting at the apical dendrites of neighbouring granule cells. This structural modification of the connections between glutamatergic granule neurons were correlated to a possible strengthening of excitation in DG. Experimental confirmation of this hypothesis has been demonstrated recently utilizing chronic epileptic animal models (Cavazos et al., 1991).

In a recent paper we described self-sustained rhythmic afterdischarges after tetanic stimulation of the EC in the isolated guinea pig brain maintained *in vitro* (Paré et al., 1992). This activity showed similarities with epileptiform events recorded in human temporal lobe epilepsy and was investigated to analyse the role played by the entorhinal-hippocampal loop in shaping the hippocampal epileptic discharges.

The isolated *in vitro* brain preparation combines the advantages of an *in vitro* preparation (mechanical stability, absence of pulsation and respiration artifacts, easy access to deep structures, control over ionic microenvironment) with the complete preservation of the limbic synaptology (de Curtis et al., 1991). It is therefore an unique and ideal preparation for the electrophysiological study of synaptic networks in the central nervous system.

Materials and methods

Brains were isolated from young adult Hartley guinea-pigs (150–200 g) after barbiturate anaesthesia. The technique of isolation and arterial perfusion have been described in detail (de Curtis et al., 1991; Muhlethaler et al., in preparation). During intracardiac perfusion with cold Ringer solution a complete craniotomy was performed to expose the whole brain, from the olfactory bulbs to the cervical spinal cord; in most of the experiments the hippocampus was exposed by carefully removing the overlying cerebral cortex by suction. The brain was then lifted from the base of the skull, the cranial nerves and the arterial vessel were cut and the isolated brain was transferred to a perfusion chamber. A thin polyethylene cannula was inserted in one of the vertebral arteries and the intra-arterial perfusion was started (6–7 ml/min flow). The major arteries (carotids and smaller leaking vessels of the brainstem) were then tied to ensure the perfusion of the brain through the circle of Willis and the vertebro-basilar system. The composition of the perfusing solution was (in mM): 126 NaCl; 26 $NaCO_3$; 3 KCl; 1.2 KH_2PO_4; 1.3 $MgSO_4$; 2.4 $CaCl_2$; 5 HEPES; 15 glucose; 0.4 thiourea; and 3% dextran (mol. wt. 70,000). The experiments were performed with a perfusate temperature of 31 °C. Extracellular and intracellular recording electrodes (tungsten microelectrodes and glass pipettes; 5–10 MΩ and 50–80 MΩ input resistance, respectively) were positioned in DG, CA3, CA1 and EC and their position were controlled electrophysiologically (orthodromically evoked responses) and histologically (tip electrode coagulation and intracellular injection with biocytin). Tungsten coaxial stimulating electrodes were positioned in the EC. Intracellular HRP was revealed after intracellular biocytin injection by histologically processing the brains at the end of the experiments with standard techniques (see de Curtis et al., 1991; Horikawa & Armstrong, 1988).

Results

The position of the recording electrodes was controlled by performing field potential profiles of the hippocampal formation after stimulation of the EC, along dorso-ventral penetrations. The field potentials were then compared to those described in literature for DG, CA1 and CA3 (Andersen et al., 1966a, 1966b; Andersen, 1975). Figure 2 illustrates a typical penetration in the septal portion of the hippocampus following EC stimulation. The reconstruction of the electrode track is shown (right) on a coronal hippocampal section. EC stimulation evoked a response in the DG with a monosynaptic latency (lower traces m and g), followed by the activation of CA1. Note the location of the reversal in polarity of the DG and CA1 field components along the reconstructed penetration.

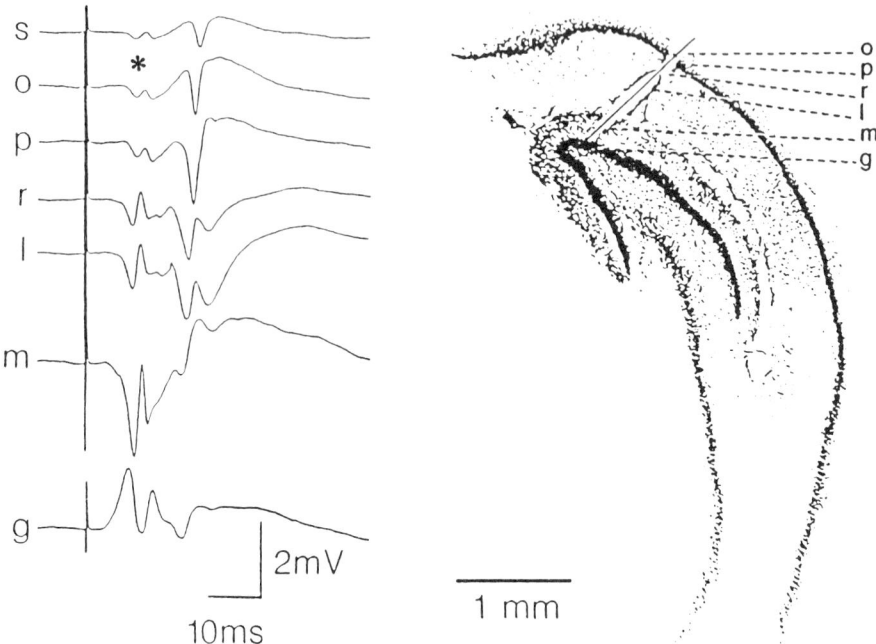

Fig. 2. Field potential profile obtained along a coronal dorso-ventral penetration in the hippocampus. The penetration illustrated on the right was reconstructed by combining micrometer readings with the location of a small electrolytic lesion made at the end of the experiment. S=surface; o=stratum oriens; p=stratum pyramidale; r=stratum radiatum; l=stratum lacunosum; m=stratum moleculare; g=stratum granulosum. In s and o, note the far field conducted from DG (asterisk). Reproduced from Paré et al. (1992) with permission.

Volume-conducted far fields reflecting the activation of CA1 and DG were evident when the electrode was positioned in the DG and CA1, respectively.

Self-sustained epileptic afterdischarges were induced by repeated EC pulse-trains (100 Hz) applied every 2 s. Spontaneous epileptiform activity was induced following afterdischarge activation. As shown in the CA1 recording displayed in Fig. 3, the temporal evolution of these epileptic discharges included an early phase (stage 1) characterized by quasi-rhythmic spikes separated by 300–700 msec (upper line in Fig. 3). This pattern of activity was observed at every level of the hippocampus except in the DG, where no sign of synchronized neuronal discharge could be found during stage 1. Approximatively 30–90 s after the beginning of stage 1, the transition to stage 2 occurred. At every level of the hippocampal-entorhinal cortex circuit this phase was characterized by 15–25 Hz rhythmic trains of population spikes lasting 0.3–4 s and separated by 1–2 s silent periods. Examination of stage 2 discharges with a higher time resolution revealed that all the population spikes observed in CA1 except the first one were preceded by a small potential, which probably reflected a volume-conducted far field due to the prior activation of DG or CA3. If this were the case, the hypothesis could be formulated that rhythmic discharges were possibly sustained by the reactivation of the hippocampal loop during stage 2.

To confirm this hypothesis, simultaneous recordings from DG, CA3, CA1 and EC were performed during the epileptic discharges (Fig. 4). These experiments demonstarted that each train of population spikes observed in the CA1 region reflects ongoing reverberant activity in the hippocampal-entorhinal loop. The earliest population spike usually occurred in the CA3 region (asterisk in Fig. 4B) and coincided with a positivity in the molecular layer of the DG. Thereafter population spikes occurred in the CA1 region, EC, DG, and in the CA3 region. The sequential nature of the activity

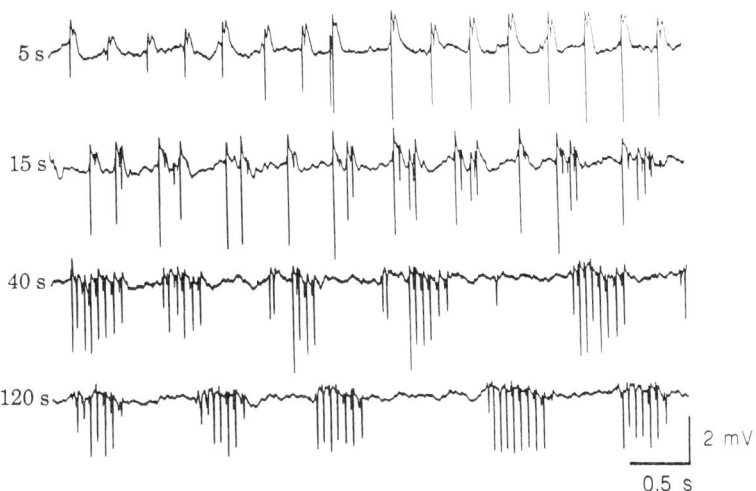

Fig. 3. Continuous recording of a typical epileptiform seizure recorded extracellularly in CA1 in the guinea-pig isolated brain. Stage 1 is illustrated in the upper line (early 5 s). The second line shows the transition to the stage 2 (40 s on). Reproduced from Paré et al. (1992) with permission.

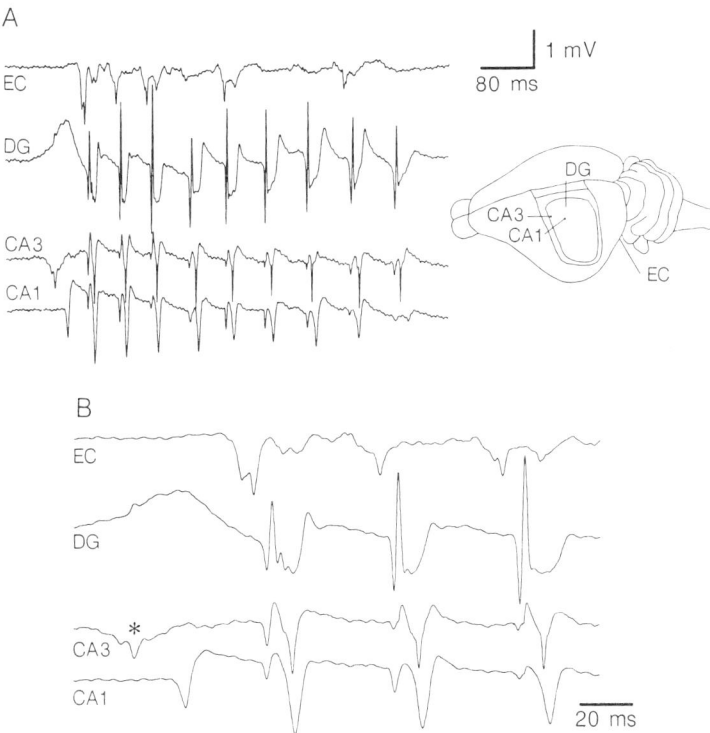

Fig. 4. Simultaneous extracellular recordings from the entorhinal cortex (EC), the dentate gyrus (DG), the areas CA3 and CA1 in the hippocampus during a stage 2 discharge. The position of the electrode in the hippocampus is illustrated in the inset. In B the early 300 ms of the event shown in A is illustrated with a different time scale. Note the sequential activation of the hippocampal subfields along the tri-synaptic pathway. The starting event (marked by an asterisk) occurs in the CA3 area. Reproduced from Paré et al. (1992) with permission.

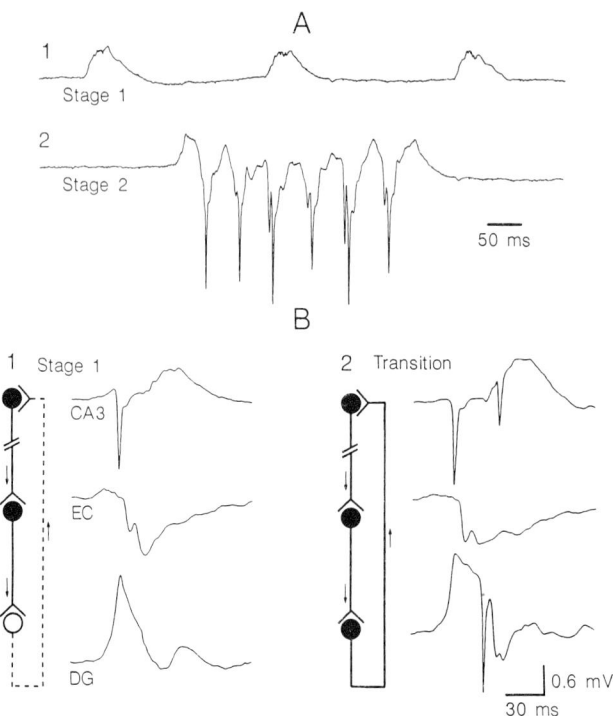

Fig. 5. A: DG extracellular recordings during stage 1 and stage 2.
B: Simultaneous recordings from CA3, EC and DG and schematic representation of the hippocampal loop activation in stage 1 (left panel) and at the beginning of stage 2 (right panel). The back projection from the EC to DG is not active in stage 1 (dotted line), while it is massively activated in stage 2. Reproduced from Paré et al. (1992) with permission.

recorded at the different levels of the hippocampal-entorhinal loop is illustrated in Fig. 4B, where the first three epileptiform cycles of a population spike train are illustrated with an extended time base. In addition, we observed that the population spikes occurring in the DG always coincided with the small potential preceding the CA1 and CA3 population spike. This highly synchronous DG potential did not occur at the onset of the stage 2 discharges, but only after a complete activation of the hippocampal-entorhinal loop.

To better understand the mechanisms involved in the transition from stage 1 to stage 2, the activity of the DG during the two stages was analysed (Fig. 5). During stage 1, only slow events were recorded in DG, probably reflecting a far field from the large population spikes occurring in CA3 or CA1 areas and/or population EPSPs subthreshold for population spike generation. During the transition from stage 1 to stage 2, this early slow activity was followed by a large population spike in DG. The necessary involvement of large synchronous events in the DG (population spikes) to initiate stage 2 discharges is better described in the experiment illustrated in Fig. 5B, where simultaneous recordings from CA3, DG and EC in both stage 1 and 2 are reported. It is clear from the left panel that the isolated events of stage 1 originate in CA3 and diffuse to the next synaptic station without occurrence of CA3 reactivation. The potential showed in the DG recording represents a far field volume-conducted from the CA3 active site (compare this DG response with that in the right panel). As shown in the right panel in Fig. 5B, the onset of the rhythmic discharge typical of stage 2 coincided with the occurrence of the first DG population spike. Only after DG synchronization the reactivation of the CA3 region occurred. The above picture was confirmed with

Chapter 8 EPILEPTOGENESIS IN THE HIPPOCAMPUS OF THE ISOLATED GUINEA PIG BRAIN

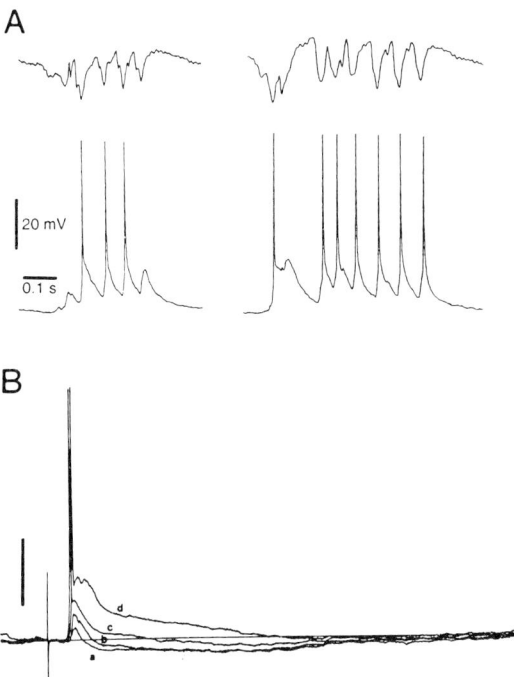

Fig. 6. A: Simultaneous extra (upper traces) and intracellular recordings (lower traces) obtained in neurons from the EC during stage 2.
B: Synaptic response evoked by EC stimulation in a CA3 cell in control conditions (a), in stage 1 (b) and during the transitory and conclamate stage 2 (c and d).

intracellular recordings from neurons from dentate granule cells, CA1 and CA3 pyramidal neurons and EC cells. At these four synaptic links neurons discharged action potentials in phase with the locally recorded population spikes. Samples of recordings are illustrated in Fig. 6 and in the original paper (Paré et al., 1992). This activity was superimposed on a gradual depolarizing shift, which could reach up to 10 mV and lasted for the duration of stage 2. In contrast, CA3 pyramidal neurons showed a bursting behaviour, which was more pronounced during stage 2 (not shown; Paré <et al., 1992). Figure 6B illustrates the synaptic response of a CA3 cell after stimulation of the EC at different times during the evolution of the seizure activity. A gradual decrease in amplitude of the inhibitory post-synaptic potential (IPSP) probably mediated by a local circuit interneuron occurred in parallel with the progressive evolution from stage 1 to stage 2.

Discussion

The present paper illustrates the characteristics of temporal evolution of epileptiform activity induced in the hippocampus of the isolated guinea pig brain by tetanic stimulation of the EC. We choose to utilize this preparation because it preserves the integrity of the synaptic connectivity and provides easy access with multiple electrodes to different areas of the limbic system, which are difficult to reach in the *in vivo* condition (de Curtis et al., 1991). These experiments constitute an attempt to identify the functional involvement of the hippocampus in the genesis of rhythmic epileptiform activity similar to that reported during the onset of seizures originating in the hippocampus of patients afflicted with temporal lobe epilepsy (Walsh & Delgado-Escueta, 1984). The epileptiform activity described in the present model of temporal lobe epilepsy was produced by high frequency stimulation of the entorhinal cortex. Laminar analysis, intracellular and extracellular simultaneous recordings performed in DG, CA3, CA1 and EC enabled us to locate the sites of generation of epileptiform activities in hippocampus and to establish the sequence of synaptic events responsible for their temporal organization. A tentative interpretation of the results will be discussed, based on the descriptive sequence of events reported. On the basis of electrophysiological criteria, we were able to divide the critical events in two stages. During stage 1 synchronous neuronal discharges (epileptiform population spikes) occurred first in the CA3 region and then spread to the EC after prior activation of the CA1 region. These data are in agreement with previous studies that demonstrated the preferential involvement of the CA3 area in the generation of hypersynchronous epileptiform activity in the hippocampus (Schwartzkroin & Prince, 1978; Wong & Traub, 1983; Traub & Miles, 1991). Although multiple events are possibly involved in the generation of such hypersynchronous events, a significant role is probably played by the decrease in the efficacy of inhibitory inputs, as is demonstrated by the progressive reduction of the IPSP's amplitude of CA3 pyramidal cells during the early stage of the epileptiform event (see Fig. 6B). We demonstrate that the CA3 region is the first structure to undergo synchronization, but it is not essential in promoting the re-entrant activation of the hippocampal-entorhinal loop. During stage 1 the structure preventing this reactivation is the DG. Indeed, no sign of synchronized activity (large population spikes) were observed in the DG during stage 1 following the activation of the EC. The transition to stage 2 coincided with the appearance of a prominent, sharp population spike in the DG. This potential probably reflects the synchronous activation of a large population of granule cells and occurs systematically after previous activation of population spikes in CA3, CA1 and the EC (see Figs. 4B & 5B). Thus, we propose that massive DG activation is the determinant event in the re-entrant activation of the hippocampal-entorhinal loop. The mechanisms that determine this transition are not completely understood. Interestingly, Stringer and collaborators (Stringer & Lothman, 1989, 1991; Stringer *et al.*, 1989) demonstrated that the DG has a critical influence in the developement of kindled seizures in hippocampus. These authors reported that a phenomenon called 'maximal DG activation' is essential for the generation of the afterdischarge implicated in the development of seizure in kindled animals. The authors conclude that the DG may restrict the spread of discharges into the hippocampus serving as a gateway to the flow of epileptiform activity to the CA3 region. In support of this hypothesis, recent studies (Sutula *et al.*, 1989; Cavazos *et al.*, 1991; Babb *et al.*, 1991) demonstrated a strong correlation between synaptic reorganization of the DG and the developement of epilepsy in the hippocampus. Even if no direct demonstration of causal relation between the proliferation of glutamatergic mossy fibres in the supragranular DG region and the development of epileptic activity was confirmed, these data suggest a functional role of the DG in the generation of hippocampal epileptic events.

We propose that epileptiform activity can be induced acutely in hippocampus through the re-entrant activation of the trisynaptic hippocampal loop. Preliminary results obtained by perfusing the isolated brain preparation with GABA receptor blockers and other convulsants (Biella & de Curtis, unpublished observations) suggest that the resonant activation of the hippocampal-entorhinal circuit may be a general modality of development and progression of epileptiform activity in the hippocampus, not related to the nature of the epileptogenic agent.

The specific cellular and circuit mechanisms relevant in the generation, spread and cease of epileptiform discharges in the hippocampal-entorhinal loop will be further investigated in this *in vitro* preparation.

References

Amaral, D.G. & Witter, M.P. (1989): The tridimensional organization of the hippocampal formation: a review of anatomical data. *Neuroscience.* **31**, 571–591.

Andersen, P. (1975): Organization of hippocampal neurons and their interconnection. In: *The hippocampus*, eds. R.L. Isaacson & K.H. Pribram, pp. 155–175. New York: Plenum Press.

Andersen, P., Holmqvist, B. & Voorhoeve, P.E. (1966a): Entorhinal activation of dentate gyrus cells. *Acta Physiol. Scand.* **66**, 448–460.

Andersen, P., Holmqvist, B. & Voorhoeve, P.E. (1966b): Excitatory synapses on hippocampal apical dendrites activated by entorhinal stimulation. *Acta Physiol. Scand.* **66**, 461–472.

Babb, T.L., Kupfer, W.R., Pretorius, J.K., Crandall, P.H. & Levesque, M.F. (1991): Synaptic reorganization by mossy fibers in human epileptic fascia dentata. *Neuroscience* **42**, 351–363.

Buzsaki, G., Hsu, M., Slamka, C., Gage, F.H. & Horvaz, Z. (1991): Emergence and propagation of interictal spikes in the subcortical denervated hippocampus. *Hippocampus* **1**, 163–180.

Cavazos, J., Goralai, G. & Sutula, T.P. (1991): Mossy fiber synaptic reorganization induced by kindling: time course of development, progression and permanence. *J. Neurosci.* **11**, 2795–2803.

de Curtis, M., Paré, D. & Llinas, R.R. (1991): The electrophysiology of the olfactory-hippocampal circuit in the isolated and perfused adult mammalian brain *in vitro*. *Hippocampus* **1**, 341–354.

Horikawa, K. & Armstrong, W.E. (1988): A versatile means of intracellular labeling: injection of biocytin and its detection with avidin conjugates. *Neuroscience* **25**, 1–11.

Liberson, W.T., Scoville, W.B. & Dunsmore, R.H. (1951): Stimulation studies of the prefrontal lobe and uncus in man. *EEG Clin. Neurophysiol.* **7**, 211–222.

McVicar, B.A. & Dudek, F.E. (1981): Electrotonic coupling between pyramidal cells: a direct demonstration in rat hippocampal slices. *Science* **213**, 782–785.

Paré, D., de Curtis, M. & Llinas, R.R. (1992): Role of the hippocampal-entorhinal loop in temporal lobe epilepsy: extra and intracellular study in the isolated guinea pig brain *in vitro*. *J. Neurosci.* (in press)

Schwartzkroin, P.A. & Prince, D.A. (1978): Cellular and field potential properties of epileptogenic hippocampal slices. *Brain Res.* **147**, 117–130.

Stringer, J.L. & Lothman, E.W. (1989): Maximal DG activation: characteristics and alterations after repeated seizures. *J. Neurophysiol.* **62**, 136–143.

Stringer, J.L., Williamson, J.M. & Lothman, E.W. (1989): Induction of paroxysmal discharges in the DG: frequency dependence and relationship to afterdischarge production. *J. Neurophysiol.* **62**, 126–135.

Stringer, J.L. & Lothman, E.W. (1991): Maximal dentate activation is critical for the appearance of an afterdischarge in the dentate gyrus. *Neuroscience* **46**, 309–314.

Sutula, T., Cascino, G., Cavazos, J., Parada, I. & Ramirez, L. (1989): Mossy fiber synaptic reorganization in the epileptic human temporal lobe. *Ann. Neurol.* **26**, 321–333.

Traub, R.D. & Miles, R. (1991): *Neuronal networks of the hippocampus*. Cambridge: Cambridge University Press.

Walsh, G.O. & Delgado-Escueta, A.V. (1984): Type II complex partial seizures: poor results of anterior temporal lobectomy. *Neurology* **34**, 1–13.

Wong, R.K.S. & Traub, R.D. (1983): Synchronized burst discharges in the dishinibited hippocampal slices. I. Initiation in the CA2–CA3 region. *J. Neurophysiol.* **49**, 459–471.

Chapter 9

Ontogenetic models of epilepsy

Maria Rita de Feo and Oriano Mecarelli

I Neurofisiopatologia, Dipartimento di Scienze Neurologiche, Università 'La Sapienza', Rome, Italy

Summary

Many electroclinical studies have pointed out that in humans, during the neonatal period and early infancy, epileptic manifestations are particularly frequent and show peculiar characteristics different from those of adults. This has been related to the anatomical and functional immaturity of the brain during the early stages of development. The experimental ontogenetic studies of epilepsy may help in the understanding of the pathogenetic mechanisms at the basis of the epileptic disorders occurring in the first periods after birth; indirectly, they may also shed light on the mechanisms of epilepsy of the adult brain.

This report discusses the experimental data derived from studies on the more common ontogenetic models of epilepsy. Only *in vivo* animal models which allow correlations between electrophysiological and behavioural epileptic manifestations have been considered. Seizures caused by the systemic or topical administration of convulsant drugs (chemically induced), seizures induced by electroshock and kindling (electrically induced) and seizures appearing in animals genetically susceptible (genetic models) are described. The electrophysiological and behavioural characteristics of the epileptic manifestations, typical for the age of the animals, and their correlations with anatomical, biochemical and functional levels of cerebral maturation, have been reported.

Introduction

Studies on the development of epilepsy in immature animals are relatively few in spite of the fact that the majority of human seizure disorders have their onset from infancy through adolescence, and that in children epilepsy presents peculiar features which are related to the immaturity of neuronal excitability, cortical connectivity and electrical impulse propagation. Thus, animal models in which seizures may be experimentally induced at various levels of cerebral maturation may supply important information about the biochemical and functional mechanisms underlying the epileptic manifestations. The low number of systematic studies investigating the development of epilepsy in immature animals may be partially due to the difficulty of the technical procedures necessary for the study. For example, the application of adult stereotaxic procedures for the implantation of acute and chronic cortical and subcortical electrodes in developing animals is difficult, sometimes impossible, because of the anatomical characteristics of the heads of the pups. In very young animals particularly, the cartilaginous skull is pliable and the auditory meat not accessible for insertion of ear bars. In addition, the pup's snout is too short to aid in positioning the head with a tooth bar or nose clamp. Thus, modified stereotaxic apparatus and specific detailed atlases supplying the coordinates for electrode implantation are necessary for electrophysiological studies (Gilbert & Cain, 1980; Cherubini *et al.*, 1982; Hoorneman, 1985; Paxinos *et al.*, 1991).

Chemically induced seizures

Systemic administration of convulsant drugs

Ontogenetic studies of epileptic patterns induced by the systemic administration of convulsant substances are relatively few and the majority of them have been carried out during the last two decades. In relation to the convulsant, generalized or partial electroclinical seizures are obtained, with different features depending on the age of the animals.

Generalized epilepsy

Only the widely studied models of epilepsy induced by pentylenetetrazol (PTZ), bicuculline and allylglycine will be here described. The activating mechanism of pentylenetetrazol is still unexplained; however, both a selective antagonist action on GABA-mediated postsynaptic inhibition and a direct excitatory effect on neuronal membrane has been suggested (Woodbury, 1980).

In developing rats it is interesting to note that: (a) during the first week of life PTZ induces a continuous behavioural pattern of hyperactivity with uncoordinated movements of the limbs, diffuse tremors, pedalling movements, loss of postural control, without any corresponding epileptic EEG changes; (b) the first clear-cut generalized epileptic response is characterized the tonic seizures with hyperextension of the limbs and flexion of the axial muscles, accompanied on the EEG by flattening of the tracing; (c) at the end of the 2nd and during the 3rd week, myoclonic jerks represent the most prominent epileptic features, usually characterized, on the EEG, by bursts of polyspikes; (d) the electrical and behavioural correlations are complete as from the 4th week onwards, with the appearance of well-organized tonic-clonic seizures. During this period, subconvulsive doses of PTZ induce sequences of spike-wave complexes, associated with a behavioural pattern of immobility and non-reactivity of the animal, similar to PM (petit mal) absences (Vernadakis & Woodbury, 1969; Ricci et al., 1984; Schicherova et al., 1984; Pohl & Mares, 1987).

Bicuculline and allylglycine are two convulsant substances which act by involving the GABAergic system at various levels (Woodbury, 1980). Their injection in rats younger than 8 days induces very atypical behavioural modifications, correlated or not to epileptic EEG changes (de Feo et al., 1985; Baram & Carter Snead, 1990). Successively, a gradual evolution of the electroclinical pattern is observed, with similar characteristics in both bicuculline- and allylglycine-treated animals. As observed in PTZ model, the only well-defined epileptic manifestation peculiar to the first 2 weeks of life is the tonic fits, accompanied by desynchronization of the tracing and marked reduction or total disappearance of the pre-existing epileptic elements. It is only from the 3rd week that electroclinical patterns similar to those of adult animals and more specific for the type of the convulsant agent appear. It is possible to hypothesize that during the first 2 weeks the degree of global immaturity of the brain structures underlies the atypical epileptic manifestations. Successively, the more advanced stage of maturation allows a better organization of the electroclinical patterns and a more selective involvement of different cerebral structures (de Feo et al., 1985).

Partial epilepsy

In the last decade the epileptogenic action of some neurotoxins has been studied in adult as well as in immature animals. Particularly, kainic acid (KA), a rigid analogue of glutamate, when systemically or intracerebrally injected in adult animals preferentially activates limbic structures inducing partial seizures resembling human temporal lobe epilepsy.

The systemic injection of KA in immature rats has been demonstrated to induce different electrographic and behavioural patterns specific for the age of the animals (Cherubini et al., 1983; Albala et al., 1984; Ben Ari et al., 1984; Tremblay et al., 1984; Holmes et al., 1988; Ricci et al., 1990).

In the first week of life, scratching movements, hypo- and hyperactivity, loss of postural control, tremors and hyperextension of the limbs are observed. Similar but more accentuated motor signs are observed when KA is administered during the 2nd week of life. On the EEG, spikes or polyspikes firstly localized in the cortex and then spreading to the hippocampus are recorded, poorly correlated with the behavioural manifestations. By the 3rd week, wet dog shakes (WDS) and typical limbic seizures begin to appear, usually leading to a status epilepticus. On the EEG, hippocampal epileptic discharges arise from the hippocampus, with possible spreading to the cortex.

The appearance of typical limbic seizures only from the 3rd week on may be related to the immaturity of the hippocampus in which both post- and presynaptic receptors are not completely developed and/or functionally mature at birth (Baudry et al., 1981). In addition, the functional immaturity of some excitatory afferent systems in the hippocampus of young animals may account for the lack of activation of presynaptic receptors by KA (Bayer & Altman, 1974; Schlesinger et al., 1975). In the first 2 weeks of life, the neocortex is the structure primarily involved in epileptic activity, suggesting that a different level of maturation between glutamergic cortical and hippocampal receptors exists at this age.

The ontogenetic KA model of epilepsy is particularly interesting because it is useful in studying possible behavioural and cognitive disturbances which may follow the occurrence of seizures at different ages. It has been reported that status epilepticus induced by KA in rats at various ages results in deficits of conditioned and spontaneous behavior of the animals later in life (de Feo et al., 1986; Holmes et al., 1988).

Pilocarpine has been recently described to induce another ontogenetic model of partial seizures (Cavalheiro et al., 1987). Pilocarpine, a cholinergic muscarinic agonist, induces in adult animals a pattern of limbic epilepsy evolving into status epilepticus. In addition, spontaneous motor seizures continue to be observed several weeks after treatment (Turski et al., 1983). In 3–9 day old rats, hyper- and hypoactivity, tremor, loss of postural control, scratching, head bobbing and myoclonic movements of the limbs follow systemic injection of the drug. No overt limbic motor seizures are observed in this age group, in which electrographic activity consists in low voltage spiking registered concurrently in the hippocampus and the cortex.

More remarkable behavioural modifications, sometimes evolving into limbic seizures and status epilepticus occur in 12-day-old animals, in which also epileptic activity localized in the hippocampus with secondary diffusion to the cortical regions progressively appears. The adult pattern of behavioural and electrographic manifestations by pilocarpine is reached in 15–21-day-old rats. Thus, both in KA and pilocarpine epilepsy models, the 3rd week is a critical period of development during which seizure susceptibility is enhanced. The different sensitivity of immature rats to the convulsant action of pilocarpine has been related to the immaturity of the cholinergic neuronal networks in the brain, engaged in the generation and spread of seizure activity.

Topical application of convulsant drugs

Strychnine, penicillin and KA are the most usual topically applied substances for experiments in ontogenetic studies of epilepsy.

The ontogenesis of cortical strychnine spikes was first described by Bishop (1950) in immature rabbits. In these animals, during the first postnatal days (PND), the spikes show triphasic morphology, extremely long duration and low frequency of occurrence. During successive days, the spike duration decreases and the frequency gradually increases following a S curve.

In developing rats, the first epileptic spikes induced by the cortical application of strychnine appear only at PND 4 (Ricci et al., 1983). Initially the spikes are rare, biphasic and of long duration (> 500 ms). In successive days the frequency increases with a critical period at PND 11. At the end of the 2nd week a plateau of about 35 spikes/min is reached. Meanwhile, the duration of the spikes diminishes, so that around the 3rd week of life the adult morphology is achieved.

By topical application of penicillin in immature rabbits, Wright & Bradley (1968) demonstrated that since PND 1 the cerebral cortex possesses a definite but limited capacity to produce epileptiform activity. The maturation of the epileptic activity shows a time course consistent with increased neuronal hypersynchrony, reaching adult characteristics by the 3rd postnatal week. Moreover, the authors supplied evidence that the penicillin focus projects to the contralateral hemisphere in a limited and inconstant manner during the postnatal week. The ability to generate sustained electrographic seizure discharges develop only by the 2nd week of life.

The anatomical, behavioural and electrographic correlations were investigated by Caveness (1969) in newborn monkeys in which the cortical application of penicillin induces delayed clinical manifestations with involvement primarily of the distal large joints, late and sustained head turning, and extension of the lower extremities. In these animals, the first spikes, usually of long duration, low amplitude and frequency, spreading to other regions in a delayed time, precede remarkably (by about 45 min) the appearance of the clinical manifestations. In pubescent monkeys, the clinical patterns are characterized by early rotatory movements of the head and early fine movements of the digits. Successively, flexo-extension movements appear contralaterally to the injection side, with a rapidly seizure generalized. The spikes, first appearing in the injected hemisphere and successively (about 20 min later) spreading to the opposite side, precede by about 18 min the first behavioural epileptic manifestations. In the adult monkeys the focal seizures show a very rapid generalization and the delay between the occurrence of the seizures and the first spikes is notably shorter (about 3 min).

The characteristics of morphology and diffusion of the spikes induced by the cortically applied penicillin have been described also in developing rats (Mares, 1973; Kudo & Yamauchi, 1988a). In rats 3–4 days old, the first slow waves or spike-wave complexes, appearing with a long latency, are isolated, very infrequent and diffuse to all the cortical areas with a reduced amplitude. In 14-day-old animals, isolated but repetitive epileptic elements appear with a shorter latency; their amplitude and frequency progressively increase until a Sustained High-frequency Discharge (SHD) is generated. At this time the spikes appear firstly in the sensorimotor cortex and then spread to the caudate putamen and the mesencephalic reticular formation, while the SHDs immediately spread to the subcortical structures. In young adult rats, the first isolated spikes are firstly localized in the sensorimotor cortex; successively they spread to the contralateral sensorimotor cortex, the caudate putamen, the homolateral thalamus and, finally, to all the other brain structures. The SHDs occur with a short latency at the injection site and then spread to the subcortical homo- and contralateral structures. It has to be noted that, in this model of epilepsy, the SHDs are absent in neonatal rats, their latency of appearance being longer and their frequency lower in younger than in adult rats (14 and 30 days, respectively). This suggests that the occurrence of SHDs, more than that of isolated spikes, is possible only when a sufficient anatomo-functional cortical development is achieved.

Locally injections of penicillin into the amygdala of neonatal rats induce SHD localized to the homolateral subcortical structures. On the contrary, in rats 10–15 days old, the SHDs rapidly spread from the injection site to the reticular bilateral formation and the medial thalamic nucleus, demonstrating that these structures play an important role in the diffusion of the epileptic discharge (Kudo & Yamauchi, 1988b)

Both cortical and hippocampal injection of KA has demonstrated to induce in rats younger than 7 days, epileptic elements simultaneously occurring in the two structures. An epileptic response, initially localized in the injection area, begins to appear at PND 7–9, but an adult electrographic pattern is observed only from the 3rd week on (Cavalheiro et al., 1983). Similar results have been obtained by Wolf & Keilhoff (1984) who demonstrated that the hippocampal neurons are sensitive to the excitotoxic action of ventricularly injected KA, only from the end of the 2nd week of life.

Electrically induced seizures

Electroshock (EKS)

The electrical stimulation of the brain may induce minimal EKS seizures (threshold seizures) or maximal EKS responses (tonic-clonic responses), depending on the intensity of the electrical applied stimulus. In maturing rats and mice, the threshold seizures (facial clonus and rhythmic movements of the vibrissae, jaw and ears) occur only after PND 8; in the successive days the threshold progressively and markedly decreases until PND 16–18, and then slowly increases somewhat thereafter (Vernadakis & Woodbury, 1969).

The maximal EKS pattern gradually evolves from PND 1 (when only hyperkinesia is observed) to PND 16 when a full tonic-clonic seizure pattern is developed.

Cortical self-sustained afterdischarges (SSADs)

The direct repetitive stimulations of cortical sensorimotor area regularly evoke SSADs.

The ontogenetic development of SSADs was studied in rats by Mares & Mares (1980) who found well organized spike-wave complexes starting from PND 15, the frequency of the complexes increasing from 2–2.5 Hz in 15–18 day old rats to 3–4 Hz in older animals.

Kindling

Kindling is a permanent increase in epileptogenicity produced by repetitive electrical or chemical stimulation of various brain structures (Racine & McIntyre, 1986). In adult rats the electrical stimulation of the limbic structures (hippocampus, amygdala) evokes focal seizure discharges typically developing through five stages (Racine, 1972).

Ontogenetic studies have demonstrated that in immature animals it is possible to obtain both amygdala and hippocampal kindling with some differences compared to adults (Moshé et al., 1983). In amygdala kindling not only the behavioural expressions of the motor convulsions in animals aged 15 days differ from those in older animals, but also the afterdischarge (AD) threshold, defined as the lowest current intensity required to trigger an AD, varies with age and is highest in the youngest animals (Moshé, 1981; Moshé et al., 1981). Moreover, while stimulations delivered at short inter-stimulation interval (ISI = 15–30 min) either markedly retard or fail to induce kindling in adult rats (Racine et al., 1973), in rat pups kindling may be obtained with shorter ISI, probably as an expression of a shorter refractory period (Moshé et al., 1983). These physiological characteristics may be related to the differential anatomical and functional development of the immature limbic structures (Jacobson, 1978; Schwartzkroin, 1982).

In developing animals hippocampus is more seizure-prone than maturated tissue. Suckling rats show a faster development of kindling, a longer duration of initial AD and prolonged wet dog shakes (WDS) without any decrease in their occurrence and duration in relation to the increase in the number of stimulation. The greatest magnitude of long-term potentiation (LTP), which is involved in the neurophysiological changing process occurring during kindling (Majrowski, 1986) is observed in 15-day-old rats and LTP magnitude is considerably larger than that produced in adults (Harris & Teyler, 1984). This increased susceptibility probably results from alterations in the balance between excitatory and inhibitory synaptic interactions during development (Michelson & Lothman, 1989). It has to be noted that the range of ages that has been studied is limited, and little is known regarding kindling in animals younger than 2 weeks of age. Gilbert & Cain (1982) found that rats younger than PND 14 cannot support the kindling phenomenon: one particular difficulty in extending 'traditional' kindling paradigms to the immature rats is that the duration of the experimental protocol (e.g. 10–14 days with amygdala kindling) becomes impractical at a time when development is occurring at such a rapid rate (Michelson & Lothman, 1991). While earlier studies of the kindling phenomenon suggest that rats younger than 2 weeks of age are resistant to kindling (Gilbert & Cain, 1982), it has been recently demonstrated that it is possible to kindle rats as young as 7 days, using the technique of rapidly recurring hippocampal seizures (RRHS)(Michelson & Lothman, 1991). This technique consists of the administration of 10 s, 20 Hz stimulus trains, every 5 min for 6 h on one day (short-interval RRHS) or every 30 min for 9 h on each of two consecutive days (long-interval RRHS). Results have shown that, even if rapid kindling occurs in 7-day-old rats, animals at this age are less capable of retaining kindling effect than are older rats.

Genetic models of epilepsy

Genetic animal models of epilepsy may provide information about the fundamental mechanisms involved in the onset and development of the epilepsies that is inaccessible with most other techniques of seizure induction.

Genetic models can be subdivided into animals with spontaneously occurring recurrent seizures, and models in which seizures are induced by specific sensory stimulation in genetically susceptible animals. However, the majority of the ontogenetic studies have been carried out in genetically epilepsy-prone rats (GEPRs), in which a genetic susceptibility to sound-induced seizures has been demonstrated (Hjeresen et al., 1987; Ribak et al., 1988; Reigel et al., 1989; Thompson et al., 1991). In both GEPR 3 (a moderate seizure colony) and GEPR 9 (a severe seizure colony), epileptic manifestations appear between PND 17 and 21. Initially only running episodes are observed followed in the successive days (PNDs 19–21) by tonic-clonic seizures, the incidence and severity of them being a function of age. By 30 days of age the epileptic manifestations approach the adult seizure pattern which is completely established only at PND 45. Similar development of susceptibility to sound-induced seizures is shown by DBA/2 mice in which susceptibility appears at PND 20 then increases rapidly reaching a peak incidence of 90 per cent between PND 30 and 34; successively it declines and finally disappears entirely from PND 80. Thus, once seizure susceptibility occurs, the GEPRs remain susceptible for life, whereas the DBA/2 mice lose seizure susceptibility with increasing age (Vicari, 1951).

The development of hearing is a critical factor in the ontogeny of sound-induced seizures in the GEPRs. In fact, the age range in which GEPRs progress from complete non-susceptibility (PND 14–15) to complete susceptibility (PND 21) to sound-induced seizures appears to parallel the maturation of hearing in rats. However, susceptibility and severity of sound-induced seizures in the adult GEPRs have been also related to widespread central defects in central neurotransmitter systems, primarily norepinephrine and serotonin (Jobe et al., 1986).

Audiogenic seizure (AGS) susceptibility can be induced during a critical developmental period in normal mice and Wistar rats by auditory deprivation as well as cochlear trauma or intoxication (Chen, 1980; Van Middlesworth & Norris, 1980; Pierson & Swann, 1988). Very recently, AGS susceptibility has been induced in Wistar rats by a single prolonged exposure, between PND 12 and 36, to high-intensity noise (Pierson & Swann, 1991). PND 14 is the age when exposure is most likely to result in eventual seizure susceptibility, measured 2 weeks later (PND 28). In this regard, PND 28 ontogenetically appears to be the age of greatest inherent susceptibility. This then decreases between PND 28 and 36, but remains stable thereafter into adulthood.

Typically, the seizures begin as wild running attacks and are followed by tonic-clonic convulsions. The greater effectiveness of the noise in inducing cochlear damage at PND 14 is probably related to the maturational time-course of the auditory function in the rat. Cochlear function in rats has its origin on PND 10 (Crowley & Hepp-Reymond, 1966), while PND 11 and 12 represents probably the onset of the auditory function at the level of the inferior colliculus, the most probable site of initiation of AGS in susceptible rodents. At PND 13 the ear canal of the rat becomes patent, although not fully so. Thereafter, the peripheral and central auditory pathways continue to mature in rats until PND 24. The coincidence of the time of opening of the ear canal (about PND 13) and the remarkable effectiveness of noise exposure when applied after PND 13, strongly suggests that onset of noise inducibility requires the opening of the rat ear canal (Pierson & Swann, 1991).

Sound-triggered seizures are probably initiated within the inferior colliculus (Ludwig & Moshé, 1987; Pierson et al., 1989). However, the behavioural manifestations of the seizures (wild running and tonic or clonic convulsions) are believed to reflect seizure generalization through the mid- and hindbrain reticular formation and possibly through cortical pathways (Browning, 1986). The presence of at least two critically sensitive periods in the genesis of AGS susceptibility, one that is specific for induction of susceptibility (PND 14) and one specific for its expression (PND 28), suppports the idea that both experiential and maturational factors are important in inducing this kind of seizures in rats.

From a clinical point of view, even if there is no direct evidence that auditory deprivation during the development of auditory pathways in humans has any consequence of epileptic type, it may be noted that an incidence of 74 per cent of abnormal EEG has been found in congenitally deaf children (Fishman et al., 1983).

References

Albala, B.J., Moshé, S.L. & Okada, R. (1984): Kainic-acid-induced seizures: a developmental study. *Brain Res.* **3**: 139–148.

Baram, T.Z. & Carter Snead, III O. (1990): Bicuculline induced seizures in infant rats: ontogeny of behavioural and electrocortical phenomena. *Dev. Brain Res.* **57**, 291–295.

Baudry, M., Arst, D., Oliver, M. & Linch, G. (1981): Development of glutamate binding sites and their regulation by calcium in rat hippocampus. *Dev. Brain Res.* **1**, 37–48.

Bayer, S.A. & Altman, J. (1974): Hippocampal development in the rat: cytogenesis and morphogenesis examined with autoradiography and low level of X-irradiation. *J. Comp. Neurol.* **158**, 55–80.

Ben Ari, Y., Tremblay, E., Berger, M. & Nitecka, L. (1984): Kainic seizure syndrome and binding sites in developing rats. *Dev. Brain Res.* **14**, 284–288.

Bishop, E.J. (1950): The strychnine spike as a physiological indicator of cortical maturity in the postnatal rabbit. *Electroencephalogr. Clin. Neurophysiol.* **2**, 309–315.

Browning, R.A. (1986): Neuroanatomical localization of structures responsible for seizures in the GEPR: lesion studies. *Life Sci.* **39**, 857–867.

Cavalheiro, E.A., de Feo, M.R., Mecarelli, O. & Ricci, G.F. (1983): Intracortical and intrahippocampal injections of kainic acid in developing rats: an electrographic study. *Electroencephalogr. Clin. Neurophysiol.* **56**, 480–486.

Cavalheiro, E.A., Silva, D.F., Turski, W.A., Calderazzo-Filho, L.S., Bortolotto, Z.A. & Turski, L. (1987): The susceptibility of rats to pilocarpine-induced seizures is age-dependent. *Dev. Brain Res.* **37**, 43–58.

Caveness, W.F. (1969): Ontogeny of focal seizures. In: *Basic mechanisms of the epilepsies*, eds. H.H. Jasper, A.A. Ward & A. Pope, pp. 517–534. Boston: Little, Brown and Co.

Chen, C.S. (1980): Rapid development of acoustic trauma-induced audiogenic seizure risk in 3 strains of seizure-resistant mice. *Experientia* **36**, 1194–1196.

Cherubini, E., de Feo, M.R., Mecarelli, O. & Ricci, G.F. (1982): A simple method for implanting electrodes in freely moving neonatal rats. *J. Neurosci. Meth.* **6**, 175–177.

Cherubini, E., de Feo, M.R., Mecarelli, O. & Ricci, G.F. (1983): Behavioural and electrographic patterns induced by systemic administration of kainic acid in developing rats. *Dev. Brain Res.* **9**, 69–77.

Crowley, D.E. & Hepp-Reymond, M. (1966): Development of cochlear function in the ear of the infant rat. *J. Comp. Physiol. Psychol.* **62**, 427–431.

de Feo, M.R., Mecarelli, O. & Ricci, G.F. (1985): Bicuculline and allylglycine-induced epilepsy in developing rats. *Exp. Neurol.* **90**, 411–421.

de Feo, M.R., Mecarelli, O., Palladini, G. & Ricci, G.F. (1986): Long-term effects of early status epilepticus on the acquisition of conditioned avoidance behavior in rats. *Epilepsia* **27**, 476–482.

Fishman, J.E., Gadoth, N. & Radvan, H. (1983): Congenital sensorineural deafness associated with EEG abnormalities, epilepsy and familial incidence. *Dev. Med. Child Neurol.* **25**, 747–754.

Gilbert, M.E. & Cain, D.P. (1980): Electrode implantation in infant rats for kindling and chronic brain recording. *Behav. Brain Res.* **1**, 553–555.

Gilbert, M.E. & Cain, D.P. (1982): A developmental study of kindling in the rat. *Dev. Brain Res.* **2**, 321–328.

Harris, K.M. & Teyler, T.J. (1984): Developmental onset of long-term potentiation in area CA1 of the rat hippocampus. *J. Physiol.* **346**, 27–41.

Hjeresen, D.L., Franck, J.E. & Amend, D.L. (1987): Ontogeny of seizure incidence, latency and severity in genetically epilepsy-prone rats. *Dev. Psychobiol.* **20**, 355–363.

Holmes, G.L., Thompson, J.L., Marchi, T. & Feldman, T.S. (1988): Behavioural effects of kainic acid administration on the immature brain. *Epilepsia* **29**, 721–730.

Hoorneman, E.M.D. (1985): Stereotaxic operation in the neonatal rat; a novel and simple procedure. *J. Neurosci. Meth.* **14**, 109–116.

Jacobson, M. (1978): In: *Developmental neurobiology*, pp. 188–199. New York: Plenum Press.

Jobe, P.C., Dailey, J.W. & Reigel, C.E. (1986): Noradrenergic and serotonergic determinants of seizure susceptibility and severity in genetically epilepsy-prone rats. *Life Sci.* **39**, 775–782.

Kudo, T. & Yamauchi, T. (1988a): An ontogenetic study of focal seizures induced by penicillin injections into sensorimotor area in rats. *Exp. Neurol.* **102**, 254–260.

Kudo, T. & Yamauchi, T. (1988b): An ontogenetic study of amygdala seizures induced by penicillin in rats. *Exp. Neurol.* **99**, 531–543.

Ludwig, N. & Moshé, S.L. (1987): Cyclic AMP derivatives injected into the inferior colliculus induce audiogenic seizure-like phenomena in normal rats. *Brain Res.* **437**, 193–196.

Majrowski, J. (1986): Kindling: a model for epilepsy and memory. *Acta Neurol. Scand.* **74**, 97–108.

Mares, P. (1973): Ontogenetic development of bioelectrical activity of the epileptogenic focus in rat neocortex. *Neuropediatrics* **4**, 434–445.

Mares, J. & Mares, P. (1980): The ontogenesis of cortical self-sustained after-discharges in rats. *Epilepsia* **21**, 111–121.

Michelson, H.B. & Lothman, E.W. (1989): An *in vivo* electrophysiological study of the ontogeny of excitatory and inhibitory processes in the rat hippocampus. *Dev. Brain Res.* **47**, 113–122.

Michelson, H.B. & Lothman, E.W. (1991): An ontogenetic study of kindling using rapidly recurring hippocampal seizures. *Dev. Brain Res.* **61**, 79–85.

Moshé, S.L. (1981): The effects of age on the kindling phenomenon. *Develop. Psychobiol.* **14**, 75–81.

Moshé, S.L., Sharpless, N.S. & Kaplan, J. (1981): Kindling in developing rats: variability of afterdischarge threshold with age. *Brain Res.* **211**, 190–195.

Moshé, S.L., Albala, B.J., Ackermann, R.F. & Engel, J.Jr. (1983): Increased seizure susceptibility of the immature brain. *Dev. Brain Res.* **7**, 81–85.

Paxinos, G., Tork, J., Tecott, L.H. & Valentino, K.L. (1991): *Atlas of the developing rat brain*. London: Academic Press.

Pierson, M.G. & Swann, J.W. (1988): The sensitive period and optimum dosage for induction of audiogenic seizure susceptibility by kanamicin in the Wistar rat. *Hearing Res.* **32**, 1–10.

Pierson, M.G., Smith, K. & Swann, J.W. (1989): Slow NMDA-mediated potential underlies seizures originating from midbrain. *Brain Res.* **486**, 381–386.

Pierson, M.G. & Swann, J.W. (1991): Ontogenetic features of audiogenic seizure susceptibility induced in immature rats by noise. *Epilepsia* **31**, 1–9.

Pohl, M. & Mares, P. (1987): Flunarizing influences metrazol-induced seizures in developing rats. *Epilepsy Res.* **1**, 302–305.

Racine, R.J. (1972): Modification of seizure activity by electrical stimulation. I. Motor seizures. *Electroencephalogr. Clin. Neurophysiol.* **32**, 281–294.

Racine, R.J., McIntyre-Burnham, W., Gartner, J.C. & Levitan, D. (1973): Rates of motor seizure development in rats subjected to electrical brain stimulation: strain and interstimulation interval effects: *Electroencephalogr. Clin. Neurophysiol.* **35**, 553–556.

Racine, R.J. & McIntyre, D. (1986): Mechanisms of kindling: a current view. In: *The limbic system: functional organization and clinical disorders*, eds. B.K. Doane & K.E. Livingston, pp. 109–121. New York: Raven Press.

Reigel, C.E., Jobe, P.C., Dailey, J.W. & Savage, D.D. (1989): Ontogeny of sound-induced seizures in the genetically epilepsy-prone rat. *Epilepsy Res.* **4**, 63–71.

Ribak, C.E., Roberts, R.C., Buyn, M.Y. & Kim, H.L. (1988): Anatomical and behavioural analyses of the inheritance of audiogenic seizures in the progeny of genetically epilepsy-prone and Sprague–Dawley rats. *Epilepsy Res.* **2**, 345–355.

Ricci, G.F., Mecarelli, O. & de Feo, M.R. (1990): Ontogenesis of gabaergic and glutamergic receptors in the developing brain, In *Neonatal seizures*, eds. C.G. Wasterlain & P. Vert, pp. 211–221. New York: Raven Press.

Ricci, G.F., Cherubini, E., de Feo, M.R. & Mecarelli, O. (1983): Development of epileptic activity and its correlation with GABAergic and glutamergic system during brain maturation in the rat. In: *Epilepsy: An update on research and therapy*, eds. G. Nisticó, R. Di Perri & H. Meinardi, pp. 77–86. New York: Alan R. Liss.

Ricci, G.F., de Feo, M.R. & Mecarelli, O. (1984): Status epilepticus and brain maturation. *Rev. EEG Neurophysiol.* **14**, 187–195.

Schicherova, R., Mares, P. & Trojan, S. (1984): Correlation between electrocorticographic and motor phenomena induced by pentamethylenetetrazol during ontogenesis in rats. *Exp. Neurol.* **84**, 153–164.

Schlesinger, A.R., Cowan, W.M. & Gottlieb, D.I. (1975): An autoradiographic study of the time of origin and the pattern of granule cell migration in the dentate gyrus of the rat. *J. Comp. Neurol.* **159**, 149–76.

Schwartzkroin, P.A. (1982): Development of rabbit hippocampus: physiology. *Dev. Brain Res.* **2**, 469–486.

Thompson, J.L., Carl, F.G. & Holmes, G.L. (1991): Effects of age on seizure susceptibility in genetically epilepsy-prone rats (GEPR-9s). *Epilepsia* **32**, 161–167.

Tremblay, E., Nitecka, L., Berger, M.L. & Ben Ari, Y. (1984): Maturation of kainic acid seizure-brain damage syndrome in the rat. I. Clinical, electrographic and metabolic observations. *Neuroscience* **13**, 1051–1072.

Turski, W.A., Cavalheiro, E.A., Schwarz, M., Czuczwar, S.J., Kleinrok, Z. & Turski, L. (1983): Limbic seizures produced by pilocarpine in rats: a behavioural electroencephalographic and neuropathological study. *Behav. Brain Res.* **9**, 315–336.

Van Middlesworth, L. & Norris., C.H. (1980): Audiogenic seizures and cochlear damage in rats after perinatal antithyroid treatment. *Endocrinology* **106**, 1686–1690.

Vernadakis, A. & Woodbury, D.M. (1969): The developing animal as a model. *Epilepsia* **10**, 163–178.

Vicari, E.M. (1951): Fatal convulsive seizures in the DBA mouse strain. *J. Psychol. (Lipz)* **32**, 79–97.

Wolf, G. & Keilhoff, G. (1984): Kainate and glutamate neurotoxicity in dependence of the postnatal development with special reference to hippocampal neurons. *Dev. Brain Res.* **14**, 15–21.

Woodbury, D.M. (1980): Convulsant drugs: mechanisms of action. In: *Antiepileptic drugs: mechanisms of action*, eds. G.H. Glaser, J.K. Penry & D.M. Woodbury, pp. 249–303. New York: Raven Press.

Wright, F.S. & Bradley, W.E. (1968): Maturation of epileptiform activity. *Electroencephalogr. Clin. Neurophysiol.* **25**, 259–265.

Chapter 10

Potassium homoeostasis and epileptogenesis in the immature hippocampus

U. Heinemann, D. Albrecht, H. Beck, E. Ficker, B. Nixdorf, J. Stabel and D. von Haebler

Institut für Neurophysiologie, Zentrum Physiologie und Pathophysiologie, Universität zu Köln, Robert-Koch-Str. 39, D-5000 Köln 41, FRG

Summary

We have studied the maturation of K^+ homoeostasis in rat hippocampal slices. During activation of afferent fibres towards area CA1, $[K^+]_o$ increases in adult animals to about 12 mM while in slices from juvenile animals larger rises can occur. The findings suggest that the maturation of glial cells in hippocampus is delayed. The increased accumulation in $[K^+]_o$ does not occur during seizures generated by lowering extracellular $[Ca^{2+}]_o$. However, abnormal increases in $[K^+]_o$ do occur during low Mg^{2+} epileptiform activity. Studies on the maturation of $[K^+]_o$ currents show a developmental time course which depends on cell type. Whether such maturational disturbances do contribute to the augmented $[K^+]_o$ is still to be seen.

Introduction

The epileptogenicity of developing cortical tissue is greater than that of adult animals. This applies to the whole animal as well as to slice preparations of the neocortex, the entorhinal cortex or the hippocampus. In rat hippocampus, entorhinal cortex and neocortex augmented epileptogenicity becomes rather marked at about 1 week after birth. This is found with a number of convulsants, but also with kindling as a chronic model of epileptogenesis. The peak of epileptogenicity is reached between 2 and 3 weeks after birth.

A number of reasons may account for the increased epileptogenicity of juvenile nervous tissue. The action potentials are often prolonged and smaller in amplitude (e.g. von Haebler *et al.*, in press) and membrane potential may be more depolarized than in adult animals. The cells may be more excitable than adult neurons. Some of these alterations may also depend on a delayed maturation of the Na-K-ATPase (Haglund *et al.*, 1985). It was also previously noted that juvenile hippocampal cells produced depolarizing IPSPs sometimes capable of eliciting action potentials (Ben-Ari *et al.*, 1989; Cherubini *et al.*, 1990) presumably because of their inability to regulate intracellular chloride concentration (Lux, 1971; Misgeld *et al.*, 1986; Müller *et al.*, 1989). In neocortex, the inhibitory system is indeed immature even at 2 weeks after birth (see contributions by Prince (Chap. 2) and Avanzini (Chap. 3), this volume). Most of these parameters mature within a few days and are near adult levels when the period with augmented epileptogenicity starts. A number of factors, however, are yet immature at this time. Thus it has been shown that NMDA receptors are overexpressed in rat juvenile hippocampus. Axons are often not fully myelinated and may therefore release more K^+ during excitation, and excitatory synaptic coupling may be larger than in adult animals.

Delayed maturation of potassium homoeostasis

The increased epileptogenicity in juvenile tissue was first described in focal models of epilepsy in intact animals (Prince & Gutnick, 1972). There it was noted that small amounts of penicillin triggered violent seizures and this often led to abnormal elevations in $[K^+]_o$ and to spreading depressions (Mutani et al., 1974). Such studies were initially done in rabbit cortex and considered to indicate specific properties of rabbit tissue. However, more recently it has been found that treatment of neocortical and hippocampal slices with GABA antagonists readily triggers seizure-like events where in adult slices spontaneous interictal discharges or some grouped discharges are seen (Swann, Brady, 1984; Swann et al., 1986; Hablitz & Heinemann, 1987, 1989). The most important factor for the generation of these sustained seizure-like events seems to be the enhanced recurrent connectivity. However, in studies both on neocortex and hippocampus it was noted that abnormal K^+ elevations do occur during such spontaneous seizure-like events. While in adult tissue, maximal rises in $[K^+]_o$ reach levels of between 10 and 12 mM (Heinemann, Lux, 1977; Lewis & Schuette, 1975) which can not readily be surpassed, it is frequently noted that in young tissue $[K^+]_o$ levels of near 18 mM can be reached (Hablitz & Heinemann, 1989; Swann et al., 1986).

We therefore started a study in which we investigated the maturation of stimulus-induced rises in $[K^+]_o$ in area CA1 of rat hippocampal slices. We either stimulated the stratum radiatum with its Schaffer collaterals and commissural fibres or the alveus, which contains some afferent fibres to pyramidal cells but otherwise axons which originate from the pyramidal cell somatas. We found that repetitive stimulation cause normal elevations in $[K^+]_o$ at about 1 week after birth. This applied both to anti- and orthodromic activation of CA1 pyramidal cells. When the animals were permitted to mature it was found that orthodromic stimulation could reach $[K^+]_o$ levels near 18 mM. This was usually observed in the 2nd postnatal week. Within the next 2 weeks the rises in $[K^+]_o$ became smaller again and at the end of postnatal week 4 the behaviour was well comparable to that of adult tissue (Fig. 1). This compares well to similar findings in neocortical slices (Hablitz & Heinemann, 1987, 1989). It seems possible that abnormal elevations in $[K^+]_o$ contribute to epileptogenesis because of the many effects which K^+ elevations have on neuronal behaviour. Thus K^+ accumulation will depolarize nerve cells, reduce the driving force for inhibitory K^+ outward currents and augment EPSPs while the efficacy of inhibitory potentials is lowered (Lux et al., 1986). Indeed, elevating K^+ may trigger epileptiform activity (Chamberlin & Dingledine, 1988; Traynelis & Dingledine, 1988; Zuckermann & Glaser, 1968), particularly in the hippocampus.

In the adult tissue the regulation of extracellular potassium depends on various factors: K^+ is cleared into glia by the Na-K-ATPase which causes reuptake also into nerve cells (Grisar, 1984). As a consequence of Na^+ uptake into nerve cells and K^+ release, the Na-K-ATPase is activated. This leads to the generation of undershoots in $[K^+]_o$ which indeed follow any activity dependent increase in $[K^+]_o$ (Heinemann & Lux, 1975). In addition, K^+ is removed from the extracellular space by a KCl-uptake into astrocytes (Ballanyi et al., 1987) and from sites of maximal neuronal activity with large accumulation of K^+ by spatial redistribution through glial cells (Orkand et al., 1966; Dietzel et al., 1980). Therefore, glial cells must be spatially extended and to some degree electrically coupled. Since the glial membrane potential is determined largely by the transmembrane K^+ concentration gradient, glial cells depolarize when extracellular potassium accumulates as predicted by the Nernst equation. Under conditions where $[K^+]_o$ rises locally at well-defined sites the glial cell depolarization will be determined by that rise in $[K^+]_o$. This depolarization will spread along the membrane surface. Hence the depolarization is at the site of maximal K^+ accumulation somewhat smaller than predicted by the Nernst equation, while at remote sites it is somewhat larger than expected. As an example, it can be shown that both anti- and orthodromic stimulation of hippocampal pyramidal cells leads to maximal rises of $[K^+]_o$ in stratum pyramidale of area CA1. The depolarization of glial cells recorded in this layer is somewhat smaller than expected from the Nernst equation. Recordings of $[K^+]_o$ and glial membrane potential at some distance show that the smaller rises in $[K^+]_o$ are associated with glial cell depolarizations larger than expected from the Nernst equation. This provides for an inward driving force into glia at sites of maximal K^+ accumulation and for an outward driving force for K^+ at remote sites. As a consequence, K^+ is more rapidly distributed in the tissue than would be expected by passive diffusion through the extracellular space alone (Nicholson et al., 1979; Gardner-Medwin, 1983). Moreover, the K^+ uptake into glia contributes to the generation of slow negative field potentials (fp) at sites of maximal K^+ accumulation and to positive field potentials at remote sites (Somjen, 1979).

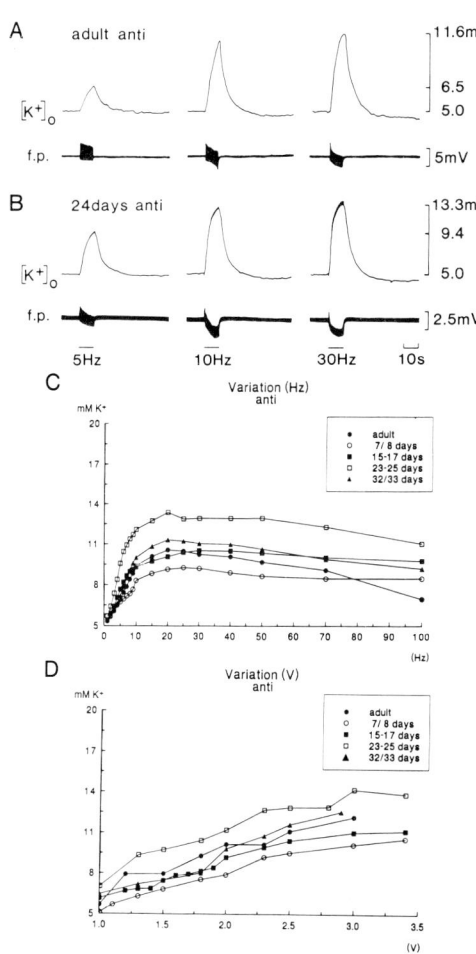

Fig. 1. Stimulus-induced changes in extracellular potassium concentration in adult and young hippocampal slices. Repetitive stimulation of the Schaffer collaterals with varying frequencies and near maximal stimulation. A: Adult animals. B: juvenile animals. C: Plot of average maximal values of $[K^+]_o$ in seven to 10 slices from each age group.

In order to obtain insight into the role of glial cells during ontogenesis we performed studies in area CA1 of rat hippocampus in which we stained astrocytes using GFAP antibodies. We counted the number of cells which showed a clear soma in the optical plane in slices from postnatal weeks 1,2,3 and 4. In the 1st week after birth most glial cells are still of the radial glia type. At the end of the 1st postnatal week more and more astrocytes become apparent. This occurs predominantly at sites where fibre tracts are formed, i.e. the alveus and the stratum moleculare lacunosum. At the end of the 2nd. week the number of astrocytes has almost reached normal levels in stratum radiatum. This is in line with the general development of astroglia throughout the nervous system (Stichel et al., 1991). However, in stratum pyramidale (SP), astrocytes have a still lower density as compared to adult animals. At the end of the 3rd week the density of glial cells is almost normal throughout all hippocampal layers.

The capability of glial cells to redistribute potassium depends also on the spatial extent of astrocyte processes and on the degree of electrical coupling. A preliminary shell analysis of astrocyte processes suggests that the spatial extension of astrocytes at the 2nd and 3rd postnatal week is somewhat below that of adult tissue.

A delayed maturation of glial cells is also suggested by the fact that the extracellular space seems to be wider in young animals than in older ones. This is suggested by superfusion experiments with Ca^{2+}- and Mg^{2+}-free solutions. The wash-out time constant for young hippocampal tissue is much faster than that for adult tissue. As an example, in adult slices, when calcium or magnesium is lowered in the ACSF (400 µm standard slices in an interface chamber) 60 min are required to achieve a near steady state. In contrast, the time to reach near equilibrium is often less than 20 min in slices obtained from 1-week-old rat pups. This implies that drug effects in young hippocampal tissue also reach equilibrium more readily. It also implies that equilibration kinetics for both convulsant and anticonvulsant drugs differ in young hippocampal tissue from adult ones (Albrecht & Heinemann, 1989).

The maturation of the extracellular space will not only depend on astrocyte and neuron maturation but also on maturation of oligodendrocytes. These develop into mature forms between weeks 1 and 2 after birth when they start myelinization in hippocampus.

The spatial redistribution of K^+ is linked to the generation of slow negative field potentials (Lothman & Somjen, 1975; Dietzel & Heinemann, 1986). In young hippocampal tissue we found that rises in $[K^+]_o$ are associated with much smaller extracellular slow potentials than expected. This is probably due to the increase in extracellular space. However, it might also be explained by a reduced capability of glial cells to spatially redistribute K^+. The time required for this parameter to reach adult levels is more than 4 weeks. Since the equilibration time course for Ca^{2+} and Mg^{2+} is near normal at 23 to 25 days after birth, we assume that this signifies a delayed maturation of K^+ homoeostasis via glial cells.

Rises in $[K^+]_o$ are usually followed by undershoots (Heinemann & Lux, 1975; Lewis & Schuette, 1975; Krnjevic & Morris, 1975). We found that the relationship between rises in $[K^+]_o$ and subsequent undershoots is augmented after the first postnatal week and then slowly approaches the behaviour in slices from adult animals. This finding may suggest that there is some overexpression of the Na-K-ATPase in week 2 to 3 after birth.

Potassium accumulation involved in low Ca^{2+} epileptogenesis

So far most reports on abnormal K^+ accumulation came from studies where GABA receptor antagonists were used to induce epileptiform activity (Mutani *et al.*, 1974; Hablitz & Heinemann, 1987, 1989; Swann *et al.*, 1986). We therefore tested whether abnormal K^+ accumulation is also associated with low Ca^{2+}-induced epileptiform activity (Dunwiddie & Lynch, 1979; Yaari *et al.*, 1983). We used pairs of Ca^{2+}- and K^+-sensitive microelectrodes in order to determine the onset of epileptiform activity in relation to the $[Ca^{2+}]_o$ and to measure changes in $[K^+]_o$ during such activity. We found that epileptiform activity began at much higher $[Ca^{2+}]_o$ levels than in adult animals. With increasing age of the animals, the level of $[Ca^{2+}]_o$ at which the epileptiform events began became lower until finally the seizure-like events commenced at a $[Ca^{2+}]_o$ level of 0.28 mM, typical for slices prepared from adult animals. Unlike in adult animals, we found that in young animals seizure-like events could be produced with a $[K^+]_o$ of 3 mM, while in adult animals 5 mM were required. Each of the seizure like events was associated with a rise in $[K^+]_o$. However, the amplitudes of such rises were smaller than those in adult animals. This suggests that fewer K^+ channels might be open during the epileptiform events, perhaps as a result of delayed maturation of K^+ outward currents. This would contribute to an augmented epileptogenesis.

Potassium accumulation in low Mg^{2+} epileptogenesis

We also studied changes in $[K^+]$ during low Mg^{2+}-induced epileptiform events (Walther *et al.*, 1986; Mody *et al.*, 1987). Comparable to the low Ca^{2+}-induced epileptiform discharges, epileptiform activity induced by low Mg^{2+} starts at higher Mg^{2+} levels than in adult animals. In slices from 1-week-old animals we found that low Mg^{2+} induced epileptiform activity at concentrations of about 1 mM, while in slices from adult animals Mg^{2+} had to be lowered to near 0.3 mM, before epileptiform discharges started. While in adult hippocampal slices, lowering of Mg^{2+} induces usually short epileptiform events of 40 to 80 ms duration, seizure-like events are induced more frequently in slices from 1-week-old animals. These seizure-like events are not yet associated with abnormal elevations in $[K^+]_o$. This is different for slices obtained 2 weeks after birth. There seizure like events are often associated with abnormally large rises in $[K^+]_o$. These may readily trigger spreading depressions. Indeed, a spreading depression is more often induced by repetitive electrical stimulation in animals of these age groups than in adult ones. Before the 4th postnatal week this behaviour disappears and at the end of the 4th postnatal week usually only short recurrent discharges are induced in 400 µm thick hippocampal slices. In appears that $[K^+]_o$ can elevate to abnormally large levels during low Mg^{2+} seizures and induce spreading depression more readily. Whether the abnormal K^+ elevation is a mere byproduct of augmented epileptogenesis or whether it contributes to enhanced epileptogenicity can not be decided on the basis of these experiments.

Maturation of potassium currents in hippocampal cells

The findings described above point to an increase in cellular excitability. This led us to study the patterns of potassium currents in hippocampal neurons obtained from area CA1, area CA3 and the dentate gyrus during development. The recordings were obtained either from cultured or from acutely isolated hippocampal neurons. The studies were complemented by an investigation of cell properties in thin slices. The recording were done in the whole cell mode with Ca^{2+} chelators present in high concentrations. Therefore an analysis of Ca^{2+}-dependent K^+ currents was not possible. The outward currents under such recording conditions can be classified into two species: (1) the fast transient A-type currents with a threshold around -50 mV, a window current between -60 and -40 mV, and a rapid time-dependent inactivation and (2) a slowly decaying delayed rectifier current with an activation threshold near -30 mV. A general observation was that the time course of inactivation of A currents in young cells was somewhat faster than in adult cells. The time course of inactivation in acutely isolated neurons from hippocampal area CA3 was particularly fast. Interestingly, we never observed such fast A currents in hippocampal cultures suggesting that disturbance of development as is certainly caused by dissociation of the cells and explanting them in culture dishes may affect the expression of K^+ current. In contrast to adult cells, A currents in young cells were also insensitive to dendrotoxine. In general the pharmacological properties of these currents were well comparable to those of adult cells. They responded to 4-aminopyridine (4 AP) and were not directly dependent on Ca^{2+} (Ficker & Heinemann, 1992).

The delayed rectifier currents showed interesting differences the different preparations. In embryonic hippocampal cells the delayed rectifier current was stable during perfusion of the cell interior. Since perfusion causes run-down if the ion channels require some metabolic regulation for their functionality, it was of interest that similar currents in the dentate gyrus (DG) displayed a certain degree of run-down. Kinetically both currents were rather similar and showed a time-dependent inactivation with two time constants, one in the order of some 100 ms and one in the order of 1 s. They displayed a window current with a maximum near -30 mV. It may well be that this steady-state current contributes to the limitation of paroxysmal depolarization shifts at this potential. Both in DG granule cells and in hippocampal pyramidal cells the delayed rectifier currents were sensitive to tetraethylammonium. However, while the currents of granule cells are poorly affected by 4 AP, they are very sensitive to this K^+ channel blocker when recorded in embryonic hippocampal cells.

In studies on embryonic hippocampal pyramidal cells we found at E18 that all cells possessed a delayed rectifier current. 50 per cent of the recorded cells did not display A-type currents (Ficker & Heinemann, 1992). Consequently, action potentials showed no rapid afterhyperpolarizations when cells were recorded in the current clamp mode. 50 per cent of neurons already had a small transient outward current at the birth of these neurons. Within the first 10 days after birth it was found that more than 90 per cent of neurons expressed transient outward currents. Adult hippocampal cells also possessed an inward rectifying current which is insensitive to barium but blocked by caesium. This current is usually well expressed in cells at postnatal day 10. Thus it appears that the investigated K^+ current maturation cannot explain the increased excitability of the hippocampal neurons in week 3 and 4 after birth. This does not however exclude that Ca^{2+}-dependent K^+ currents show a delayed developmental time course.

The ontogenetic time course in the expression of K^+ currents in dentate granule cells is quite different from that of embryonic hippocampal pyramidal cells (Beck, Ficker and Heinemann, 1992). Current clamp recordings in these cells revealed that the first action potential induced by depolarizing current injection reached near normal amplitude, and recovered rapidly with an afterhyperpolarization while subsequently induced action potentials were small, broad and not followed by afterhyperpolarization. Indeed, voltage clamp recordings in these cells reveal that they possessed predominantly transient outward currents. With ongoing maturation, the transient A type currents become less important while delayed rectifier currents become more so. This became obvious in an analysis where the relative contribution of the two current components of the outward currents were plotted in relation to each other from all recorded cells in the different age groups. Based on this analysis, dentate granule cells could be grouped into three classes depending on whether transient or delayed rectifier currents dominated. At 2 to 3 weeks after birth the neurones with a prominent delayed rectifier current dominated. Thus it appears that the electrophysiological maturation of dentate granule cells differs profoundly from that of CA1 cells.

We also found that most dentate granule cells recorded at P4 to 5 displayed a rather depolarized resting membrane potential which normalized when the cells were perfused with high K^+-containing electrolyte. The membrane potential usually normalized within 2 days after the birth of dentate granule cells; e.g. at P6–7.

Properties of horizontal cells in the DG

In studies on current development in the DG we discovered a cell type located near the fissure in the outer stratum moleculare of the DG. These cells are of interest, since many forms of early onset epilepsies, particularly those with a suspected genetic disposition, are characterized by the survival of an increased number of horizontal and ectopic cells in the tissue. We therefore became rather interested in the ontogenetic behaviour of such horizontal cells. These cells are present at P2 (we did not look for earlier stages of development) and seem to disappear at P14. The largest number of cells was found in P5. The development of the hippocampus is following a certain timetable. The entorhinal cortexas well as areas CA1 and CA3 are developed before the DG, which is the connecting structure. The peak of cell formation in the DG lies somewhere around P4. The entorhinal cortex superficial cells project to the DG and the hippocampal CA1 region through the perforant path. Thus, the problem exists that the ready CA1 area is already developed long before the DG matures. We suspect that the horizontal cells are axon-guiding cells which receive part of the later innervation from the entorhinal cortex for the DG. These cells have a low membrane potential. This might be due to a delayed expression of the Na-K-ATPase. Upon perfusion with high K^+ solutions, the membrane potentials reaches normal hyperpolarized levels, as expected if due to low pumping activity the intracellular K^+ concentration is low. Thus, we conclude that due to a reduced pumping capability of these cells the intracellular potassium concentration may be low. These cells possess both transient and delayed rectifier currents. However, their amplitude is much smaller than those of dentate granule cells. As a consequence of low expression of K^+ currents, the TTX-sensitive action potentials recorded in these cells are very long lasting. During a series of action potentials they can reach a duration of more that 25 ms. Unlike dentate granule cells the horizontal cells possess a pronounced inward rectifying current. In response to glutamate they develop bursting membrane potential changes of rather drastic appearance. We suspect that these cell properties can contribute to epileptogenesis in young hippocampal tissue.

Conclusions

Our present studies show that K^+ regulation displays a delayed maturation in rat hippocampal slices.

Part of this delayed maturation is due to delayed development of astrocytes and presumably also to oligodendrocytes. The resulting abnormal K⁺ accumulation will support development of convulsant activity and particularly sponsor the generation of spreading depressions. The described large expression of NMDA receptors which are crucial for the generation of spreading depression (SD) at postnatal week 2 in stratum radiatum (SR) will contribute to this behaviour (Hamon & Heinemann, 1988). Abnormal K⁺ accumulation is however not obligatorily linked to augmented epileptogenicity during ontogenesis since low Ca^{2+}-induced epileptiform activity is not linked to abnormal K⁺ elevations. Since the low Ca^{2+}-induced epileptiform activity persists in the absence of evoked chemical neurotransmission it is unlikely that recurrent synaptic excitation accounts for the augmented epileptogenicity. However, the maturation of transient and delayed rectifier currents seems to be largely finished at 1 week after birth. This implies presumably that Ca^{2+}-dependent K⁺ currents are less well expressed. The properties of DG granule cells mature rapidly after birth of the neurons. However, cells seem to exist in this area which could readily provide lateral excitation and thereby overcome the normal gating properties of the DG. Survival of these cells under conditions of disturbed maturation of the temporal cortex may be a factor contributing to temporal lobe epileptogenesis under such conditions.

Acknowledgements

This research was supported by DFG-grants He 1128/6–2 and a grant from the SFB 194. We are indebted to M. Bullmann, G. Heske and A. Specht for skilful assistance in the preparation of the experiments, figures and the manuscripts.

References

Albrecht, D. & Heinemann, U. (1989): Low calcium-induced epileptiform activity in hippocampal slices from infant rats. *Dev. Brain Res.* **48**, 316–320.

Ballanyi, K., Grafe, P. & ten Bruggencate, G. (1987): Ion activities and potassium uptake mechanisms of glial cells in guinea-pig olfactory cortex slices. *J. Physiol. (Lond)* **382**, 159–174.

Beck, H., Ficker, E. & Heinemann, U. (1992): Properties of the voltage-activated potassium currents in acutely isolated juvenile rat dentate gyrus granule cells. *J. Neurophysiol.* **68**, 2086–2099.

Ben Ari, Y., Cherubini, E., Corradetti, R. & Gaiarsa, J.-L. (1989): Giant synaptic potentials in immature rat CA3 hippocampal neurones. *J. Physiol. (Lond)* **416**, 303–325.

Chamberlin, N.L. & Dingledine, R. (1988): GABAergic inhibition and the induction of spontaneous epileptiform activity by low chloride and high potassium in the hippocampal slice. *Brain Res.* **445**, 12–18.

Cherubini, E., Rovira, C., Gaiarsa, J.L., Corradetti, R. & Ben-Ari, Y. (1990): GABA mediated excitation in immature rat CA3 hippocampal neurons. *Int. J. Dev. Neurosci.* **8**, 481–490.

Dietzel, I., Heinemann, U., Hofmeier, G. & Lux, H.D. (1980): Transient changes in the size of the extracellular space in the sensorimotor cortex of cats in relation to stimulus-induced changes in potassium concentration. *Exp. Brain Res.* **40**, 432–439.

Dietzel, I. & Heinemann, U. (1986): Dynamic variations of the brain cell microenvironment in relation to neuronal hyperactivity. *Ann. NY Acad. Sci.* **481**, 72–86.

Dunwiddie, T.V. & Lynch, G. (1979): The relationship between extracellular calcium concentration and the induction of hippocampal long-term potentiation. *Brain Res.* **169**, 103–110.

Ficker, E. & Heinemann, U. (1992): Slow and fast transient potassium currents in cultured rat hippocampal cells. *J. Physiol. (Lond)* **445**, 431–455.

Gardner-Medwin, A.R. (1983): Analysis of potassium dynamics in brain tissue. *J. Physiol. (Lond)* **335**, 393–426.

Grisar, T. (1984): Glial and neuronal Na-K-pump in epilepsy. *Ann. Neurol.* **16**, 128–134.

Hablitz, J.J. & Heinemann, U. (1987): Extracellular K⁺ and Ca^{2+} changes during epileptiform discharges in the immature rat neocortex. *Dev. Brain Res.* **36**, 299–303.

Hablitz, J.J. & Heinemann U. (1989): Alterations in the microenvironment during spreading depression associated with epileptiform activity in the immature neocortex. *Dev. Brain Res.* **46**, 243–252.

Haglund, M.M., Stahl, W.L., Kunkel, D.D. & Schwartzkroin, P.A. (1985): Developmental and regional differences in the localization of Na,K- ATPase activity in the rabbit hippocampus. *Brain Res.* **343**, 198–203.

Hamon, B. & Heinemann, U. (1988): Developmental changes in neuronal sensitivity to excitatory amino acids in area CA1 of the rat hippocampus. *Dev. Brain Res.* **38**, 286–290.

Heinemann, U. & Lux, H.D. (1975): Undershoots following stimulus-induced rises in extracellular potassium concentration in cerebral cortex of cat. *Brain Res.* **93**, 63–76.

Heinemann, U. & Lux, H.D. (1977): Ceiling of stimulus-induced rises in extracellular potassium concentration in the cerebral cortex of cat. *Brain Res.* **120**, 231–249.

Krnjevic, K. & Morris, M.E. (1975): Factors determining the decay of K^+ potentials and focal potentials in the central nervous system. *Can. J. Physiol. Pharmacol.* **53**, 923–934.

Lewis, D.V. & Schuette, W.H. (1975): NADH fluorescence and extracellular K^+ changes during hippocampal electrical stimulation. *J. Neurophysiol.* **38**, 405–417.

Lothman, E.W. & Somjen, G.G. (1975): Extracellular potassium activity, intracellular and extracellular potential responses in the spinal cord. *J. Physiol. (Lond)* **252**, 115–136.

Lux, H.D. (1971): Ammonium and chloride extrusion: hyperpolarizing synaptic inhibition in spinal motoneurons. *Science* **173**, 555–557.

Lux, H.D., Heinemann, U. & Dietzel, I. (1986): Ionic changes and alterations in the size of the extracellular space during epileptic activity. *Basic mechanisms of the epilepsies: molecular and cellular approaches (Advances in neurology)*, Vol. 44, eds. A.V. Delgado-Escueta, A.A. Ward, D.M. Woodbury & R.J. Porter, pp. 619–639. New York: Raven Press.

Misgeld, U., Deisz, R.A., Dodt, H.U. & Lux, H.D. (1986): The role of chloride transport in postsynaptic inhibition of hippocampal neurons. *Science* **232**, 1413–1415.

Mody, I., Lambert, J.D.C. & Heinemann, U. (1987): Low extracellular magnesium induces epileptiform activity and spreading depression in rat hippocampal slices. *J. Neurophysiol.* **57**, 869–888.

Mutani, R., Futamachi, K.J. & Prince, D.A. (1974): Potassium activity in immature cortex. *Brain Res.* **75**, 27–39.

Müller, W., Misgeld, U. & Lux, H.D. (1989): Gamma-aminobutyric acid-induced ion movements in the guinea pig hippocampal slice. *Brain Res.* **484**, 184–191.

Nicholson, C., Phillips, J.M. & Gardner-Medwin, A.R. (1979): Diffusion from an iontophoretic point source in the brain: role of tortuosity and volume fraction. *Brain Res.* **169**, 580–584.

Orkand, R.K., Nicholls, J.G. & Kuffler, S.W. (1966): Effects of nerve impulses on the membrane potential of glial cells in the central nervous system of amphibia. *J. Neurophysiol.* **29**, 788–806.

Prince, D.A. & Gutnick, M.J. (1972): Neuronal activities in epileptogenic foci of immature cortex. *Brain Res.* **45**, 455–468.

Somjen, G.G. (1979): Extracellular potassium in the mammalian central nervous system. *Ann. Rev. Physiol.* **41**, 159–177.

Stichel, C.C. Müller, C.M. & Zilles, K. (1991): Distribution of glial fibrillary acidic protein and vimentin immunoreactivity during rat visual cortex development. *J. Neurocytol.* **20**, 97–108.

Swann, J.W., Smith, K.L. & Brady, R.J. (1986): Extracellular K^+ accumulation during penicillin-induced epileptogenesis in the CA3 region of immature rat hippocampus. *Dev. Brain Res.* **30**, 243–255.

Swann, J.W. & Brady, R.J. (1984): Penicillin-induced epileptogenesis in immature rat CA3 hippocampal pyramidal cells. *Dev. Brain Res.* **12**, 243–254.

Traynelis, S.F. & Dingledine, R. (1988): Potassium-induced spontaneous electrographic seizures in the rat hippocampal slice. *J. Neurophysiol.* **59**, 259–276.

von Haebler, D., Stabel, J., Draguhn, A., Heinemann, U. (in press): Properties of horizontal cells transiently appearing in the rat dentate gyrus during ontogenesis. *Exp. Brain Res.*

Walther, H., Lambert, J.D.C., Jones, R.S.G., Heinemann, U. & Hamon, B. (1986): Epileptiform activity in combined slices of the hippocampus, subiculum and entorhinal cortex during perfusion with low magnesium medium. *Neurosci. Lett.* **69**, 156–161.

Yaari, Y., Konnerth, A. & Heinemann, U. (1983): Spontaneous epileptiform activity of CA_1 hippocampal neurons in low extracellular calcium solutions. *Exp. Brain Res.* **51**, 153–156.

Zuckermann, E.C. & Glaser, G.H. (1968): Hippocampal epileptic activity induced by localized ventricular perfusion with high-potassium cerebrospinal fluid. *Exp. Neurol.* **20**, 87–110.

Chapter 11

Postnatal development of EAA-mediated excitation in rat neocortex

S. Franceschetti, S. Buzio, F. Panzica, G. Sancini and G. Avanzini

Department of Neurophysiology, Istituto Neurologico C. Besta, Milan, Italy

Summary

Maturational changes in excitatory neurotransmission and in EAA-induced responses were studied on neocortical slices obtained from rats with ages ranging between postnatal days P3 and P21. Intracellular recordings were performed on pyramidal neurons lying in layer V. Under P10, an APV-sensitive, NMDA-mediated component considerably contributes to the long decay time of the EPSP evoked by low-rate stimulation of the white matter. This late component is conspicuous at resting V_M, and is reduced but not suppressed by membrane hyperpolarization. Multiphasic late EPSPs have been often elicited between P8 and P13 neurons. They were blocked by APV, and converted to a paroxysmal depolarization shift during the perfusion of the GABA antagonist, bicuculline.

The apparent increase in input resistance which characterizes the response to NMDA in adult pyramidal neurons is undetectable in neocortical neurons during the first 10 days of life. In addition under P15 we never observed the tendency to bursting behaviour that can be elicited by adequate NMDA administration in mature neocortical neurons. The observed developmental changes in NMDA-mediated neurotransmission can play an important role in brain maturation and plasticity and may be correlated with some specific changes of the epileptogenesis in the immature brain.

Introduction

In rat neocortex both morphological and functional organization are immature at birth and substantial maturational processes develop during the 1st month of the postnatal life. In fact at birth the layer differentiation is rudimentary in the immature somatosensory cortex (Rice *et al.*, 1985; see also Spreafico & Frassoni, Chap. 6, this volume). Subsequently the process of layer differentiation rapidly progresses during the 1st week of life, coincident with the invasion of cortical plate from thalamocortical afferents (Wise & Jones, 1976). The morphogenetic processes involving cell body growth, dendritic development, axon extent and branching, and synaptic connections, proceed for a protracted period.

Experimental evidence shows that, concurrently with the postnatal morphogenesis, significant functional modifications develop, concerning both intrinsic neuronal properties (Purpura *et al.*, 1965; McCormick & Prince, 1987; Huguenard *et al.*, 1988; Perkins & Teyler, 1988) and synaptic activities (Sutor & Hablitz, 1989; Luhmann & Prince, 1990, 1991).

In particular chemical neurotransmission undergoes both quantitative and qualitative changes during the first 3–4 weeks of postnatal life as demonstrated by anatomical and biochemical evidence concerning both inhibitory (Wolff et al., 1984; Miller, 1988) and excitatory neurotransmitters (Bode-Gruel & Singer, 1989; Insel et al., 1990). Electrophysiological studies have confirmed the existence of important maturational processes in chemical transmission, during early postnatal life. One crucial piece of evidence concerns the maturational changes of the GABA-mediated neurotransmission (Luhmann & Prince, 1991). In fact during the 1st week of life, inhibitory postsynaptic potentials (IPSPs) are not detectable in most neocortical neurons (Luhmann & Prince, 1991). This immaturity can be explained by anatomical studies showing that local circuit neurons form synapses only at the end of the 1st postnatal week (Miller, 1986). Significant maturational changes occur also in excitatory neurotransmission, that in neocortex is primarily mediated by excitatory amino acids (EAA). In fact, synaptically mediated excitation can by elicited at all postnatal ages, but during the first week of life the excitatory postsynaptic potential (EPSP) is extremely fatigable and shows a very long duration (Kriegstein et al., 1987; Avanzini et al., 1990); the evolution toward a mature behaviour and shape is progressively expressed during the 2nd week of life. Moreover a considerable proportion of neurons shows a transient expression of polysynaptic EPSPs (Luhmann & Prince, 1990). The present paper is aimed to analyse developmental changes in neocortical EAA-mediated neurotransmission during the first 3 weeks of postnatal life.

Materials and methods

Experiments were carried out on coronal neocortical slices prepared from Wistar rats aged between postnatal day (P)3 and P21; control experiments were performed in mature Wistar rats ranging from P30 to P90. Rats were decapitated under deep ether anaesthesia. The brain was removed and submerged in cold (4 °C) standard artificial cerebrospinal fluid (ACSF) of the following composition (in mM): NaCl, 126; KCl, 3.5; $CaCl_2$, 2; $MgSO_4$, 2; NaH_2PO_4, 1.2; $NaHCO_3$, 26, and glucose, 10 (pH 7.3–7.4) bubbled with 95 per cent O_2 and 5 per cent CO_2. From each hemisphere, four to five slices, 400–450 µm thick, were cut by a vibratome starting 3–5 mm caudal to the frontal pole. The slices were transferred to an interface chamber, perfused by ACSF (2.5 ml/min) and oxygenated by the gas mixture. The temperature was maintained at 35 °C, and slices were allowed to equilibrate for 1–1.5 h before starting electrophysiological recording.

Intracellular recordings were mainly obtained in layer V, by glass electrodes filled with biocytin (3–4 per cent biocytin Sigma, in 1–2 M potassium acetate, buffered by Tris HCl at pH 7.5–8; resistance 80–150 MΩ). Holding hyperpolarizing current was passed through the electrode for a few minutes after the impalement and was withdrawn before starting recording. Only neurons with stable resting membrane potential (V_M) exceeding –55 mV, stable firing level and overshooting action potential were included in the study. Postsynaptic potentials were evoked by electrical stimulation with bipolar electrodes placed in the white matter underlying the recording point. Square current pulses, 60–600 ms in duration and DC hyperpolarizing and depolarizing currents were applied to evaluate passive proprieties, firing characteristics and voltage dependency of postsynaptic potentials. Signals were stored on magnetic tape and/or digitized on a Micro PDP 11/73 Digital computer for further analysis.

N-Methyl-D-aspartate (NMDA) 50 mM, L-glutamic acid (Glu) 1 M, and quisqualic acid (QUIS) 50 mM (Sigma), were dissolved in 150 mM NaCl, titrated to pH 7.5–8 with NaOH and applied by current balanced microiontophoresis. 2-Amino-5-phosphonovaleric acid (APV, Sigma) 100 µM, 6-cyano-7-nitroquinoxaline-2,3-dione (CNQX RBI) 10 µM, and bicuculline methiodide 10 µM (Sigma) were administered via the superfusion medium.

At the end of electrophysiological experiments the slices containing biocytin-injected cells were fixed overnight by submersion in cold (4 °C) 4 per cent paraformaldehyde in phosphate-buffered saline (PBS), pH 7.3, embedded in agarose (6 per cent in distilled H_2O,) and cut by a vibratome in 50–80 µm thick sections. Sections were rinsed in PBS, pretreated for 1 h in 0.4 per cent Triton-

X100 in PBS, incubated for 2–4 h in ABC complex (Vector Labs) and reacted with 0.075 per cent diaminobenzidine and 0.002 per cent H_2O_2 in 0.05 M Tris HCl.

Results

The analysis has been carried out on 94 neurons, most of which were successfully injected with biocytine. All the labelled cells were identified as pyramidal neurons laying in layer V. They were distributed according to the following age groups: P3–P7, 10 neurons; P8–P14, 34 neurons; P15–P21, 16 neurons; adults 34 neurons.

Exogenously administered EAA

Iontophoretic applications of Glu, QUIS and NMDA were all effective in inducing membrane depolarization and sustained spike firing. The firing frequency showed an irregular trend to increase with age. Pyramidal neurons recorded during the first days of life often showed a more gradual onset of EAA-induced effect as compared with the 'older' ones. Beside this we did not find any detectable age-dependent difference in the EAA-induced depolarization. In particular, the intensity or duration of microiontophoretic ejection pulses needed to reach the threshold for the depolarizing response and firing activation were comparable at all ages. In neurons from mature animals (Fig. 1) adequate NMDA administration was often associated with bursting discharge. This response was never observed below P15 and was inconstant during the 3rd postnatal week. Figure 1 shows a typical response to iontophoretic administration (10 s pulse) of NMDA in four pyramidal neurons respectively recorded in P7, P9, P13 and in an adult control rat.

In addition we observed an age-dependent character of the NMDA-induced changes in input resistance (R_N). In fact R_N was typically increased during NMDA application in mature animals, due to the effect of the voltage-dependent Mg^{2+} block of current flow through NMDA channels. On

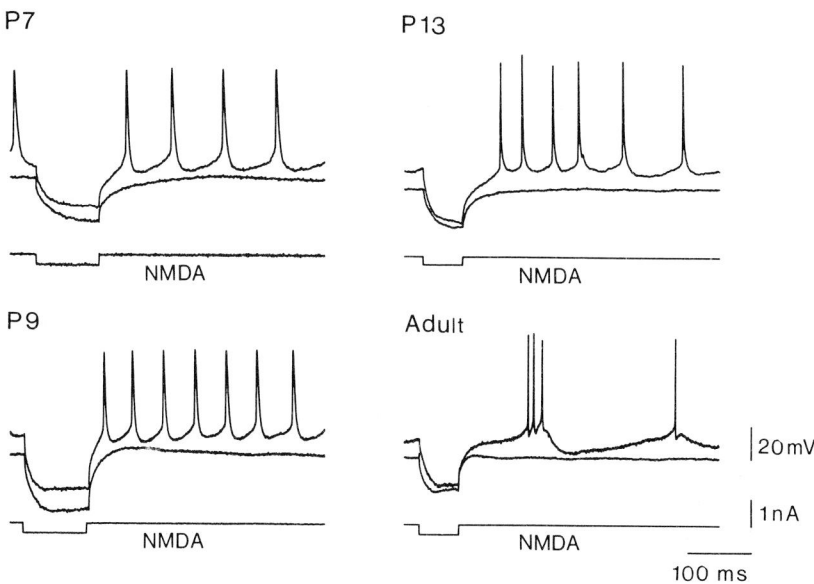

Fig. 1. Response to iontophoretic administration of NMDA (5–15 nA) in four pyramidal neurons recorded respectively in a P7, P9, P13 and in an adult animal. A sweep sample during the NMDA depolarizing effect is plotted superimposed to a basal sample. Note in the P13 neuron the apparent increase in input resistance, measured on the basis of membrane deflection induced by the administration of hyperpolarizing current pulse, and the obvious bursting behaviour in the adult cell.

the contrary, under P10 R_N was usually unchanged or slightly decreased during all the time-course of NMDA effect, as shown in Fig 1.

Synaptic activities

From P3 to P10 low frequency (0.1–0.2 Hz) stimulation of white matter consistently evoked long lasting EPSPs. The total duration of the immature EPSP was primarily due to a very long time to decay, which showed a progressive trend to decrease with the increasing age. In Table 1 the calculated mean value of total duration (T), half time to decay (T/2) and time constant of the EPSPs at different ranges of postnatal age are reported.

Table 1. *EPSPs parameters in different postnatal age*

Age	3–7	8–10	11–21
Amplitude (mV)	11 ± 3	8 ± 2	9 ± 3
T/2 (ms)	50 ± 22	15 ± 8	12 ± 8
T (ms)	179 ± 51	85 ± 60	50 ± 23

Table 2. *Effect of APV on EPSPs parameters*

	Resting V_M basal	Resting V_M APV	
Amplitude (mV)	9.3 ± 1.9	9.2 ± 2.8	0.1989
T/2 (ms)	54.6 ± 32.1	27.7 ± 19.7	0.0058
T (ms)	212.7 ± 101.1	126.2 ± 84.4	0.0085
TC (ms)	90.4 ± 42.3	55.6 ± 38.6	0.0090
	Hyperpolarized basal	Hyperpolarized APV	
Amplitude (mV)	12.3 ± 2.1	11.5 ± 2.9	0.1365
T/2 (ms)	48.8 ± 23.2	28.5 ± 18.2	0.0038
T (ms)	182.6 ± 72.9	124.2 ± 65.2	0.0068
TC (ms)	73.5 ± 26.6	51.0 ± 29.0	0.0066

The late EPSP component was only partially voltage sensitive, since it was shortened but not suppressed by membrane hyperpolarization. To prove a possible NMDA-mediated origin of the slowly decaying EPSPs component, we tested a subset of the recorded neurons by perfusing the slices with the NMDA receptor antagonist APV. As shown in Fig. 2, the NMDA antagonist consistently shortened the immature EPSP decay phase, without effect on the EPSP amplitude. On the contrary the non-NMDA antagonist CNQX is obviously effective in reducing EPSP amplitude, leaving a low-amplitude slow component possibly mediated by NMDA receptors. As shown in Fig. 3 in P4 and P9 neurons, the shortening effect of a long-lasting EPSP decay was evident at resting V_M and persisted when the V_M was held hyperpolarized until –90 mV. The effect of APV on decay phase of immature EPSPs is expressed in Table 2 as mean values for T/2 and total time duration relatively in 11 neurons recorded between P4 and P9. The APV effect was still present when V_M was hyperpolarized 10–15 mV under the resting V_M.

From P8 to P15 the antidromic stimulation evoked in a subset of neurons, identified as pyramidal, long-lasting multiphasic responses following the early EPSP (Fig. 4). Late components of postsynaptic potentials were enhanced when V_M were shifted toward hyperpolarized levels. The complex response was reversibly abolished by 100 μM APV added to ACSF (not shown). On the contrary

Chapter 11 POSTNATAL DEVELOPMENT OF EAA-MEDIATED EXCITATION IN RAT NEOCORTEX

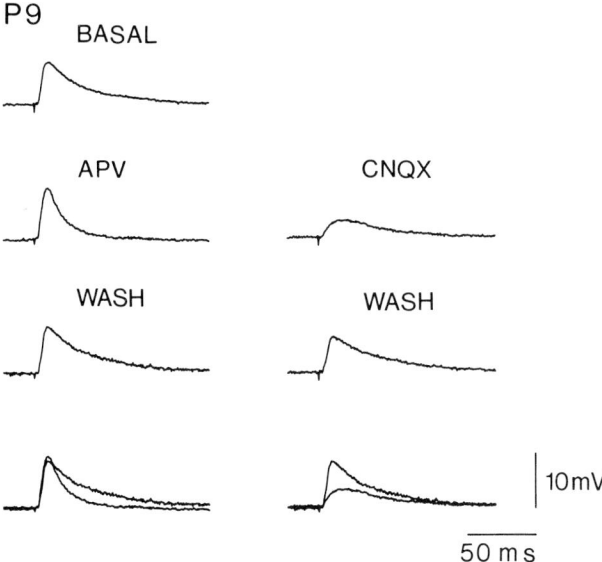

Fig. 2. *EPSPs evoked by electrical stimulation of the white matter underlying the cortex in a P9 neuron. The effect of APV in shortening EPSP decay time is compared to CNQX effect (every sample is obtained by five averaged sweeps).*

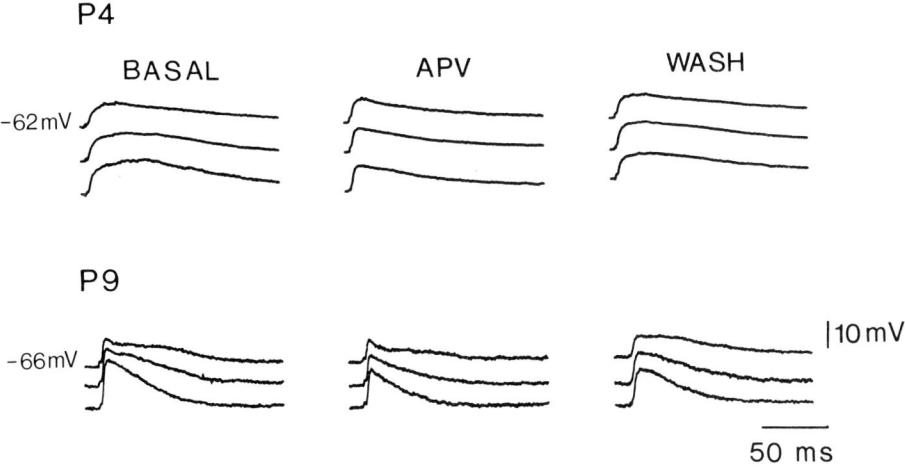

Fig. 3. *EPSPs evoked at different membrane hyperpolarization (from V_M to about -90 mV) are plotted for a P4 and a P9 neuron in basal condition, during perfusion with APV and at the wash time (every sample is obtained by five averaged sweeps).*

administration of the GABA antagonist bicuculline methiodide did not block the late depolarizing response (Fig. 4), thus ruling out the possibility that they consisted of a depolarizing IPSPs.

Discussion

The results of this study indicate that, during the postnatal ontogenesis, important maturational

111

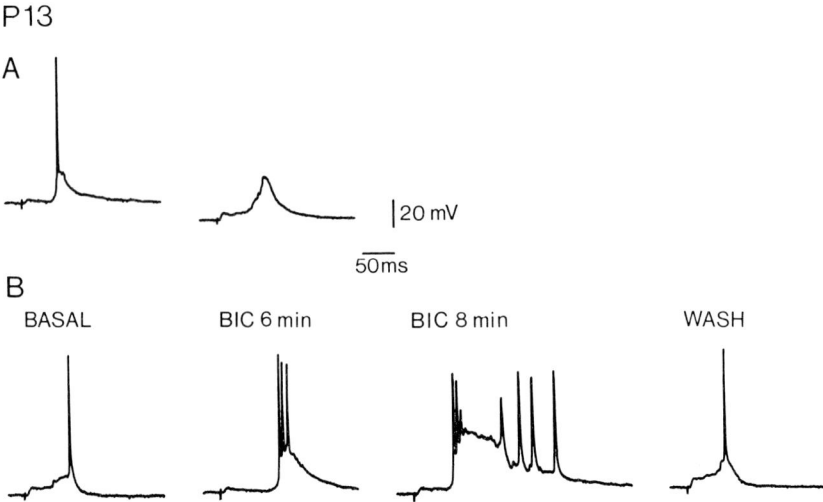

Fig 4. A: Polysynaptic EPSP evoked in a P13 pyramidal neuron. Membrane hyperpolarization (15 mV under the resting level) under the threshold for action potential enhances the amplitude of the late 'giant' EPSP. B: Effect of bicuculline methiodide on long latency multiphasic EPSP in a P12 neuron. Note that the paroxysmal depolarizing shift develops earlier on the late polysynaptic response than on the monosynaptic response to orthodromic stimulation.

changes occur in EAA-mediated neurotransmission in rat neocortex. The most significant changes affect the NMDA-mediated transmission that appears to be immature under P10 and evolves progressively to a mature pattern which is completely expressed at the end of the 3rd week of life.

The main characteristics of the immature NMDA-mediated responses can be summarized as follows. Long-lasting EPSPs that can be evoked by white matter stimulation in neurons lying in the intermediate neocortical layers, comprehend, under P10, an APV-sensitive, NMDA-mediated component that considerably contributes to the long decay time. This late NMDA-mediated component is conspicuous at resting V_M, and is reduced but not suppressed by membrane hyperpolarization. The apparent increase in R_N which regularly occurs during membrane depolarization induced by NMDA in adult pyramidal neurons (Dingledine, 1983; Flatman et al., 1986) is undetectable in neocortical neurons during the first 10 days of life and can be gradually detected only after this age.

Under P15 we never observed the tendency to bursting behaviour that in mature neurons characterize the response to adequate NMDA administration (Flatman et al., 1986). In mature animals the activation of NMDA receptors induces an inward current, carried by Na^+ and Ca^{2+} ions, which drives the V_M toward more depolarized levels (Dingledine, 1983). The NMDA-induced depolarization is associated with an apparent increase in R_N, that can be evaluated by intracellular injection of hyperpolarizing current pulses. This reflects a negative slope of the current/voltage relationship due to a voltage-dependent Mg^{2+} block of current flow through NMDA channels (MacDonald et al., 1982; Mayer et al., 1984; Flatman et al., 1986). As a result of the voltage-dependent Mg^{2+} block in mature animals, the NMDA-mediated component of the EPSPs is hardly detectable at resting V_M (Thomson, 1986). This was also found true in our study for neurons recorded from animals after P10, but never before this age.

Both the characteristics of the response of microiontophoretically administered NMDA and the peculiar behaviour of the APV-sensitive component of the EPSP may be accounted for by a less developed voltage sensitivity of the NMDA-mediated excitation in immature neocortex. It should be noted that the NMDA component of the EPSP cannot result from the less slightly negative values of resting V_M (Kriegstein *et al.*, 1987; Avanzini *et al.*, 1990) since it persisted when the membrane was hyperpolarized up to –90 mV.

Experimental results suggesting a less consistent voltage-dependence of the NMDA receptor activation in immature pyramidal cells, as compared with adult ones, have been reported by Ben Ari *et al.* (1988) and King *et al.* (1989) in immature CA3 hippocampal neurons where NMDA currents appeared to be less consistently voltage dependent than in adult animals. The immature responsiveness to NMDA of both hippocampal and neocortical pyramidal neurons can be ascribed to the activation of immature receptors which generate an inward current that is less voltage-dependent than in mature neurons. The underlying mechanisms cannot be clarified at present, suffice to say that the hypothesis that it may involve the Mg^{2+} channel interaction is not supported by recent results obtained by Lo Turco *et al.* (1991) with voltage clamp recordings. This is also supported by preliminary results obtained in our laboratory in neocortical slices perfused by higher Mg^{2+} concentration (5–7 mM) where the shortening of EPSP during membrane hyperpolarization became more evident. Whichever are the involved mechanisms, the incomplete voltage-dependence of the NMDA-operated conductance results in a facilitated NMDA-mediated neurotransmission which accounts for the prolonged time course of monosynaptic EPSPs. In addition polysynaptic NMDA-mediated EPSPs have been often elicited between P8 and P13. As previously reported by Luhmann & Prince (1990) they are blocked by APV and enhanced by the GABA antagonist bicuculline and are therefore considered to result from an incomplete effectiveness of the immature GABA system (Luhmann & Prince, 1990). Additional factors which may increase this probability to occur are the above-mentioned facilitation of NMDA transmission and transient over-expression of NMDA receptors, demonstrated by autoradiographic studies, which peak in the same period (Insel *et al.*, 1990). Since Ca^{2+} influx into the cells is an important factor of growth and differentiation the activation of Ca^{2+}-dependent, NMDA-operated channels may play a crucial biological role in brain maturation and plasticity.

On the contrary the immature response of exogenous administered NMDA, characterized by the absence of bursting behaviour and by a less expressed voltage dependence, can be interpreted as a limiting phenomenon for the hyperexcitability of the immature neocortex. It is noteworthy that a similar significance can be attributed to the delayed maturation of the physiological bursting behaviour in layer V pyramidal neurons (Avanzini *et al.*, 1992) which are thought to support cortical synchronization (Chagnac-Amitai & Connors, 1989).

The present observations can have some physiopathological implications for the peculiar expression of spontaneous human epilepsies. In fact the enhancement of NMDA-mediated excitatory neurotransmission can contribute to explain the high susceptibility of the immature nervous system to epileptogenic agents (Hablitz, 1987), on the other hand the delayed expression of burst-generating mechanisms may result in the asynchronous epileptic discharges that characterize the epileptic patterns in infancy.

References

Avanzini, G., Buzio S., Franceschetti, S. & Panzica, F. (1990): Developmental changes in excitatory amino acid (EAA) mediated responses in rat neocortical slices. Abstract 13th Annual Meeting of the European Neuroscience Association, Stockholm, p. 123.

Avanzini, G., Franceschetti, S., Panzica, F. & Buzio, S. (1992): Age-dependent changes in excitability of rat neocortical neurons studied *in vitro*. In: *Molecular neurobiology of epilepsy*, eds. G. Avanzini, E.A. Cavalheiro, U. Heinemann, C. Westerlain & J. Engel, pp. 95–105. Amsterdam: Elsevier.

Ben Ari, Y., Cherubini, E. & Krnjevic, K. (1988): Changes in voltage dependence of NMDA currents during development. *Neurosci. Lett.* **94**, 88–92.

Bode-Gruel, K. & Singer, W. (1989): The development of N-methyl-D-aspartate receptors in cat visual cortex. *Dev. Brain Res.* **46**, 197–204.

Chagnac-Amitai, Y. & Connors, B.W. (1989): Synchronized excitation and inhibition driven by intrinsically bursting neurons in neocortex. *J. Neurophysiol.* **62**, 1149–1162.

Dingledine, R. (1983): *N*-Methylaspartate activates voltage-dependent calcium conductance in rat hippocampal pyramidal cells. *J. Physiol.* **343**, 385–405.

Flatman, J.A., Schwindt, P.C. & Crill, W.E. (1986): The induction and modification of voltage-sensitive responses in cat neocortical neurons by *N*-dimethyl-D-aspartate. *Brain Res.* **363**, 62–77.

Franceschetti, S., Buzio, S., Panzica, F., Spreafico, R. & Avanzini, G. (1990): Membrane properties and synaptic responses analysis in neocortical slices from developing rats. Abstract 13th Annual Meeting of the European Neuroscience Association, Stockholm, p. 283.

Hablitz, J.J. (1987): Spontaneous ictal-like discharges and sustained potential shifts in the developing rat neocortex. *J. Neuroscience* **58**, 1052–1065.

Insel, T.R., Miller, L.P. & Gelhard R.E. (1990): The ontogeny of excitatory aminoacid receptors in rat forebrain. I. *N*-methyl-D-aspartate and quisqualate receptors. *Neuroscience* **35**, 45–52.

Huguenard, J.R., Hamill, O.P. & Prince D.A. (1988): Developmental changes in Na^+ conductances in rat neocortical neurons: apparence of a slowly inactivating component. *J. Neurophysiol.* **59**, 778–795.

King, A.E., Cherubini, E. & Ben-Ari, Y. (1889): *N*-methyl-D-aspartate induces recurrent synchronized burst activity in immature CA3 neurons *in vitro*. *Dev. Brain Res.* **46**, 1–8.

Kriegstein, A.R., Suppes, T. & Prince, D.A. (1987): Cellular and synaptic physiology and epileptogenesis of developing rat neocortical neurons *in vitro*. *Dev. Brain Res.* **34**, 161–171.

Lo Turco, J.J., Blanton, M.G. & Kriegstein A.R. (1991): Initial expression and endogenous activation of NMDA channels in early neocortical development. *J. Neurosci.*, **11**, 792–799.

Luhmann H.J. & Prince D.A. (1990): Transient expression of polysynaptic NMDA receptor-mediated activity during neocortical development. *Neurosci. Lett.* **111**, 109–115.

Luhmann, H.J. & Prince, D.A. (1991): Postnatal maturation of the GABAergic system in rat neocortex. *J. Neurophysiol.* **65**, 247–263.

Mayer, M.L., Westbrook, G. & Guthrie, P.B. (1984): Voltage dependent block by Mg^{2+} of NMDA responses in spinal cord neurones. *Nature* **309**, 261–263.

McCormick, D.A. & Prince, D.A. (1987): Post-natal development of electrophysiological properties of rat cerebral cortical pyramidal neurones. *J. Physiol.* **393**, 743–762.

MacDonald, J.F., Porietis, A.V. & Wojtowicz, J.M. (1982): L-Aspartic acid induces a region of negative slope conductance in the current-voltage relationship of cultured spinal cord neurons. *Brain Res.* **237**, 248–253.

Miller, M.W. (1986): Maturation of rat visual cortex. III. Postnatal morphogenesis and synaptogenesis of local circuit neurons. *Dev. Brain Res.* **25**, 271–285.

Miller, M.W. (1988): Development of projection and local circuit neurons in neocortex. In: *Cerebral cortex*, Vol. 7, Development and maturation of cerebral cortex, eds. A. Peters, E.G. Jones, pp. 133–175. New York: Plenum Press.

Perkins IV, A.T. & Teyler, T.J. (1988): A critical period for long-term potentiation in the developing rat visual cortex. *Brain Res.* **439**, 222–229.

Purpura, D.P., Shofer, R.J. & Scarff, T. (1965): Properties of synaptic activities and spike potentials of neurons of immature neocortex. *J. Neurophysiol.* **28**, 925–942.

Rice, F.L., Gomez, C., Barstow, C., Burnet, A. & Sands, P. (1985): A comparative analysis of the development of the primary somatosensory cortex: interspecies similarities during barrel and laminar development. *J. Comp. Neurol.* **236**, 477–495.

Spreafico, R. & Frassoni, C. (1993): Morphological aspects of neocortical maturation. In: *Epileptogenic and excitotoxic mechanisms*, eds. G. Avanzini, R. Fariello, U. Heinemann & R. Mutani, pp. 59–66. London: John Libbey.

Sutor, B. & Hablitz, J.J. (1989): EPSPs in rat neocortical neurons *in vitro*. II. Involvement of *N*-methyl-D-aspartate receptors in generation of EPSPs. *J. Neurophysiol.* **61**, 621–634.

Thomson, A.M. (1986): A magnesium-sensitive post-synaptic potential in rat cerebral cortex resembles neuronal responses to *N*-methylaspartate. *J. Physiol.* **370**, 531–549.

Wise, S.P. & Jones, E.G. (1987): Developmental studies of thalamocortical and commissural connections in the rat somatic sensory cortex. *J. Comp. Neurol.* **178**, 187–208.

Wolff, J.R., Bottcher, H., Zetzsche, T., Oertel, W.H. & Chronwall, B.M. (1984): Development of GABA ergic neurons in rat visual cortex as identified by glutamate decarboxylase-like immunoreactivity. *Neurosci. Lett.* **47**, 207–212.

Chapter 12

GABA excites immature rat CA3 hippocampal neurones

Enrico Cherubini

Biophysics Laboratory, International School for Advanced Studies, Via Beirut 2/4, 34014 Trieste, Italy

Summary

In the adult CNS, GABA is the main inhibitory transmitter. It inhibits neuronal firing by increasing a Cl⁻ conductance. In neonatal CA3 hippocampal neurons, GABA responses exhibit several electrophysiological characteristics different from the adult ones: (i) During the first postnatal week, synaptically released or exogenously applied GABA depolarizes and excites neuronal membranes. This effect which is mediated by GABA$_A$ receptors, coupled to Cl⁻ channels seems to be due to a different Cl⁻ gradient; (ii) GABA responses show little desensitization; (iii) GABA responses are not potentiated by benzodiazepines. Furthermore GABA-mediated responses are presynaptically modulated by NMDA and non NMDA receptors and are potentiated by glycine in a strychnine-insensitive manner.

These observations suggest that during the first week of life, GABA provides most of the excitatory drive on pyramidal cells. GABA-mediated depolarization may induce a raise in intracellular calcium and therefore may play an important role in cell growth and differentiation.

Introduction

In the adult hippocampus, as in many other brain structures, excitatory and inhibitory events are mediated by glutamate and γ-aminobutyric acid (GABA) respectively. In CA3 pyramidal neurones, the electrical stimulation of the mossy fibres evokes an excitatory postsynaptic potential (EPSP) followed by an inhibitory postsynaptic potential (IPSP). The EPSP is mediated by the activation of a non-*N*-methyl-D-aspartate (NMDA) receptor (Neuman *et al.*, 1988a). The NMDA-mediated component of the EPSP cannot be revealed at resting membrane potential because the NMDA channel is blocked by Mg^{2+} ions present in the extracellular fluid (Collingridge *et al.*, 1988). This component can be evidentiated by removing magnesium from the extracellular medium (Neuman *et al.*, 1988b), by depolarizing the cell membrane or by blocking the GABA$_A$-mediated inhibition. The IPSP is primarily mediated by GABA: the fast IPSP by GABA acting on bicuculline-sensitive GABA$_A$ receptors, coupled to Cl⁻ channels; the slow IPSP by GABA acting on bicuculline-insensitive GABA$_B$ receptors, coupled to K⁺ channels.

The morphological substrate for these inhibitory events is provided by GABAergic interneurons which are usually activated by recurrent collaterals of the pyramidal cells and by hippocampal excitatory afferents (Frotscher & Leranth, 1988). In contrast to adult neurons, little is known about the circuitry and the transmitters involved in the synaptic excitation and inhibition early in postnatal life. This period is of interest, because a synaptic rearrangement occurs in the CA3 hippocampal region: towards the end of the first postnatal week, the mossy fibres originating from the granule cells in the gyrus dentatus reach their target and consolidate their excitatory synaptic contacts with CA3 pyramidal cells (Amaral & Dent, 1981). Moreover the early postnatal period is characterized by important and abrupt changes in brain receptor distribution. In the hippocampal formation, a transient increase in the expression of NMDA receptors has been observed during the first postnatal week. This and other considerations (i.e. the role of NMDA receptors in developmental plasticity – see Tsumoto et al., 1987; Kleinschmidt et al., 1987) have prompted us to study the developmental profile of synaptic activity in the CA3 hippocampal region. We have found that the predominant form of synaptic activity in immature animals is excitation which is mediated by GABA acting on $GABA_A$ receptors. GABA therefore at this period of development is depolarizing and excitatory.

Previous immunocytochemical studies, using tritiated thymidine, have shown that GABAergic neurons have an early neurogenesis, being generated between E13 and E15 embryonic age (Amaral & Kurz, 1985), 2 days before pyramidal neurons. Using an immunocytochemical approach with GABA antibodies in semithin sections, Rozenberg et al. (1989) have studied the developmental changes in GABA distribution in early postnatal life. According to these authors: (i) GABA immunolabelling is observed 2–4 days after the last mitosis (E18); (ii) GABAergic boutons around the cell bodies of pyramidal neurons are observed only starting from P6.

Spontaneous synaptic activity

Intracellular recordings were made from CA3 hippocampal neurons in slices obtained from 0–18-day-old Wistar rats. As previously described (Ben Ari et al., 1989), the spontaneous synaptic activity was characterized by giant depolarizing potentials (GDPs). These consisted of large (25–50 mV) depolarizations (lasting 300–500 ms) which triggered action potentials and were followed by an afterhyperpolarization. GDPs were due to the synchronous activation of a network. In fact: (i) they were synchronous with field potentials recorded with extracellular electrodes positioned in the stratum radiatum; (ii) they were synchronous in pairs of CA3 neurons recorded simultaneously with intracellular electrodes; (iii) they were blocked by TTX (1 µM) or by a low calcium (0.1 mM) high magnesium (6 mM) solution; (iv) their frequency was independent of the membrane potential.

GDPs were mediated by GABA acting on $GABA_A$ receptors since they reversed polarity at the same potential of the response to exogenously applied GABA or the $GABA_A$ agonist isoguvacine (about –50 mV, in any case always positive to the resting membrane potential) and they were blocked by the specific $GABA_A$ antagonist bicuculline (10 µM). The most striking demonstration of changes taking place in the role of $GABA_A$ receptors in early postnatal life comes from the experiments with bicuculline. Before P6–P8 bicuculline had a paradoxical effect: it blocked the spontaneous GDPs and induced a membrane hyperpolarization. After P6–P8, bicuculline blocked the GABAergic inhibitory drive and induced, as in adults, interictal discharges.

During the the 2nd postnatal week GDPs were often replaced by spontaneous large hyperpolarizing potentials. As already mentioned, the slow hyperpolarizing potentials were blocked by bicuculline which at this stage induced interictal bursts. Comparing to GDPs, interictal bursts had a faster rising phase and reversed polarity near 0 mV, suggesting that an excitatory amino acid was involved in their generation.

Evoked synaptic activity

Electrical stimulation of the hilar region at P1–P5 evoked GDPs. These were similar to spontaneous GDPs in terms of amplitude, duration and afterhyperpolarization. Like the spontaneous GDPs, the evoked synaptic potentials were generated by a polysynaptic circuit, since: (i) they were not graded and usually responded to hilar stimulation in an all or nothing manner; (ii) they were synchronous with intra- and extracellular recordings; (iii) they were reversibly abolished by TTX and by a low calcium, high magnesium medium. Evoked GDPs were often preceded by a small depolarizing potential which frequently appeared only as a small inflexion on the initial phase of the GDP. Evoked GDPs reversed polarity at the same potential as the spontaneous ones, around −50 mV and were reversibly blocked by bicuculline (10 µM). Bicuculline also blocked the small depolarizing potential that often preceded the GDP, whereas neither AP–50 (50 µM) nor CNQX (10 µM) blocked it.

Previous electrophysiological data of the synaptic responses in the CA1 area of the hippocampus *in vivo* (Michelson & Lothman, 1989) or *in vitro* (Harris & Teyler, 1983) have emphasized the relatively slow maturation of the GABAergic inhibitory system in early postnatal life. Thus the paired-pulse inhibition, that probably represents inhibition by basket cells on CA1 pyramidal neurons has never been observed before P6 (Harris & Teyler, 1983). Intracellular recordings from cortical and hippocampal neurons have confirmed that the predominant form of synaptic activity in immature animals is excitation. Several differences between adult and neonatal GABA responses have been described:

(i) As confirmed by cytometric techniques (Fiszman *et al.*, 1990), GABA depolarizes neonatal neurons. GABA depolarization may be due to a modified Cl^- gradient that results from the reversed operation of the Cl^- membrane pump. Alternatively, if GABA-activated channels are also permeable to bicarbonate ions (HCO_3^-), the reversal potential will deviate significantly from the Cl^- equilibrium potential toward the HCO_3^- equilibriium potential which is more positive than that of Cl^-. HCO_3^- may be produced by changes in cell metabolism during development.

(ii) In neonatal neurons, GABA responses show little desensitization (Cherubini *et al.*, 1990).

(iii) GABA responses are almost linearly related to the membrane potential in the range between −80 and −40 mV (Ito & Cherubini, 1991).

(iv) GABA responses are potentiated by barbiturates but are insensitive to benzodiazepines (Rovira & Ben Ari, 1991).

Developmental changes in $GABA_A$ receptor structure may underline changes in GABA responses observed in immature neurons. The $GABA_A$ receptor is a hetero-oligomeric protein composed of several distinct polypeptide types (α, β, γ, δ). When expressed in heterologous cells, these polypeptides produce GABA-activated Cl^- channels. The functional characteristics of the receptor is determined by the structure and assembly of different subunits. For instance, the γ_2 subunit is responsible for the potentiating effect of the benzodiazepines while the β_2 subunit is responsible for the desensitization and outward rectification of the GABA current. It has been recently shown that the α_1 subunit of the GABA receptor, which constitutes also a part of the benzodiazepine type I receptor appears later in development (MacLennan *et al.*, 1991).

Spontaneous and evoked GDPs are presynaptically modulated by NMDA and non-NMDA receptors

In the rat hippocampus a transient increase in the density of NMDA receptor binding sites strictly parallels the development of GDPs in early postnatal life (Trembley *et al.*, 1988). We therefore tested the effects of NMDA-receptor antagonists and NMDA channel blockers on spontaneous and evoked GDPs.

Spontaneous GDPs were reduced in frequency or blocked either by NMDA receptor antagonists AP-5, AP-7 (50 µM), CPP (30 µM) or the NMDA channel blocker ketamine (20 µM, Ben Ari *et al.*, 1989). Furthermore, bath application of low concentrations of NMDA (0.5–2 µM) enhanced the frequency of spontaneous GDPs. This effect was blocked by AP–5, AP–7 or bicuculline.

Since the NMDA receptor complex has an allosteric facilitatory site, activated by nanomolar concentrations of glycine (Johnson & Ascher, 1987) we have investigated the effects of glycine on

GDPs. Glycine at low concentrations (10–30 μM) increased the frequency of GDPs from 0.14 to 0.29 Hz. This effect which was mimicked by D-serine (10–30 μM) was insensitive to strychnine and was blocked by the NMDA-receptor antagonist AP-5, suggesting that NMDA-receptor activation is required for the action of glycine (Gaiarsa et al., 1990). Glycine also potentiated the effects of bath application of NMDA (0.1–1 μM). In the presence of TTX (1 μM) glycine failed to potentiate the inward current induced by NMDA. However glycine was able to antagonize the inhibitory effect of 7-Cl-kynurenate (10–20 μM) on NMDA-induced currents. These observations suggest that, although a glycine modulatory site is present on the pyramidal cell, the facilitatory effects of glycine on GDPs are not mediated by a direct action but through the activation of NMDA receptors located on GABAergic interneurons.

NMDA receptors in hippocampal neurons, are usually co-localized with non-NMDA receptors. Therefore we have investigated the possible role of non-NMDA receptors in the modulation of GABA-mediated synaptic events in the CA3 region of neonatal rats. CNQX (10 μM), a rather selective non-NMDA antagonist, blocked GDPs. This effect persisted when glycine (5 μM) was added to the perfusing solution in order to prevent the antagonistic effect of CNQX on the allosteric glycine site of the NMDA receptor. Low concentrations of quisqualate (300 nM) increased the synaptic noise and the frequency of GDPs. CNQX blocked the action of quisqualate, suggesting that the observed effect was mediated through an ionotropic type of receptor. The activation of an ionotropic receptor was confirmed by the experiments with AMPA that like quisqualate increased the frequency of GDPs. Also kainate (100 nM) increased the frequency of GDPs. The effect of kainate was blocked by CNQX and bicuculline but not by AP-5 (Gaiarsa et al., 1991). In the presence of TTX (1 M), quisqualate (100–300 nM), AMPA (100–500 nM) and kainate (100 nM) failed to induce any change in membrane potential, input resistance or synaptic noise, indicating that the effects on GDPs were indirect, mediated through the activation of receptors localized on GABAergic interneurones.

Like spontaneous synaptic potentials, NMDA receptor activation also contributed to the evoked GDPs. The NMDA-receptor antagonists AP-5, AP-7 and CPP (30–50 μM) reduced the amplitude and the duration of the evoked GDPs. The possible role of NMDA receptors in the evoked GDPs was further examined following changes in the strength or in the frequency of stimulation. After blockade of GDPs by bicuculline, increasing the strength of stimulation revealed a depolarizing potential followed by a hyperpolarization. Both the bicuculline-insensitive component and the following hyperpolarization were abolished by the NMDA receptor antagonist AP-5. An AP-5-sensitive component of the evoked postsynaptic potential could also be revealed in the presence of bicuculline by a brief, high frequency train of stimuli. In these conditions a depolarizing component was revealed which was blocked by AP-5 (Ben Ari et al., 1989).

To explain the generation of GDPs we propose the following scheme. The GABAergic interneuron oscillates in response to the activation of NMDA receptors by glutamate released by axon collaterals of pyramidal cells. The calcium influx, induced by the activation of the NMDA channel will activate a calcium-dependent potassium conductance which will repolarize the cell. The oscillating GABAergic interneuron would release GABA. The depolarization induced by GABA will promote a positive feedback loop through which the synchronous discharge of a population of pyramidal cells might be produced. These oscillatory events which are modulated by NMDA and non-NMDA receptors are important signals during synaptogenesis.

The functional significance of the depolarizing action of GABA and the high sensitivity of GABAergic interneurons to glutamate agonists is presently unknown. Nevertheless extensive investigations in cultures indicate that a rise in intracellular calcium is essential for neuronal growth and differentiation (Mattson et al., 1988). This can be produced either by activation of voltage dependent calcium channels or excitatory amino acid receptors. GABA may have a similar effect increasing intracellular calcium concentration. This has been shown in neonatal but not adult cerebellar and cortical neurons (Connor *et al.*, 1987; Yuste & Katz, 1991). It therefore seems possible that GABA plays a trophic role in early postnatal life.

Acknowledgements

The work presented in this review was done at INSERM U. 29, in Paris (France) in collaboration with Y. Ben Ari, J.L. Gaiarsa, C. Rovira and R. Corradetti.

References

Amaral, D.G. & Dent, J.A. (1981): *J. Comp. Neurol.*, **195**, 51–86.

Amaral, D.G. & Kurtz, J. (1985): *Neurosci. Lett.* **59**, 33–39.

Ben Ari, Y., Cherubini, E., Corradetti, R. & Gaiarsa, J.L. (1989): *J. Physiol.* **416**, 303–325.

Cherubini, E., Rovira, C., Gaiarsa, J.L., Corradetti, R. & Ben Ari, Y. (1990): *Int. J. Dev. Neurosci.* **8**, 481–490.

Collingridge, G.L., Herron, C.E. & Lester, R.A.J. (1988): *J. Physiol.* **399**, 283–300.

Connor, J.A., Tseng, H. & Hockberger, P.E. (1987): *J. Neurosci.* **7**, 1384–1400.

Fiszman, M.L., Novotny, E.A., Lange, G.D. & Barker, J.L. (1990): *Dev. Brain Res.* **53**, 186–193.

Frotscher, M. & Leranth, C. (1988): *Histochemistry* **88**, 313–319.

Gaiarsa, J.L., Corradetti, R., Cherubini, E. & Ben Ari, Y. (1990): *Proc. Natl. Acad. Sci. USA* **87**, 343–346.

Gaiarsa, J.L., Corradetti, R., Cherubini, E. & Ben Ari, Y. (1991): *Eur. J. Neurosci.* **3**, 301–309.

Harris, K.M. & Teyler, T.J. (1983): *Brain Res.* **268**, 339–343.

Ito, S. & Cherubini, E. (1991): *J. Physiol.* **440**, 67–83.

Johnson, J.W. & Ascher, P. (1987): *Nature* **325**, 529–531.

Kleinschmidt, A., Bean, M. & Singer, W. (1987): *Science* **328**, 355–358.

Mattson, M.P., Don, P. & Kater, S.B. (1988): *J. Neurosci.* **8**, 2087–2100.

MacLennan, A.J., Brecha, N., Khrestchatisky, M., Sternini, C., Tillakaratne, N.K.J., Chang, M.Y., Anderson, K., Lai, M. & Tobin, A.J. (1991): *Neuroscience* **43**, 369–380.

Michelson, H.B. & Lothman, E.W. (1989): *Dev. Brain Res.* **47**, 113–122.

Neuman, R.S., Ben Ari, Y., Gho, M. & Cherubini E. (1988a): *Neurosci. Lett.* **92**, 64–88.

Neuman, R.S., Cherubini, E. & Ben Ari, Y. (1988b): *Neuroscience* **28**, 393–399.

Rovira, C. & Ben Ari, Y. (1991): *Neurosci. Lett.* **130**, 157–161.

Rozenberg, F., Robain, O., Jardin, L. & Ben Ari, Y. (1989): *Dev. Brain Res.* **50**, 177–187.

Trembley, E., Roisin, M.P., Represa, A., Charriaut-Marlangue, C. & Ben Ari, Y. (1988): *Brain Res.* **461**, 393–396.

Tsumoto, T., Hagihara, K., Sato, H. & Hata, Y. (1987): *Nature* **327**, 513–514.

Yuste, R. & Katz, L.C. (1991): *Neuron* **6**, 333–344.

Chapter 13

Kindling in developing animals

L.S. Velíšek[*], E.F. Sperber[*†] and S.L. Moshé[*†‡]

*Departments of *Neurology, †Neuroscience and ‡Pediatrics, Albert Einstein College of Medicine, Bronx, NY, USA*

Summary

Kindling is an established model of progressive epileptogenesis. It was initially described in adult animals, but it is more powerful in developing animals. In this review, the age-related differences will be emphasized. Immature animals are more susceptible to the development of kindled convulsions than adult animals. The manifestations of certain kindled seizures have age-specific characteristics. The substrates of kindled seizures differ as a function of age and these differences may account for decreased ability of immature animals to resist the development of prolonged, repetitive or multifocal seizures. Kindling, once established, is permanent at all ages. Developmental kindling studies may be important in understanding the emergence, establishment and treatment of developmental human seizure disorders.

Introduction

Mature animals

While most kindling reviews attribute the initial era of kindling to the late 1960s, the decrease of the afterdischarge (AD) threshold with repeated stimulations in the hippocampus was described by Delgado & Sevillano in 1961. In 1967, Graham Goddard noticed that when weak electrical stimuli were daily delivered in the amygdala, behavioural seizures appeared and were followed by persistent motor convulsions. Goddard called this phenomenon 'kindling' from 'kindling a fire'. Since then, kindling was demonstrated to be a valuable model of epileptogenesis. It was shown that almost all sites in the limbic system and the entire forebrain including neocortex could be kindled. On the contrary, midbrain structures and the cerebellum could not be kindled (Goddard *et al.*, 1969; Racine, 1978; Pinel & Rovner, 1978; Le Gal La Salle, 1979; Ono, 1983). Later studies demonstrated that repeated local administration of chemical convulsants may also lead to the same results, i.e. persistent motor convulsions. To elicit chemical kindling various drugs were used, such as pentylenetetrazol (Mason & Cooper, 1972; Diehl *et al.*, 1984), penicillin (Collins, 1978), carbachol (Vosu & Wise, 1975; Cain, 1983), lidocaine and cocaine (Post *et al.*, 1975; Post, 1977; Stripling & Ellingwood, 1977). The same effect was also produced by systemic administration of subconvulsive doses of convulsant drugs as pentylenetetrazol (Piredda *et al.*, 1986). In contrast, the neurotoxin kainic acid did not induce kindling and resulted in hippocampal cell loss (Holmes & Thompson, 1988). It is possible that only drugs with a low neurotoxicity/neuroexcitatory ratio (Fagg *et al.*, 1986) can induce kindling.

Developing animals

Kindling studies in developing animals appeared in the early 1980s (Moshé, 1981; Moshé et al., 1981, 1983; Gilbert & Cain, 1982). These studies revealed the exquisite sensitivity of the immature brain to external stimuli. The current literature on kindling in developing animals deals predominantly with electrical kindling in rats and cats (Moshé et al., 1981; Holmes & Weber, 1986; Lee et al., 1986; Holmes & Thompson, 1988; Shouse et al., 1990). The only study which attempted to induce chemical kindling with kainic acid in rat pups failed (Holmes & Thompson, 1988), so successful chemical kindling in developing animals has not yet been demonstrated.

Stimulation parameters and afterdischarges:
Basis for amygdala and hippocampal electrical kindling

Mature animals

As a rule, an AD is required before subsequent kindling develops (Racine, 1972a,b). Thus, sites where repeated stimulations fail to produce ADs are considered to be resistant to kindling. The induction of repeated ADs can be considered as an initial stage of kindling (Mareš & Marešová, 1987). Detailed studies from the prekindling and kindling era describe sites inside and outside the limbic system which respond to stimulation with ADs (Kaada, 1951; Green & Shimamoto, 1953; Mareš et al., 1980, 1982, 1983; Mareš et al., 1985; Pohl et al., 1986; Marešová & Mareš, 1988; Pohl & Mareš, 1990).

To elicit an AD and subsequent kindling, certain stimulation parameters must be maintained. Stimuli are delivered periodically with an interstimulation interval which varies from 20 min to 48 h or longer (Goddard et al., 1969). Intervals longer than 1 h are more effective in inducing kindling (Goddard et al., 1969; Peterson et al., 1981; McIntyre et al., 1987). Interstimulation intervals shorter than 20 min are probably associated with post-AD inhibition which hinders the development of kindling. Thus kindling stimulations delivered with short interstimulation intervals are significantly less effective in adult animals and often fail to induce kindling (Racine et al., 1973; Mucha & Pinel, 1977; Peterson et al., 1981; Moshé et al., 1983). Lothman et al. (1985) used both low (10 Hz) and high (60 Hz) frequency stimuli delivered at 5 min intervals. The experiments resulted in periodic alternating motor seizures and depression. During the 1st day of stimulation the depression following a motor seizure lasted between 25–30 min, whereas during the 2nd day it lasted only 10–15 min.

Commonly, sine wave or rectangular pulses trains with 50–60 Hz frequency lasting 1–2 s (rectangular pulse duration 0.2–1 ms) are used. The stimulation parameters were originally used in maximal electroshock models and were derived from power net frequency (Holmes, 1983). Lower frequencies can also induce kindling (about 10 Hz), as long as the current intensity is increased and the stimulus is delivered for a long period, usually 10–60 s (Corcoran & Cain, 1980; Cain & Corcoran, 1981). There are no studies expressing the efficacy of stimulation as a function of electrical charge (i.e. effective current multiplied by the duration of delivery). From the available data, it appears that the total charge may be the most important factor influencing the progression of kindling (Corcoran & Cain, 1980; Cain & Corcoran, 1981; Lothman et al., 1985; Minabe et al., 1986).

In adult animals, the amygdala AD threshold is substantially higher than the hippocampal AD threshold (Racine, 1978; Dyer et al., 1979). For both hippocampal and amygdala kindling, the current intensity commonly used is suprathreshold for ADs. During the course of kindling, the ADs increase in amplitude and duration and propagate to other brain sites. In amygdala-kindled animals, the ADs occur in other ipsilateral limbic sites and in the contralateral amygdala. Eventually, ADs spread to the basal ganglia, including the substantia nigra and the neocortex. This spread correlates with the occurrence of generalized seizures (Wada et al., 1975; Bonhaus et al., 1986). During the course of kindling the metabolic activity of brain tissue can be revealed by 2-deoxyglucose autoradiography (Ackermann et al., 1986). In amygdala kindling, the increased metabolic rate corresponds well with the AD propagation recorded on EEG (Engel et al., 1978). Hippocampal kindling involves the amygdala and then proceeds the same way as amygdala kindling (Aihara et al., 1982). In hippocampal-kindled animals, the destruction of the amygdala results in retardation of kindling (McIntyre et al., 1982; Araki et al., 1985). This suggests that either amygdala has an active inhibitory role in hippocampal kindling or it is an obstacle to seizure spread. Nevertheless, the common output pathway may involve the piriform cortex (McIntyre & Kelly, 1990).

Immature animals

Conventional stimulation parameters (i.e. 60 Hz sine wave current for 1 s) can be used to elicit ADs and kindling in pups. Amygdala kindling was first demonstrated in rat pups, 15 days old (Moshé, 1981). In this age group, the AD threshold is higher than in adult rats (Moshé et al., 1981; Stark et al., 1986). The current intensity of 400 µA is commonly used for amygdala stimulation of rat pups (Moshé & Albala, 1982; Thompson et al., 1988). However, for 21–39-day-old (prepubescent and pubescent) rats, the AD threshold is lower than in younger or older rats (Moshé et al., 1981; Gilbert & Cain, 1982). Prepubescent pups require a greater number of stimulations than other age groups (Moshé et al., 1981). In 15-day-old pups, kindling occurs with 15 min intervals as well as 60 min intervals (Moshé et al., 1983; Lee et al., 1986; Stark et al., 1986). Twenty-four-hour intervals are also effective (Stark et al., 1986).

In rat pups, hippocampal kindling has a similar profile as amygdala kindling (Haas et al., 1990). Pups can be kindled with either short (15 min), or long (60 min) intervals using 60 Hz, 1 s long stimulation trains. Holmes & Thompson (1987) elicited both hippocampal and amygdala kindling using 10 Hz stimulation for 10 s every 5 min in 30-day-old pups. Michelson & Lothman (1991) demonstrated that rat pups aged 7 to 28 days can develop seizures when stimulated in the hippocampus with low frequency currents every 30 min.

Rat pups, 15–18 days old, are more susceptible to kindling than adult animals (Moshé et al., 1983), i.e. they develop seizures more rapidly. Indeed in the immature rat, the 2nd and 3rd week of postnatal life represents a period of increased sensitivity to seizures as shown by the increased efficacy of amygdala and hippocampal stimulations, although the AD threshold is much higher than in adult rats. Younger animals (7 days old) are more resistant to hippocampal stimulation (Velíšek & Mareš, 1991). It is possible, however, to elicit hippocampal ADs in this age group, although AD threshold is more than 10 times greater than that of adult rats (Mikolášová et al., unpublished). The study of Michelson & Lothman (1991) demonstrated successful hippocampal kindling in 7-day-old rat pups; however this age group was less capable of retaining the kindled effect than older rats. In amygdala kindling, the basolateral amygdala appears to be the initial kindling pacemaker (Ackermann et al., 1990). The amygdala ADs propagate to the contralateral amygdala and the striatum. Although electrographic ADs can be recorded in the substantia nigra, 2-deoxyglucose studies do not show any increase in glucose utilization in this structure. Hippocampal ADs (usually longer and often containing secondary AD) also propagate bilaterally, and to the substantia nigra and striatum. Even in the case of severe seizures, the metabolic activity remains restricted to limbic areas (Ackermann et al., 1989, 1990).

Motor expression of kindled seizures

Mature animals

The motor phenomena occurring during amygdala and hippocampal kindling in rats are best described by the five-point scale designed by Racine (1972b). Stages 0–2 (Table 1) represent focal seizures. By the time stage 3 (unilateral clonic seizures of the forelimb) occurs, the seizure activity involves the ipsilateral hemisphere including motor structures and/or paths. Stages 4 and 5 are characterized by bilateral clonic seizures; in stage 5, falling also occurs. In amygdala kindling, 10–14 stimulations are generally required before a stage 5 seizure occurs. Stage 5 is commonly considered to be the endpoint of kindling; the number of stimulations to reach this stage is referred to as the kindling rate. Pinel & Rovner (1978) proceeded with stimulations beyond stage 5 to demonstrate more severe seizures (Stages 6–8). They observed tonic-clonic seizures and eventually spontaneous seizures in animals receiving approximately 350 stimulations. These stages (6–8) are included in Table 1. Similar data were provided by Taber et al. (1977) in mice, where repeated hippocampal stimulations (60 Hz for 1 s, each 1 min) led to the alternating depression for 10–50 min, after which continuous status epilepticus lasting 165–195 min appeared.

Table 1. *Kindled seizures in adult rats and rat pups*

Stage	Adults	Pups
1	Chewing	Facial movements
2	Head nodding	Rhythmic head movements or turning of the body to stimulated site
3	Contralateral forelimb clonus	Unilateral forelimb clonus and ± hindlimb clonus; wet dog shakes
3.5		Alternating forelimb clonus
4	Bilateral symmetrical forelimb clonus, rearing	Bilateral forelimb clonus or rotatory movements of tonically extended forelimbs, rearing not consistent
5	Bilateral forelimb clonus rearing and falling over	Bilateral forelimb clonus, rearing, rare falling
6	Wild running and jumping with vocalization	Wild running and jumping with or without vocalization
7	Tonus	Tonus
8	Spontaneous seizures	Spontaneous seizures

Modified from Moshé et al. (1991).

It has been suggested that stages 0–5 involve forebrain and midbrain structures (Browning, 1985; Gale, 1988) whereas stages 6–8 involve further generalization of epileptiform activity to the lower brainstem (Browning, 1985; Browning & Nelson, 1986). The motor phenomena appearing during hippocampal kindling can also be scored according to the same five-point scale as amygdala kindling (Racine, 1972b). The kindling rate, however, is much slower; usually requiring 30–40 hippocampal stimulations (Racine et al., 1977).

Wet dog shakes are an interesting phenomenon that accompany both amygdala and hippocampal kindling (Lerner-Natoli et al., 1984). There is a difference in the frequency of wet dog shakes and the temporal profile of their appearance between amygdala and hippocampal kindling. In amygdala kindling, the number of wet dog shakes is a function of the AD duration (Squillance et al., 1980), whereas in hippocampal kindling the number of wet dog shakes decreases with repeated stimulations. Common for both kindled sites is that wet dog shakes disappear with generalizing of the epileptiform activity. Thus, wet dog shakes can be considered to be a measure of seizure generalization (Handley & Singh, 1986; Rondouin et al., 1987).

Immature animals

In prepubescent and pubescent rats (25–35 days old), the behavioural manifestations are the same as in adult rats. The behavioural phenomena seen in rat pups during amygdala kindling are age specific. Rat pups (15–18 days old) spend much less time in stages 0–2 than older rats. In stage 3.5, pups exhibit bilateral, alternating forelimb clonus; this may be a unique stage occuring in developing animals. Pups also display frequent wet dog shakes during the seizure. In stage 4, rat pups exhibit rotatory movements of rigidly held forelimbs and/or bilateral clonus; rearing is not consistent and falling is rare (Moshé et al., 1981). The pups remain for a long time in stage 4 (Moshé, 1981). Further stimulations result in the rapid emergence of stages 6 and 7 (Haas et al., 1990). Stage 6 is characterized by wild running and jumping with or without vocalization. The onset of stage 6 is of an explosive nature ('popcorn seizures', Haas et al., 1990). Stage 7 is represented by tonic seizures as in adults (Table 1). Spontaneous seizures have been reported but they are rare (Sperber et al., 1991). In rat pups, stages 6–8 can occur with 40 stimulations (Haas et al., 1990; Sperber et al., 1991).

In rat pups, hippocampal kindling elicits nearly the same pattern of seizures as amygdala kindling. During seizures frequent wet dog shakes occur. Although their number decreases with seizure generalization, they do not completely disappear. Wet dog shakes can be reliably induced in 7-day-old and older rats by hippocampal stimulation. In younger pups (5 days old) only non-coordinated, slow rotatory movements of the head were observed (Marešová & Mareš, 1988).

Immature rats (15 days old) have short refractory periods to kindling stimuli during and after the establishment of kindling (Moshé et al., 1983; Moshé & Albala, 1984). Consequently, these rats are more sensitive to the development of repetitive seizures and status epilepticus than adults. With maturation, the intensity of postictal refractoriness increases to adult levels, irrespective of any previous history of kindled convulsions (Moshé & Albala, 1984). The age-related changes in postictal refractoriness may reflect the maturational changes of the substantia nigra GABA-mediated seizure suppressing system (Moshé & Sperber, 1990).

Cellular level changes in the kindled focus

There are two principal questions concerning cellular changes in the kindling process in adult and developing animals:

(1) Which neuronal (circuit, neurotransmitter, receptor, etc.) changes are the substrates for the development and permanence of kindling? (for extensive review, see Racine & McIntyre, 1986);

(2) Which neuronal changes are responsible for the different course of kindling in immature animals?

Mature animals

Early morphological studies of the kindled focus failed to reveal any damage other than that associated with the insertion of the electrodes (Goddard et al., 1969; Goddard & Douglas, 1975). In an ultrastructural morphological study, Hovorka et al. (1989) demonstrated that there is a redistribution of synaptic vesicles in the presynaptic terminals of excitatory synapses in the dentate gyrus of entorhinal cortex kindled rats compared to controls. The vesicles were concentrated close to the presynaptic membrane instead of being randomly distributed throughout the synaptic bouton. This may increase the amount of neurotransmitter available for neurotransmission. Unfortunately, the study did not deal with the character of neurotransmitter involved. In a recent paper, Geinisman et al. (1990) demonstrated an increased ratio of perforated to nonperforated synapses in stimulated axons in dentate gyrus following perforant path kindling. The dimensions of postsynaptic densities of perforated synapses were also increased.

The hypothesis that kindling may be associated with long-term potentiation (LTP) has not been substantiated. Several studies have revealed that structures prone to kindling provide no LTP to target sites. For example, the hippocampus is kindled slowly whereas it displays strong LTP. The development of kindling requires ADs, whereas LTP can be induced without ADs (McIntyre & Racine, 1986). There are several neurotransmitter systems which were shown to be changed in the kindled focus. Burchfiel et al. (1979) demonstrated that electrically-induced hippocampal ADs produce a state of supersensitivity to microiontophoretically applied acetylcholine. Subconvulsive doses of cholinergic agents potentiate electrical kindling (Vosu & Wise, 1975; Wasterlain & Jonec, 1983). Moreover, atropine (a muscarinic cholinergic antagonist) causes an increase in the rate of electrical kindling.

Catecholamines may have both promoting and suppressing effects on kindling. Spehlmann & Norcross (1984) found that the depression of glutamate-induced firing elicited by catecholamines was significantly reduced after an AD. Depletion of norepinephrine enhances the development of generalized kindled seizures (McIntyre et al., 1979; McIntyre, 1980; Corcoran & Mason, 1980; Albala et al., 1986). Furthermore, systemic epinephrine causes retardation of amygdala-kindled seizures (Welsh & Gold, 1986).

The role of GABA has also been investigated. Kamphuis et al. (1986) demonstrated a decrease in the number of GABA immunoreactive-positive cell bodies in the CA1 region of the kindled hippocampus. Morimoto & Goddard (1986) suggested that kindling propagation may be associated with collapsed GABAergic recurrent inhibition. However, Burchfiel et al. (1979) did not find any changes in GABAergic transmission following an AD.

There is little data on the role of glutamate and aspartate in kindling. Leach et al. (1985) demonstrated that under veratridine stimulation, slices from previously kindled cortex release more glutamate and aspartate than controls.

Opiates when repeatedly injected to the hippocampus and amygdala elicit ADs and subsequently kindling (Cain & Corcoran, 1984). On the other hand, systemic administration of morphine (opiate agonist) or naloxone (opiate antagonist) did not change AD thresholds (Frenk et al., 1979).

Immature animals

Immature neurons exhibit different properties than mature neurons. Neurons of immature rats have high input resistance, as well as specific resistivity, and generate long action potentials (Schwartzkroin, 1984; Swann et al., 1990). Their membranes may contain limited number of voltage dependent channels causing the inward and outward currents to be of equal strength. This may account for the high AD thresholds (Prince & Gutnick, 1972; Kriegstein et al., 1987).

Synapses may play also an important role in the developmental differences of kindling. Electrical synapses are abundant in the young CNS and their number decreases with age (Connors et al., 1983; Kriegstein et al., 1987). There is also evidence that early in life asymmetric (presumably excitatory) synapses prevail whereas symmetric (presumably inhibitory) synapses increase during development. The biological markers of the inhibitory transmitter GABA increase during the development although there are regional differences (Schwartzkroin, 1982; Schwartzkroin et al., 1982; Seress & Ribak, 1988; Swann et al., 1989).

The late development of inhibitory processes may account in part for the rapid emergence of kindled seizures in 15–18-day-old pups. The difference in motor patterns observed between rat pups and adults may be caused by incomplete myelination, which occurs first in phylogenetically older parts of the brain and later in the callosal fibres and frontopontine tract (Davison, 1970; Agrawal & Davison, 1973). Appearance of stage 5 seizures is rare in pups as well as in adults with prefrontal lesions (Corcoran et al., 1976). This suggests that the prefrontal cortex may be involved in the expression of stage 5 seizures.

Depletion of norepinephrine accelerates kindling in adults (McIntyre et al., 1979) as well as in pubescent rats (Michelson & Butterbaugh, 1985; Konkol et al., 1990). The acceleration affects early kindling stages reminiscent of the rapid progression of kindling in 15–18-day-old pups, where the levels of norepinephrine are lower than in adults (Moshé et al., 1981; Konkol et al., 1990). In a recent paper, Gorter et al. (1990) demonstrated that norepinephrine supersensitivity, elicited by repeated clonidine (norepinephrine agonist) administration to newborn rats, retards kindling in adulthood. Hormonal influences may also play a role. Holmes & Weber (1984, 1986) demonstrated that steroid hormones (including gonadal) may suppress kindling as a function of age.

Role of substantia nigra in kindling

Iadarola & Gale (1982) reported that pharmacological treatments that increase the GABA transmission in the substantia nigra can suppress a variety of experimentally induced seizures in adult rats. Kindled seizures can be also controlled by substantia nigra (Le Gal La Salle *et al.*, 1983; McNamara *et al.*, 1984). Are there any age related differences?

Mature animals

Utilizing 2-deoxyglucose mapping, Engel *et al.* (1978) demonstrated the involvement of substantia nigra in kindling. Bonhaus *et al.* (1986) showed that during an electrographic AD, the firing pattern of the substantia nigra pars reticulata neurons changes dramatically. The cells fire in bursts, but the overall firing rate diminishes during the electrographic seizure. This suggests that there is increased GABA release which results in decreased activity of the GABA-sensitive nigral outputs (for review see Moshé & Sperber, 1990). This decrease of nigral outputs is similar to that observed with local microinfusions of the GABA agonists, muscimol and gamma-vinyl-GABA, which can suppress kindled seizures (Le Gal La Salle *et al.*, 1983; McNamara *et al.*, 1984). Electrical stimulation of the substantia nigra has been also reported to decrease the severity of kindled seizures (Morimoto & Goddard, 1987). Thus the substantia nigra appears to be a crucial site for the expression and control of kindled seizures in adult rats.

Immature animals

Deoxyglucose autoradiographic studies have not revealed increased metabolic activity in the substantia nigra of amygdala or hippocampal kindled pups (Ackermann *et al.*, 1982, 1989; Moshé 1989). Recent studies demonstrated that there are differences in the functional activity of the nigral GABA system between adults and 15–16-day-old pups. In rat pups, there is a site-specific paucity of high-affinity muscimol ($GABA_A$) binding sites in substantia nigra while there are no differences in the number of low-affinity muscimol ($GABA_A$) binding sites in comparison to adult rats (Wurpel *et al.*, 1988). Furthermore, in the immature substantia nigra, there is an increased density of $GABA_B$ receptors (Garant *et al.*, in press). Accordingly, the effects of various GABA agonists on seizures are age-specific (Moshé & Sperber, 1990). Recent data suggest that there may also be developmental differences in the composition of the nigral $GABA_A$ receptors in terms of functional isoforms. These isoforms may account, in part, for maturational differences in $GABA_A$-mediated substantia nigra based seizure control (Xu *et al.*, 1991 a,b). The abundance of nigral $GABA_B$ receptors early in life may also account for the ability of baclofen to suppress the development of kindling and kindled seizures in 15-day-old rat pups (Wurpel *et al.*, 1990).

Permanence of kindling and kindling antagonism

Mature animals

Kindling, once established, appears to be permanent (Goddard *et al.*, 1969; McIntyre & Racine, 1986). Several factors have been implicated, although the precise mechanism has not been identified. There are long-lasting changes in several neurotransmitter systems such as decreased activity of tyrosine-hydroxylase, the catecholamine synthesis enzyme in the kindling focus (Farjo & Blackwood, 1978); changes in somatostatin receptors (Higuchi *et al.*, 1986) and also alterations in calcium-dependent enzymes in the hippocampus (Wasterlain *et al.*, 1986). Amygdala kindling selectively decreases PCP/sigma receptors in the hippocampus (Sircar *et al.*, 1988); however, PCP receptor ligands can suppress fully kindled seizures without affecting the AD threshold (McNamara *et al.*, 1990). Several neuroanatomical changes have been also demonstrated. Hovorka *et al.* (1989)

highlighted the increased density of synaptic vesicles in the area adjacent to the synaptic cleft in rats following kindling. It is not clear, however, whether this phenomenon represents a basis for the kindling process or its consequences, which help to maintain kindling permanence. Another morphological approach is represented by the Timm-Haug Silver Stain (Timm, 1958; Danscher et al., 1976). It is used to demonstrate synaptic sprouting of mossy fibre terminals in the hippocampus. In adult amygdala-kindled rats, Timm staining revealed synaptic reorganization in the dentate area (Feldblum & Ackermann, 1987; Sutula et al., 1988; Sperber et al., 1990). A similar reorganization was revealed in the hippocampus of patients with complex partial seizures (Babb et al., 1988; Sutula et al., 1989).

It appears that the permanence of kindling is maintained by a combination of complex mechanisms. Once established, it is extremely difficult to abolish, suggesting that the vulnerability of all complex kindling mechanisms together is extremely low (Hiyoshi & Wada, 1990). This conclusion is supported by the study of Handforth (1982). He found that during the course of kindling the electroshock treatments increase the kindling rate from 7.6 to 22.2 stimulations whereas in fully kindled animals only an increase in seizures threshold (of 150–200 µA) was observed. This suggests that it may be easier to stop the kindling process before it is fully established. This conclusion is also supported by another phenomenon: kindling antagonism. In adult rats, Burchfiel et al. (1982) described that concurrent kindling of two limbic foci by alternating stimulations, results in the suppression of generalized seizures from one or both sites. Additional studies established a principal role for norepinephrine in kindling antagonism (Applegate et al., 1986, 1987; Applegate & Burchfiel, 1990). The influence of other transmitter systems, however, cannot be excluded.

Immature animals

Kindling in young animals persists into adulthood. Rats, kindled as pups, are more susceptible to the development of kindled or pentylenetetrazol seizures as adults (Moshé & Albala, 1982; Holmes & Weber, 1983). In adult animals, kindled seizures can be easily elicited from a previously kindled site (Moshé & Albala, 1982) or from the contralateral site (Moshé & Albala, 1983). This enhancement of seizures in adulthood following postnatal kindling is not due to neuronal trauma or glial scarring, as demonstrated with sham-operated controls (Moshé & Albala, 1982, 1983). Furthermore, in developing rats, the permanence of kindling is not associated with synaptic reorganization in the dentate area (Sperber et al., 1990). The persistence of kindling into adulthood appears to be related to the number of kindled seizures in infancy. The critical number is probably four seizures of mild symptomatology, i.e. stages 0–2 (Moshé & Albala, 1982).

A recent paper of Shouse et al. (1990) describes the development of spontaneous epilepsy in immature kindled kittens: the younger the animal the higher the probability of appearance of spontaneous seizures. These results are in concordance with the data showing that rat pups do not demonstrate kindling antagonism to the development of generalized seizures when stimulated between amygdala and ipsi- or contralateral hippocampus or between two amygdala (Haas et al., 1990; Sperber et al., 1991).

Why it is important to study kindling during development

Kindling represents a valuable model for understanding the basic mechanisms of progressive epileptogenesis and for testing new anticonvulsant drugs. Kindling, however, is rare in man: only three reports of kindling in humans have been reported (Monroe, 1970; Šramka et al., 1977; Dhuna et al., 1991). However, newly formed synaptogenesis similar to that observed in kindled animals was observed in patients with partial complex seizures (Babb et al., 1988; Sutula et al., 1989). Epileptogenesis is much more pronounced in young people (Gibbs & Gibbs, 1963) and kindling studies may in part answer why. Kindling studies can bypass some of the difficulties of pharmacokinetics resulting from systemic administration of convulsants. Kindling should be critically assessed when used to study the effect of antiepileptic drugs because of a possible change of cerebral pharmacokinetics resulting from a damaged blood–brain barrier. Nevertheless, unlike *in vitro* studies in cultured neurons and/or cerebral tissue slices, kindling preserves the integrity of the entire brain circuitry. This difference is extremely important because drug neurotransmitter and/or receptor system effects may be substantially different in the single neuron, in the limited circuits present in the slice and in the entire brain.

Acknowledgements

Supported by American Epilepsy Society Research Fellowship (L.S.V.), American Epilepsy Society Research Grant (E.F.S.) and NIH Grant NS-20253 from the NINDS (S.L.M.)

References

Ackermann, R.F., Chugani, H.T., Handforth, A., Moshé, S.L., Caldecott-Hazard, S. & Engel, J.Jr. (1986): Autoradiographic studies of cerebral metabolism and blood flow in rat amygdala kindling. In: *Kindling 3*, ed. J.A. Wada, pp. 73–87. New York: Raven Press.

Ackermann, R.F., Moshé, S.L. & Albala, B.J. (1989): Restriction of enhanced [^{14}C]-2-deoxyglucose utilization to rhinencephalic structures in immature amygdala-kindled rats. *Exp. Neurol.* **104**, 73–81.

Ackermann, R.F., Moshé, S.L., Albala, B.J. & Engel, J.Jr. (1982): Anatomical substrates of amygdala kindling in immature rats demonstrated by 2-deoxyglucose autoradiography. *Epilepsia* **23**, 434–435.

Ackermann, R.F., Sperber, E.F., Haas, K.Z. & Moshé, S.L. (1990): Anatomical substrates of severe kindled seizures in immature rats: a radiolabeled deoxyglucose and glucose study. *Epilepsia* **31**, 676.

Agrawal, H.C. & Davison, A.N. (1973): Myelination and aminoacid imbalance in the developing brain. In: *Biochemistry of the developing brain*, Vol. 1, ed. W. Himwich. pp. 143–168. New York: Marcel Dekker.

Aihara, H., Araki, H. & Ohzeki, M. (1982): Hippocampal kindling and effects of antiepileptic drugs. *Jap. J. Pharmacol.* **32**, 37–45.

Albala, B.J., Moshé, S.L., Cubells, J.F., Sharpless, N.S., & Makman, M.H. (1986): Unilateral perisubstantia nigra catecholaminergic lesion and amygdala kindling. *Brain Res.* **370**, 388–392.

Applegate, C.D. & Burchfiel, J.L. (1990): Evidence for a norepinephrine-dependent brainstem substrate in the development of kindling antagonism. *Epilepsy Res.* **6**, 23–32.

Applegate, C.D., Burchfiel, J.L., & Konkol, J.L. (1986): Kindling antagonism: effects of norepinephrine depletion on kindled seizure suppression after concurrent, alternate stimulation in rats. *Exp. Neurol.* **94**, 379–390.

Applegate, C.D., Konkol, R.J., & Burchfiel, J.L. (1987): Kindling antagonism: a role for hindbrain norepinephrine in the development of site suppression following concurrent alternate stimulation. *Brain Res.* **407**, 212–222.

Araki, H., Aihara, H., Watanabe, S., Yamamoto, T. & Ueki, S. (1985): Role of the amygdala in the hippocampal kindling effect of rats. *Jap. J. Pharmacol.* **37**, 173–179.

Babb, T.L., Kupfer, W.R. & Pretorius, J.K. (1988): Recurrent excitatory circuits by 'sprouted' mossy fibers into the fascia dentata of human hippocampal epilepsy. *Epilepsia* **29**, 674.

Bonhaus, D.W., Walters, J.R. & McNamara, J.O. (1986): Activation of substantia nigra neurons: role in the propagation of seizures in kindled rats. *J. Neurosci.* **6**, 3024–3030.

Browning, R.A. (1985): Role of the brain-stem reticular formation in tonic-clonic seizures: lesion and pharmacological studies. *Fed. Proc.* **44**, 2425–2431.

Browning, R.A. & Nelson, D.K. (1986): Variation in threshold and pattern of electroshock-induced seizures in rats depending on site of stimulation. *Life Sci.* **37**, 2205–2211.

Burchfiel, J.L., Duchowny, M.S. & Duffy, F.H. (1979): Neuronal supersensitivity to acetylcholine induced by kindling in the rat hippocampus. *Science* **204**, 1096–1098.

Burchfiel, J.L., Serpa, K.A. & Duffy, F. (1982): Further studies of antagonism of seizure development between concurrently developing kindled limbic foci in the rat. *Exp. Neurol.* **73**, 476–489.

Cain, D.P. (1983): Bidirectional transfer of electrical and carbachol kindling. *Brain Res.* **260**, 135–138.

Cain, D.P. & Corcoran, M.E. (1981): Kindling with low frequency stimulation: generality, transfer and recruiting effects. *Exp. Neurol.* **73**, 219–232.

Cain, D.P. & Corcoran, M.E. (1984): Intracerebral beta-endorphin, Met-enkephalin and morphine: kindling of seizures and handling-induced potentiation of epileptiform effects. *Life Sci.* **34**, 2535–2542.

Collins, R.C. (1978): Kindling of neuroanatomic pathways during recurrent focal penicillin seizures. *Brain Res.* **150**, 503–517.

Connors, B.W., Bernardo, L.S. & Prince, D.A. (1983): Coupling between neurons of the developing rat neocortex. *J. Neurosci.* **3**, 773–782.

Corcoran, M.E. & Cain D.P. (1980): Kindling of seizures with low frequency electrical stimulation. *Brain Res.* **196**, 262–265.

Corcoran M.E., & Mason, S.T. (1980): Role of forebrain catecholamines in amygdaloid kindling. *Brain Res.* **190**, 473–484.

Corcoran, M.E., Urstad, H., McCaughran, J.A. & Wada, J. (1976): Frontal lobe and kindling in the rat. In: *Kindling*, ed. J. Wada, pp. 215–225. New York: Raven Press.

Danscher, G., Fjerdingstad, E.J., Fjerdingstad, E. & Fredens, K. (1976): Heavy metal content in subdivisions of the rat hippocampus (zinc, lead and copper). *Brain Res.* **112**, 442–446.

Davison, A.N. (1970): The biochemistry of the myelin sheath. In: *Myelination*, eds. A.N. Davison & A. Peters, pp. 80–161. Springfield, IL: Charles C. Thomas.

Delgado, J.M.R. & Sevillano, M. (1961): Evolution of repeated hippocampal seizures in the cat. *Electroencephalogr. Clin. Neurophysiol.* **13**, 722–733.

Dhuna, A., Pascual-Leone, A. & Langendorf, F. (1991): Chronic, habitual cocaine abuse and kindling: a case report. *Epilepsia* **32**, 890–894.

Diehl, R.G., Smialowski, A. & Gotwo, T. (1984): Development and persistence of kindled seizures after repeated injections of pentylenetetrazol in rats and guinea pigs. *Epilepsia* **25**, 506–510.

Dyer, R.S., Swartzwelder, H.S., Eccles, C.U. & Annau, Z. (1979): Hippocampal afterdischarges and their post-ictal sequelae in rats: a potential tool for assessment of CNS neurotoxicity. *Neurobehav. Toxicol.* **1**, 5–19.

Engel, J.Jr., Wolfson, L. & Brown, L. (1978): Anatomical correlates of electrical and behavioural events related to amygdaloid kindling. *Ann. Neurol.* **3**, 538–544.

Fagg, G.E., Foster, A.C. & Ganong, A.H. (1986): Excitatory amino acid synaptic mechanism and neurological function. *Trends Pharmacol. Sci.* **7**, 357–363.

Farjo, I.B. & Blackwood, D.H. (1978): Reduction in tyrosine hydroxylase activity in the rat amygdala induced by kindling stimulation. *Brain Res.* **153**, 423–426.

Feldblum, S. & Ackermann, R.F. (1987): Increased susceptibility to hippocampal and amygdala kindling following intraperitoneal kainic acid. *Exp. Neurol.* **97**, 255–269.

Frenk, H., Engel, J.Jr., Ackermann, R.F., Shavit, Y. & Liebeskind, J.C. (1979): Endogenous opioids may mediate postictal behavioural depression in amygdaloid-kindled rats. *Brain Res.* **167**, 435–440.

Gale, K. (1988): Progression and generalization of seizure discharge: anatomical and neurochemical substrates. *Epilepsia* **29**, (Suppl. 2), S15–S34.

Garant, D.S., Sperber, E.F. & Moshé, S.L. The density of GABA(B) binding sites in the substantia nigra is greater in rat pups than in adults. *Eur. J. Pharmacol.*, in press.

Geinisman, Y., Morrell, F. & deToledo-Morrell, L. (1990): Alterations of synaptic ultrastructure induced by hippocampal kindling. In: *Kindling*, Vol. 4, ed. J.A. Wada, pp. 75–92. New York: Plenum Press.

Gibbs, F.A. & Gibbs, E.L. (1963): Age factor in epilepsy. *N. Engl. J. Med.* **269**, 1230–1236.

Gilbert, M.E. & Cain, D.P. (1982): A developmental study of kindling in the rat. *Develop. Brain Res.* **2**, 321–328.

Goddard, G.V. (1967): Development of epileptic seizures through brain stimulation at low intensity. *Nature* **204**, 1020–1021.

Goddard, G.V. & Douglas, R.M. (1975): Does the engram of kindling model the engram of long-term memory? *Can. J. Neurol. Sci.* **2**, 385–394.

Goddard, G.V., McIntyre, D.C. & Leech, C.K. (1969): A permanent change in brain function resulting from daily electrical stimulation. *Exp. Neurol.* **25**, 295–330.

Gorter, J.A., Kamphuis, W., Huisman, E., Bos, N.P. & Mirmiran, M. (1990): Neonatal clonidine treatment results in long-lasting changes in noradrenaline sensitivity and kindling epileptogenesis. *Brain Res.* **535**, 62–66.

Green, J.D. & Shimamoto, T. (1953): Hippocapal seizures and their propagation. *A.M.A. Arch. Neurol. Psychiat.* **70**, 687–702.

Haas, K.Z., Sperber, E.F. & Moshé, S.L. (1990): Kindling in developing animals: expression of severe seizures and enhanced development of bilateral foci. *Develop. Brain Res.* **56**, 275–280.

Handforth, A. (1982): Postseizure inhibition of kindled seizures by electroconvulsive shock. *Exp. Neurol.* **78**, 483–491.

Handley, S.L. & Singh, L. Neurotransmitters and shaking behaviour – more than a 'gut-bath' for the brain. *Trends Pharmacol. Sci.* **7**, 324–328.

Higuchi, T., Kato, N., Noguchi, T., Friesen, H.G. & Wada, J.A. (1986): Kindling and somatostatin, In: *Kindling*, Vol. 3, ed. J.A. Wada, pp. 349–359. New York: Raven Press.

Hiyoshi, T. & Wada, J.A. (1990): Failure of nine-month phenobarbital administration to reverse amygdaloid-kindled seizure susceptibility in cats. *Ann. Neurol.* **28**, 568–573.

Holmes, G.L. (1983): Effect of serial seizures on subsequent kindling in the immature brain. *Dev. Brain Res.* **6**, 190–192.

Holmes, G.L. & Thompson, J.L. (1987): Rapid kindling in the prepubescent rat. *Dev. Brain Res.* **36**, 281–284.

Holmes, G.L. & Thompson, J.L. (1988): Effects of serial administratrion of kainic acid on the developing brain. *Neuropharmacology* **27**, 209–212.

Holmes, G.L. & Weber, D.A. (1983): Increased susceptibility to pentylenetetrazol-induced seizures in adult rats following electrical kindling during brain development. *Dev. Brain Res.* **11**, 312–314.

Holmes, G.L. & Weber, D.A. (1984): The effect of progesterone on kindling: a developmental study. *Dev. Brain Res.* **16**, 45–53.

Holmes, G.L. & Weber, D.A (1986): Effects of ACTH on seizure susceptibility in the developing brain. *Ann. Neurol.* **20**, 82–88.

Hovorka, J., Langmeier, M. & Mareš, P. (1989): Are there morphological changes in presynaptic terminals of kindled rats? *Neurosci. Lett.* **107**, 179–183.

Iadarola, M.J. & Gale, K. (1982): Substantia nigra: site of anticonvulsant activity mediated by gamma-aminobutyric acid. *Science* **218**, 1237–1240.

Kaada, B.R. (1951): Somato-motor, autonomic and electrocorticographic responses to electrical stimulation of 'rhinencephalic' and other structures in primates, cat and dog. *Acta. Physiol. Scand.* **24** (Suppl. 83), 1–285.

Kamphuis, W., Wadman, W.J., Buijs, R.M. & Lopes da Silva, F.H. (1986): Decrease in number of hippocampal gamma-aminobutyric acid (GABA) immunoreactive cells in the rat kindling model of epilepsy. *Exp. Brain Res.* **64**, 491–495.

Konkol, R.J., Holmes, G.L. & Thompson, J.L. (1990): The effect of regional differences in noradrenergic neuron growth patterns on juvenile kindling. *Dev. Brain Res.* **52**, 25–29.

Kriegstein, A.R., Suppes, T. & Prince, D.A. (1987): Cellular and synaptic physiology and epileptogenesis of the developing rat neocortical neurons in vitro. *Dev. Brain Res.* **34**, 161–171.

Leach, M.J., Marden, C.M., Miller, A.A., O'Donnell, R.A. & Weston, S.B. (1985): Changes in cortical amino acids during electrical kindling. *Neuropharmacology* **24**, 937–940.

Lee, S., Kawawaki, H., Matsuoka, O. & Murata, R. (1986): Effects of Ca-antagonist (flunarizine) on kindling seizures in suckling rats. *No To Hattatsu* **18**, 292–298.

Le Gal La Salle, G. (1979): Kindling of motor seizures from the bed nucleus of stria terminalis. *Exp. Neurol.* **66**, 309–318.

Le Gal La Salle, G., Kaijima, M. & Feldblum, S. (1983): Abortive amygdaloid kindled seizures following microinjection of gamma-vinyl-GABA in the vicinity of substantia nigra in rats. *Neurosci. Lett.* **36**, 69–74.

Lerner-Natoli, M., Rondouin, G. & Baldy-Moulinier, M. (1984): Evolution of wet dog shakes during kindling in rats: comparison between hippocampal and amygdala kindling. *Exp. Neurol.* **83**, 1–12.

Lothman, E.W., Hatlelid, J.M., Zorumski, C.F., Conry, J.A., Moon, P.F. & Perlin, J.B. (1985): Kindling with rapidly recurring hippocampal seizures. *Brain Res.* **360**, 83–91.

Mason, C.R. & Cooper, R.M. (1972): A permanent change in convulsive threshold in normal amd brain damaged rats with repeated small doses of pentylenetetrazol. *Epilepsia* **13**, 663–674.

McIntyre, D.C. (1980): Amygdala kindling in rats: facilitation after local amygdala norepinephrine depletion with 6-hydroxydopamine. *Exp. Neurol.* **69**, 395–407.

McIntyre, D.C. & Kelly, M.E. (1990): Is the pyriform cortex important for limbic kindling? In: *Kindling*, Vol. 4, ed. J.A. Wada, pp. 21–31. New York: Plenum Press.

McIntyre, D.C. & Racine, R.J. (1986): Kindling mechanisms: Current progress on an experimental epilepsy model. *Prog. Neurobiol.* **27**, 1–12.

McIntyre, D.C., Rajalla, J. & Edson, N. (1987): Supression of amygdala kindling with short interstimulus intervals: effect of norepinephrine depletion. *Exp. Neurol.* **95**, 391–402.

McIntyre, D.C., Saari, M. & Pappas, B.A. (1979): Potentiation of amygdala kindling in adult or infant rats by injection of 6-hydroxydopamine. *Exp. Neurol.* **63**, 527–544.

McIntyre, D.C., Stuckey, G.N. & Stokes, K.A. (1982): Effects of amygdala lesions on dorsal hippocampus kindling in rats. *Exp. Neurol.* **75**, 184–190.

McNamara, J.O., Bonhaus, D.W., Nadler, J.V. & Yeh, G.C. (1990): *N*-methyl-D-apsartate (NMDA) receptors and the kindling model. In: *Kindling*, Vol. 4, ed. J.A. Wada, pp. 197–208. New York: Plenum Press.

McNamara, J.O., Galloway, M.T., Rigsbee, L.L. & Shin, C. (1984): Evidence implicating substantia nigra in regulation of kindled seizure threshold. *J. Neurosci.* **4**, 2410–2417.

Mareš, J., Mareš, P. & Trojan, S. (1980): The ontogenesis of cortical self-sustained after-disharges in rats. *Epilepsia* **21**, 111–121.

Mareš, J., Mareš, P. & Trojan, S. (1982): Ontogenesis of cortical self-sustained after-discharges (SSADs) elicited by 50-Hz stimulation in rats. *Physiol. Bohemoslov.* **31**, 270–271.

Mareš, J., Beneš, P., Mareš, P. & Trojan, S. (1983): Influence of certain stimulation parameters on the character of the cortical self-sustained after-discharge. *Physiol. Bohemoslov.* **32**, 30–37.

Mareš, P., Chocholová, L. & Langmeier, M. (1985): Epileptic after-discharges induced by hippocampal stimulation in rats. *Physiol. Bohemoslov.* **34** (Suppl.), 109–112.

Mareš, P. & Marešová, D. (1987): Piracetam blocks initial kindling in the rat. *Activ. Nerv. Super. (Praha)* **29**, 218–219.

Marešová, D. & Mareš, P. (1988): Ontogenetic development of wet dog shakes accompanying hippocampal epileptic after-discharges in rats. *Activ. Nerv. Super. (Praha)* **30**, 254.

Michelson, H.B. & Butterbaugh, G.G. (1985): Amygdala kindling in juvenile rats following administration of 6-hydroxydopamine. *Exp. Neurol.* **90**, 588–593.

Michelson, H.B. & Lothman, E.W. (1991): An ontogenetic study of kindling using rapidly recurring hippocampal seizures. *Dev. Brain Res.* **61**, 79–85.

Minabe, Y., Tanii, Y., Kadono, Y., Tsutsumi, M. & Nakamura, I. (1986): Low frequency kindling as a new experimental model of epilepsy. *Exp. Neurol.* **94**, 317–323.

Monroe, R.R. (1970): *Episodic behavioural disorders: a psychodynamic and neurophysiological analysis*, pp. 76–77. Cambridge: Harvard University Press.

Morimoto, K. & Goddard, G.V. (1986): Kindling induced changes in EEG recorded during stimulation from the site of stimulation: collapse of GABA-mediated inhibition and onset of rhythmic synchronous burst. *Exp. Neurol.* **94**, 571–584.

Morimoto, K. & Goddard, G.V. (1987): The substantia nigra is an important site for the containment of seizure generalization in the kindling model of epilepsy. *Epilepsia* **28**, 1–10.

Moshé, S.L. (1981): The effects of age on the kindling phenomenon. *Dev. Psychobiol.* **14**, 75–81.

Moshé, S.L. (1989): Ontogeny of seizures and substantia nigra modulation. In: *Problems and concepts in developing neurophysiology*, eds. P.K. Kellaway, J.L. Noebels & D.P. Purpura, pp. 247–262. Baltimore: Johns Hopkins Press.

Moshé, S.L. & Albala, B.J. (1982): Kindling in developing rats: persistence of seizures into adulthood. *Dev. Brain Res.* **4**, 67–71.

Moshé, S.L. & Albala, B.J. (1983): Maturational changes in postictal refractoriness and seizure susceptibility in developing rats. *Ann. Neurol.* **13**, 552–557.

Moshé, S.L., Albala, B.J., Ackermann, R.F. & Engel, J.Jr. (1983): Increased seizure susceptibility of the immature brain. *Dev. Brain Res.* **7**, 81–85.

Moshé, S.L. & Albala, B.J. (1984): Nigral muscimol infusions facilitate the development of seizures in immature rats. *Dev. Brain Res.* **13**, 305–308.

Moshé, S.L., Sharpless, N.S. & Kaplan, J. (1981): Kindling in developing rats: variability of afterdischarge thresholds with age. *Brain Res.* **211**, 190–195.

Moshé, S.L. & Sperber, E.F. (1990): Substantia nigra-mediated control of generalized seizures. In: *Generalized epilepsy: cellular, molecular and pharmacological approaches*, eds. P. Gloor, R. Kostopoulos, R. Naquet & M. Avoli, pp. 355–367. Boston: Birkhauser Inc.

Moshé, S.L., Sperber, E.F. & Albala, B.J. (1991): Kindling as a model of epilepsy in developing animals. In: *Kindling and synaptic plasticity. The legacy of Graham Goddard,* ed. F. Morrell, pp. 177–194. Boston: Birkhauser Inc.

Mucha, R.F. & Pinel, J.P.J. (1977): Postseizure inhibition of kindled seizures. *Exp. Neurol.* **54**, 266–282.

Ono, K. (1983): Dynamic propagation of seizure discharges in the motor cortical kindling. *Int. J. Neurosci.* **21**, 175–182.

Peterson, S.L., Albertson, T.E. & Stark, L.G. (1981): Intertrial intervals and kindled seizures. *Exp. Neurol.* **71**, 144–153.

Pinel, J.P.J. & Rovner, L.I. (1978): Electrode placement and kindling-induced experimental epilepsy. *Exp. Neurol.* **58**, 335–346.

Piredda, S., Yonekawa, W., Whittingham, T.S. & Kupferberg, H.J. (1986): Enhanced bursting activity in the CA3 region of the mouse hippocampal slice without long-term potentiation in the dentate gyrus after systemic pentylenetetrazole kindling. *Exp. Neurol.* **94**, 659–669.

Pohl, M. & Mareš, P. (1990): Localization of the origin of self-sustained after-discharges (SSADs) in the rat: the serrated wave (SerW) type of SSAD. *Physiol. Bohemoslov.* **39**, 335–342.

Pohl, M., Mareš, P. & Langmeier, M. (1986): Localization of the origin of self-sustained after-discharges (SSADs) in the rat. I. The spike-and-wave (S+W) type of SSAD. *Epilepsia* **27**, 516–522.

Post, R.M. (1977): Progressive changes in behavior and seizures following chronic cocaine administration: relationship to kindling and psychosis. *Adv. Behav. Biol.* **21**, 353–372.

Post, R.M., Kopanda, R.T. & Lee, A. (1975): Progressive behavioural changes during chronic lidocaine administration: relationship to kindling. *Life Sci.* **17**, 943–950.

Prince, D.A. & Gutnick, M.J. (1972): Neuronal activities in epileptogenic foci of immature cortex. *Brain Res.* **45**, 455–468.

Racine, R.J. (1972a): Modification of seizure activity by electrical stimulation: I. after-discharge threshold. *Electroencephalogr. Clin. Neurophysiol.* **32**, 269–279.

Racine, R.J. (1972b): Modification of seizure activity by electrical stimulation: II. motor seizures. *Electroencephalogr. Clin. Neurophysiol.* **32**, 281–294.

Racine, R.J. (1978): Kindling: the first decade. *Neurosurgery* **3**, 234–252.

Racine, R.J., Burnham, M.W., Gartner, J.G. & Levitan, D. (1973): Rates of motor seizure development in rats subjected to electrical brain stimulation: strain and interstimulus interval effects. *Electroencephalogr. Clin. Neurophysiol.* **55**, 553–556.

Racine, R.J. & McIntyre, D. (1986): Mechanisms of kindling: a current view. In: *The limbic system: functional organization and clinical disorders,* eds. B.K. Doane & K.E. Livingston. pp. 109–121. New York: Raven Press.

Racine, R.J., Rose, P.A. & Burnham, W.M. (1977): Afterdischarge thresholds and kindling rates in dorsal and ventral hippocampus and dentate gyrus. *Can. J. Neurol. Sci.* **4**, 273–278.

Rondouin, G., Lerner-Natoli, M. & Hashizume, A. (1987): Wet dog shakes in limbic versus generalized seizures. *Exp. Neurol.* **95**, 500–505.

Schwartzkroin, P.A. (1982): Development of rabbit hippocampus; physiology. *Dev. Brain Res.* **2**, 469–486.

Schwartzkroin, P.A. (1984): Epileptogenesis in the immature CNS. In: *Electrophysiology of epilepsy,* eds. P.A. Schwartzkroin & H.V. Wheal, pp. 389–412. New York: Academic Press.

Schwartzkroin, P.A., Kunkel, D.D. & Mathers, L.H. (1982): Development of rabbit hippocampus; anatomy. *Dev. Brain Res.* **2**, 452–468.

Seress, L. & Ribak, C.E. (1988): The development of GABAergic neurons in the rat hippocampal formation: an immunocytochemical study. *Dev. Brain Res.* **44**, 197–210.

Shouse, M.N., King, A., Langer, J., Vreeken, T., King, K. & Richkind, M. (1990): The ontogeny of feline temporal lobe epilepsy: kindling a spontaneous seizure disorder in kittens. *Brain Res.* **525**, 215–224.

Sircar, R., Ludvig, N., Moshé, S.L. & Zukin, S.R. (1988): Modulation of the N-methyl-D-aspartate-phencyclidine receptor complex following amygdala kindling. In: *Recent advances in excitatory aminoacid research,* ed. J. Lehmann, pp. 251–254. New York: Alan R. Liss.

Spehlmann, R. & Norcross, K. (1984): Decreased sensitivity of neurons in the basolateral amygdala to dopamine and noradrenaline iontophoresis after a kindling stimulus. *Exp. Neurol.* **83**, 204–210.

Sperber, E.F., Haas, K.Z. & Moshé, S.L. (1991): Presence of spontaneous seizures and lack of kindling antagonism in rat pups. *Epilepsia* **32** (Suppl. 3), 33.

Sperber, E.F., Sutula, T.P. & Moshé, S.L. (1990): Synaptic sprouting following kindled seizures is age related. *Epilepsia* **31**, 633.

Squillance, K.M., Post, R,M. & Pert, A. (1980): Development of wet dog shakes during amygdala kindling in the rat. *Exp. Neurol.* **70**, 487–497.

Šramka, M., Sedlák, P. & Nádvorník, P. (1977): Observation of the kindling phenomenon in treatment of pain by stimulation in thalamus. In: *Neurosurgical treatment in psychiatry, pain, and epilepsy*, eds. W.H. Sweet, S. Obrador & J.G. Martin-Rodriguez, pp. 651–654. Baltimore: University Park Press.

Stark, L.G., Albertson, T.E., Joy, R.M., He, P. & Streisand, J. (1986): The acquisition of a kindled response in developing rats using 24-hour intertrial interval. *Dev. Brain Res.* **24**, 291–294.

Stripling, J.S. & Ellingwood, E.H. Jr. (1977): Augmentation of behavioural and electrophysiologic responses to cocaine by chronic adminsitration in the rat. *Exp. Neurol.* **54**, 546–564.

Sutula, T., Cascino, G., Cavazos, J. & Parada, I. (1989): Mossy fiber synaptic reorganization in the epileptic human temporal lobe. *Ann. Neurol.* **26**, 321–330.

Sutula, T., Xiao-Xian, H., Cavazos, J. & Scott, G. (1988): Synaptic reorganization in the hippocampus induced by abnormal functional activity. *Science* **239**, 1147.

Swann, J.W., Brady, R.J. & Martin, D.L. (1989): Postnatal development of GABA mediated synaptic inhibition in rat hippocampus. *Neuroscience* **28**, 551–562.

Swann, J.W., Smith, K.L. & Brady, R.J. (1990): Neural networks and synaptic transmissions in immature hippocampus. In: *Excitatory amino acids and neuronal plasticity. Advances in experimental medicine and biology*, ed. Y. Ben-Ari. pp. 161–171. New York: Putnam Press.

Taber, K.H., McNamara, J.J. & Zornetzer, S.F. (1977): Status epilepticus: a new rodent model. *Electroencephalogr. Clin. Neurophysiol.* **43**, 707–724.

Thompson, J.L., Bryan, M., Bates, T. & Holmes, G.L. (1988): Failure of kindling to alter susceptibility to kainic acid. *Dev. Brain Res.* **38**, 149–151.

Timm, F. (1958): Zur Histochemie der Schwermetalle. Das Sulfid-Silber Verfahren. *Dtsch. Z. Gesamte Gerichtl. Med.* **47**, 428–481.

Velíšek, L. & Mareš, P. (1991): An increased epileptogenesis in the hippocampus of developing rats. *Exp. Brain Res. Ser.* **20**, 183–185.

Vosu, H. & Wise, R.A. (1975): Cholinergic seizure kindling in the rat: comparison of caudate, amygdala and hippocampus. *Behav. Biol.* **13**, 491–495.

Wada, J.A., Sato, M. & McCaughran, J.A.Jr. (1975): Cortical electrographic correlates on convulsive seizure development induced by daily electrical stimulation of the amygdala in rats and cats. *Fol. Psychiat. Neurol. Jap.* **29**, 329–339.

Wasterlain, C.G. & Jonec, V. (1983): Chemical kindling by muscarinic amygdaloid stimulation in the rat. *Brain Res.* **271**, 311–323.

Wasterlain, C.G., Fairchild, M.D., Bronstein, J.M. & Farber, D.B. (1986): Molecular changes in the synaptic apparatus associated with septal kindling. In: *Kindling*, Vol. 3, ed. J.A. Wada, pp. 55–69. New York: Raven Press.

Welsh, K.A. & Gold, P.E. (1986): Epinephrine proactive retardation of amygdala-kindled epileptogenesis. *Behav. Neurosci.* **100**, 236–245.

Wurpel, J.N.D., Sperber, E.F. & Moshé, S.L. (1990): Baclofen inhibits amygdala kindling in immature rats. *Epilepsy Res.* **5**, 1–7.

Wurpel, J.N.D., Tempel, A., Sperber, E.F. & Moshé, S.L. (1988): Age-related changes of muscimol binding in the substantia nigra. *Dev. Brain Res.* **43**, 305–307.

Xu, S.G., Garant, D.S., Sperber, E.F. & Moshé, S.L. (1991a): Effects of substantia nigra gamma-vinyl-GABA infusions on flurothyl seizures in adult rats. *Brain Res.* **566**, 108–114.

Xu, S.G., Sperber, E.F. & Moshé, S.L. (1991b): Is the anticonvulsant effect of substantia nigra infusion of gamma-vinyl-GABA (GVG) mediated by the GABA(A) receptor in rat pups? *Dev. Brain Res.* **5**, 17–21.

Chapter 14

Excitotoxicity and the developing brain

Claude G. Wasterlain and Raman Sankar*

Epilepsy Research Laboratory, VA Medical Center, Sepulveda, CA 91343, USA; Departments of Neurology and Pediatrics*, and The Brain Research Institute, UCLA School of Medicine, Los Angeles, CA 90024, USA

Summary

The occurrence of certain seizure types in the developing human brain is associated with poor developmental outcome, but the significance of that association is not clear. Brain damage and/or poor brain development could be the direct result of seizures, or seizures and poor development could be independent results of the same cause. Experimental studies have begun to give us some basic principles which may eventually help us to resolve this dilemma. The bulk of brain damage resulting from seizures appears to be mediated by so called 'excitotoxic' mechanisms, in which excitatory amino acid neurotransmitters such as glutamate open ionic channels permeable to calcium, which can reach lethal concentrations in the cytoplasm. The NMDA receptor is a subtype of glutamate receptor coupled to a calcium ionophore. It is fully expressed at birth in most mammals and is transiently overexpressed above the adult level in several species during infancy and childhood. This receptor appears to have a very active role in mediating brain damage from status epilepticus. By contrast, kainic acid receptors, representing another subtype of glutamate receptors, are poorly developed in the immature brain and become fully expressed much later than NMDA receptors. Severe experimental neonatal seizures inhibit brain growth, DNA and protein synthesis and may curtail the development of cell to cell connections. A number of factors such as a low transport capacity of the blood–brain barrier for glucose, reduced vascular reactivity of cortical vessels at certain ages, very slow mobilization of glycogen reserves, and overexpression of NMDA receptors represent liabilities for the seizing immature brain. Other factors such as better lactate transport out of brain, or immaturity of the presynaptic glutamatergic terminals, make the immature brain relatively resistant to seizure-induced damage. Direct stimulation of excitatory amino acid receptors can produce lesions which are larger in the immature brain than in the adult, reflecting the overexpression of those receptors. However, some seizure types are associated with a remarkable lack of histological brain damage. Recent data from our laboratory suggest that this protection is not absolute and that stimulation of the perforant path in 15-day-old rats does produce neuronal necrosis in the hippocampus. The relative importance of these various factors and their applicability to the human brain are currently unresolved questions under active investigation.

Introduction

Information regarding the effects of epilepsy on brain development in humans is complicated by the fact that it is often difficult to distinguish the disturbances in development caused by the epileptic condition itself from the deterioration in development caused by the underlying disease that caused the epileptic condition. Patients are invariably treated with antiepileptic medications which can themselves have effects on development, and the natural history of the condition without treatment is impossible to study. Some of the epileptic syndromes that are associated with severe developmental difficulties, such as infantile spasms and Lennox–Gastaut syndrome, are not specific pathophysiological entities, but rather, they represent the nonspecific response of the maturing brain to injury at a particular stage in development. Thus far, such syndromes appear to be unique to the human and no animal models exist. The impact of epilepsy on development is not only a function of the type of epilepsy and the severity of that condition but is also critically affected by the time when epilepsy and/or seizures intervene.

It is possible that both recurrent ictal discharges, and perhaps even interictal discharges may contribute to the intellectual and psychosocial decline sustained by children with catastrophic epilepsy (Till, 1967; Reynolds, 1981; Engel & Shewmon, 1991). Woodruff (1974) observed that regions of epileptic irritability tend to produce greater functional deficits than corresponding ablative lesions. Shewmon & Erwin (1988) have demonstrated that interictal spikes that are followed by prominent inhibitory afterpotentials can transiently disrupt cortical function; thus very frequent interictal spikes could interfere with modality-specific learning.

Aicardi & Chevrie (1970), in a study of 239 cases of status epilepticus (SE) in patients under 15 years of age, concluded that mental deterioration followed SE in 114 (48 per cent), and that 78 of them had developed normally prior to their first bout of SE. Of these 78 children, 55 had cryptogenic SE and the remaining had diseases such as meningitis, encephalitis etc. Prolonged convulsions were more devastating in young babies and even cryptogenic status had a worse prognosis in children less than 3 years of age. Similar results were reported by Fujiwara et al. (1979). Pathological evidence showing brain damage as a consequence of SE presented by Corsellis & Bruton (1983) suggests that such damage is more common in children. Aicardi has presented radiological evidence of haemiatrophia cerebri as a result of unilateral SE (Aicardi & Baraton, 1971; Aicardi, 1986). Dunn's study (1988) found that the outcome after SE was related to the aetiology and duration of SE and that the age at the time of SE was a minor factor. He found sequelae mainly in symptomatic cases and not in idiopathic or febrile SE. It is likely that the difference between the two studies in terms of the outcome is at least in part reflective of improvements in management strategies over the intervening period. A more recent report that evaluated cases between 1985 and 1987 concluded that the morbidity of aggressively treated SE in children, in the absence of an acute neurological insult or progressive neurological disorders, is low (Maytal et al., 1989). Dodrill & Wilensky (1990) have summarized the available studies on intellectual impairment as an outcome of SE.

Studies exist for complex partial seizures of temporal lobe origin that compare a group of patients with medically refractory partial seizures with a second group with similar seizures treated successfully by surgery, (Currie et al., 1971; Lindsay et al., 1979a, b, c, 1984a). These studies demonstrated marked improvements in psychosocial functioning after early temporal lobe resections. These results have been corroborated by other studies on the surgical treatment of complex partial seizures (Falconer, 1972; Jensen & Vaernet, 1977) and contrast with long-term studies of children with intractable complex partial seizures that did not undergo surgery (Lindsay et al., 1984b; Kotagal et al., 1987). However, Whittle et al. (1981) noted that even though attitude toward schooling and academic performance improved postoperatively, there was no objective improvement in IQ.

A recent study describes very favourable outcome with surgery for extratemporal partial epilepsy that began in childhood in terms of seizure control (Adler et al., 1991). However, the data provided described seizures control in much greater detail than the developmental outcome. Forty-three percent of the patients from this heterogeneous group had improvement in their 'performance rating' after surgery, which may relate at least in part to the fact that more than 50 per cent of the patients required less anticonvulsant medication.

As stated earlier, age-specific epilepsies of childhood such as infantile spasms and Lennox–Gastaut syndrome are associated with significant disturbance in development. Significant numbers of these patients demonstrate underlying focal lesions (Chugani & Engel, 1986; Chugani et al., 1988, 1990; Cusami et al., 1988). The strongest evidence that the progressive intellectual decline observed in association with cryptogenic infantile spasms can result from the epileptic disturbance itself, derives from observations of dramatic developmental improvement following resective surgery of a focal lesion that was not apparent by magnetic resonance imaging or x-ray computed tomography but was identified by functional neuroimaging employing 2-fluorodeoxyglucose positron emission tomography (Shields et al., 1990; Shields, 1991). Histopathological investigations on the resected tissue often reveal focal areas of congenital cytoarchitectural abnormalities (cortical dysplasia) (Vinters et al., 1990). Detailed results of the pre- and postsurgical developmental assessments of children who have undergone resections for intractable infantile spasms are not yet available. While our experience at UCLA suggests that patients with heterotopias and intractable seizures show improvement in both seizure control and development after resection, we have also encountered a relatively normal patient without seizures in whom heterotopias were incidentally discovered by magnetic resonance imaging during a workup for headaches (personal observation), once again suggesting that this lesion itself does not cause developmental regression unless it gives rise to a severe seizure disorder. Several lines of clinical evidence are suggestive of an adverse effect of seizures/epilepsy *per se* on neurodevelopment, but at the present time convincing demonstration of this notion must derive from animal studies. The concept is of high clinical relevance, as approaches to surgical intervention in intractable epilepsies with focal pathologies raise the hope for changing the developmental outcome of children with such lesions.

The excitotoxic hypothesis

Lucas & Newhouse (1956) were the first to identify a toxic effect of systemic glutamate on the newborn mouse retinal neurons. Olney, studying this phenomenon, noted that these mice were extremely short and obese. He found neuronal degeneration in their brains in the areas not protected by the blood–brain barrier (1969). Neuronal lesions induced by glutamate were characterized by rapid swelling located near dendrosomal synaptic receptors, which led to the hypothesis that the damage was the result of glutamate-induced depolarization (Olney, 1978, 1986). Rothman (1984), working with hippocampal cultures, noted that young cultures were much less vulnerable to hypoxia than mature cultures which had established synaptic connections. He demonstrated that hypoxic cell death in that situation resulted from synaptic activity, and found that glutamate was the predominant transmitter released by those cultures under hypoxic conditions (Rothman, 1984). He found that ionic conditions altered the injury, and that γ-D-glutamylglycine (GDGG), which blocks all types of glutamate receptors, reduced hypoxic damage in these preparations (Rothman & Olney, 1986). Magnesium, which blocks both presynaptic transmitter release and the ionic channel associated with post-synaptic NMDA receptors, also afforded hypoxic protection (Rothman et al., 1987). Kass & Lipton (1982), studying hypoxic injury in the hippocampal slice, suggested its dependence on the failure of calcium pumps associated with energy depletion. Choi (1985) found that exposure of cultured rat neocortical neurons to glutamate for a brief period caused delayed cell death, a phenomenon already described *in vivo* by Kirino et al. (1981). Choi and his collaborators in a series of elegant studies showed that delayed cell death induced by glutamate is mimicked by calcium ionophores (Choi, 1987), and is attenuated by NMDA antagonists (Choi et al., 1988) and dissociative anaesthetics (Choi, 1987; Choi et al., 1987; Rothman et al., 1987). Sloviter & Dempster (1985) demonstrated that neuronal injury induced in the hippocampus by stimulation of the perforant path shares many of the characteristics of excitotoxic injury, suggesting that seizures also damage neurons through excitotoxic mechanisms. Many studies have demonstrated that excitotoxins such as kainic acid or domoic acid induce seizures in animals and man which can result in extensive brain damage, in specific cell populations (Campochiaro & Coyle, 1978; Tremblay et al., 1988; Nitecka et al., 1984). In models of status epilepticus, protection from neuronal necrosis was obtained with NMDA blockers (Fujikawa et al., in press; Penix et al., 1991) and different populations of hilar interneurons were protected in the perforant path model by non-NMDA blockers (Penix et al., 1991) suggesting that both NMDA and non-NMDA receptors participate in the mechanisms of seizure-induced brain damage (Wieloch, 1985). The current formulation of the excitotoxic hypothesis states that seizures induce neuronal necrosis by releasing large amounts of excitatory amino acids transmitters at a time when transmitter reuptake is weakened by energy depletion, resulting in the opening of several ligand-gated ionic channels. Neuronal necrosis follows the prolonged opening of kainate or AMPA-type channels in a few regions such as CA3, but in most regions it follows the calcium influx resulting from opening of the NMDA receptor-associated ionic channels.

Table 1. Excitatory amino acid receptors*

Receptor class	Function	Agonists	Antagonists
NMDA			
NMDA recognition site	Opening of cationic ionophore	NMDA, L-glutamate, L-aspartate, ibotenate	CCP, D–AP5, D–AP7
Ionophore	Influx of Na^+ and Ca^{2+}		Phencyclidine, TCP, MK–801, ketamine, dextromethorphan
Glycine site	Positive allosteric modulation on NMDA recognition site	Glycine, D-serine	HA–966, 7-Cl-kynurenate, felbamate
Polyamine site	Positive recognition site	Spermine	
Mg^{2+} binding site	Noncompetitive inhibition of ionophore	Mg^{2+}	
Zn^{2+}	Noncompetitive inhibition of ionophore (?)	Zn^{2+}	
AMPA	Influx of Na^+, Ca^{2+}	AMPA, quisqualate, L-glutamate	CNQX, DNQX, NBQX
ACPD (metabotropic)	Hydrolysis of PI; generation of IP3 and DG; mobilization of intracellular Ca^{2+} and activation of protein kinase C	Trans-ACPD, quisqualate, L-glutamate, ibotenate, L-aspartate	L-AP3
Kainate			
Ionophore-linked	Influx of Na^+, Ca^{2+}	Kainate, L-glutamate, L-aspartate	CNQX, DNQX, NBQX
AP4			
Presynaptic (?) autoreceptor	Negative feedback	L-AP4, L-glutamate, L-aspartate	

*A summary of functions, agonists, and antagonists of the four EAA receptor classes. An endogenous excitatory amino acid neurotransmitter, L-glutamate, acts on one of four receptor classes. (This table is not all-inclusive.)

Abbreviations:
ACPD	= 1-amino-cyclopentyl-1,3-dicarboxylate;
AMPA	= α-amino-3-hydroxy-5-methyl-4-isoxazolepropionate;
AP3	= 2-amino-3-phosphonopropionate;
AP4	= 2-amino-4-phosphonobutyrate;
AP5	= 2-amino-5-phosphonopentanoate;
APV	= 2-amino-5-phosphonovalerate;
CNQX	= 6-cyano-7-nitroquinoxaline-3-dione;
CCP	= 3-((±)-2-carboxypiperazin-4-yl)propyl-1-phosphonate;
DG	= diacylglycerol;
DNQX	= 6,7-dinitroquinoxaline-2,3-dione;

Chapter 14 EXCITOTOXICITY AND THE DEVELOPING BRAIN

HA-966 = 3-amino-1-hydroxy-2-pyrrolidone;
IP3 = inositol-1,4,5-triphosphate;
MK-801 = (+)-5-methyl-10,11-dihydro-5H-dibenzo[a,d]cyclohepten-5,10-imine maleate;
NBQX = 2,3-dihydroxy-6-nitro-7-sulphamoyl-benzo[F]quinoxaline;
NMDA = N-methyl-D-aspartate;
PI = phosphoinositide;
TCP = N-[1(2-thienyl)cyclohexyl]-piperidine

The NMDA receptor complex

Endogenous excitatory amino acids (EAAs), such as glutamate and aspartate, act as excitatory neurotransmitters in most parts of the central nervous system (Fagg & Foster, 1983; Fonnum, 1984). The actions of those neurotransmitters are mediated through binding to several types of postsynaptic receptors (Table 1), which are defined by their artificial pharmacological ligands, namely N-methyl-D-aspartate (NMDA) (MacLennan, 1983; Watkins & Evans, 1983), kainate and amino-hydroxy-methyl-isoxazolopropionate (AMPA).

These receptor subtypes vary considerably in distribution throughout the central nervous system (Monaghan & Cotman, 1985). In the hippocampus, NMDA and AMPA receptors predominate in the perforant path-dentate granule cell synapses and the Schaffer collateral-CA1 synapses, while kainate receptors predominate in the mossy fibre CA3 synapses. Those receptors are ligand-gated ionic channels, which in the case of NMDA are permeable to calcium and sodium (Fig. 1), and in the case of AMPA and kainate can be permeable to either sodium alone or sodium and calcium, depending on their subunit composition (Verdoorn et al., 1991). The receptors have been cloned (Egebjerg et al., 1991; Werner et al., 1991; Moriyoshi et al., 1991). The NMDA receptor has a binding site for glutamate, which is probably its natural ligand, and a number of competitive inhibitors of that site have been developed (AP5, AP7, CPP, CGS 19755; Watkins & Olverman, 1987). The NMDA receptor complex also has a binding site for glycine (Reynolds et al., 1987) which is strychnine-insensitive and completely different from the classical glycine receptor (Kishimoto et al., 1991). Through this receptor, glycine potentiated the action of NMDA, glutamate and PCP. Several specific inhibitors of that site (HA966, 7-chlorokynurenic acid, felbamate) are avail-

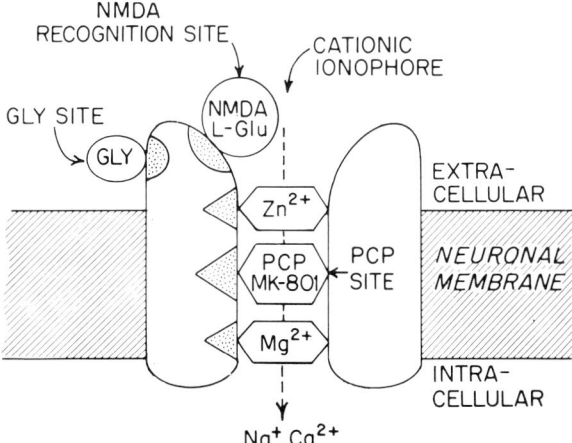

Fig. 1. A schematic structure of an NMDA receptor complex. It primarily consists of the NMDA neurotransmitter recognition site and the cationic ionophore. Activation of the NMDA recognition site by agonists, such as NMDA and L-glutamate, along with positive allosteric modulation by glycine, opens the ionophore which allows Na^+ and Ca^{2+} influx. Open channel blockade of the PCP site by PCP or MK-801 inhibits the cationic influx. The Mg^{2+} or Zn^{2+} ion binds the cationic binding site and noncompetitively inhibits the influx of Na^+ and Ca^{2+}.

able. Another allosteric site located on the ionic channel associated with the NMDA receptor binds PCP with high affinity (Foster & Wong, 1987; Wong et al., 1986). There is also a polyamine-binding site, a voltage-dependent magnesium-binding site inside the channel, and a zinc-binding site in this complex, highly regulated receptor.

Ontogeny of the excitatory amino acid system

Presynaptic ontogeny

The excitatory amino acid (EAA) system is presynaptically immature early in life, so that both in rodents and humans, a large portion of the development of axonal growth cones and dendritic ramifications occurs postnatally. The concentration of glutamate in the immature rat brain is low (Campochiaro & Coyle, 1978) and so is the concentration of glutamate-related enzymes (Barca & Toledano, 1982; Rothe et al., 1983; Kvamme et al., 1985). Hippocampal slices from immature rats have low presynaptic release of EAAs (Minc-Golomb et al., 1987) and low sodium-dependent high-affinity uptake of glutamate and aspartate into presynaptic terminals and into glial cells (Schmidt & Wolf, 1988).

Postsynaptic ontogeny

There is marked heterogeneity in the postnatal ontogeny of EAA receptors. The NMDA recognition site is abundant at birth and in the rat is overexpressed during early postnatal life. In the rat hippocampus, for example, the NMDA receptor reaches 150–200 per cent of the adult value at the age of 6 to 14 days (Tremblay et al., 1988; McDonald et al., 1989a; Peterson et al., 1989) and a similar overexpression of NMDA receptors has been found in the human brain (Represa et al., 1989). As a result, the NMDA receptor density of the term human newborn is higher than the adult's. Other studies have confirmed the transient overexpression of glutamate binding sites in immature postnatal rat brain (Barks et al., 1988; Baudry et al., 1981). Physiological development parallels this biochemical maturation. The population spike elicited by NMDA application to CA1 cells of the hippocampus peaks at 10 days, long-term potentiation in those same CA1 cells peaks around 15 days of age in the rat (Harris & Teyler, 1984; Hammon & Heinemann, 1988; Ben Ari et al., 1988). In the human brain, the NMDA recognition site and the ionic channel associated with it appear to develop concomitantly. The PCP receptor density of frontal cortex is transiently elevated in early childhood with peak density at about age 2 years (Kornhuber et al., 1989). Allosteric sites of the NMDA receptor may also show transient increases in early postnatal life (McDonald et al., 1989a).

The AMPA receptor follows a similar curve, characterized by its transient overexpression in both rat and human during early postnatal life. In the globus pallidus, for example, the AMPA-quisqualate receptor transiently exceeds the adult concentration in the 7-day-old rat, and in the 2–6-week-old human brain (Greenamyre et al., 1987). Kainate receptors follow a completely different ontogenic curve. They are scarce in the rat brain during the first 10 days of postnatal life, and only attain sizable numbers after the 3rd week of life (Campochiaro & Coyle, 1978; Berger et al., 1984). In the human hippocampus, this receptor is detected as early as 21 week gestation, and is transiently enhanced during the newborn period in discrete regions, such as a stratum lucidum of the CA3 sector of the hippocampus, and the supragranular layer of the dentate gyrus (Represa et al., 1986).

Developmental plasticity in the EAA system

The developmental significance of the transiently enhanced EAA system appears to be its age-related critical role in plasticity of the immature brain. EAA receptor activation is crucial in long-term potentiation and other models of cortical learning (Collingridge & Bliss, 1987). It also plays an essential role in brain development. For example, the NMDA receptor antagonist AP5 inhibits the physiological segregation of the retinal ganglion cell axons in the optic tecta of three-eyed tadpoles

(Cline et al., 1987). The NMDA blocker ketamine impairs ocular dominance shifts (Rauschecker & Hahn, 1987). In parallel with the overexpression of NMDA receptors in the immature brain, the potency of NMDA blockers in disrupting learning processes is age dependent. AP5 impedes visual response of cortical neurons more effectively in kittens than in adult cats (Tsumoto et al., 1987). Chronic administration of AP5 inhibits the development of early olfactory learning in rats (Lincoln et al., 1988; Coopersmith & Leon, 1984).

Early morphogenesis

The EAA system also plays an important role in early morphogenesis. Small amounts of glutamate in the extracellular space promote the growth and differentiation of cultured neurons (Aruffo et al., 1987a). Small amounts of glutamate acting on the NMDA receptor stimulate growth cones and neurite expansion in cultured neurons (Aruffo et al., 1987b). However, a vigorous stimulation of calcium influx through NMDA receptors inhibits growth cones and stimulation of non-NMDA receptors can mediate the retraction of dendritic outgrowth (Brewer & Cotman, 1989; Mattson et al., 1988). A high level of NMDA receptor stimulation, resulting in even greater calcium influx into growth cones, leads to pruning and retraction of growth cones and to the death of their neurons (Cunningham, 1982; Mattson et al., 1989; Letourneau et al., 1991). Thus the control of neurite extension and the control of the formation of connections between neurons appear to depend on the balance of excitatory and inhibitory neurotransmitters acting on growth cones and on similar dendritic structures. In the absence of any stimulation, growth cones are quiescent. A mild stimulation results in an expansion and formation of synaptic connections. Higher excitatory influences, particularly of the glutamate type, result in stabilization of growth cones; very high levels of stimulation such as could occur during seizures result in regression, pruning, and elimination of growth cones and synaptic connections, and in neuronal death. The full significance of those principles for our understanding of the effect of seizures on the developing human brain have yet to be fully explored. However, they undoubtedly constitute an important aspect of the complex relationship between seizures and brain development.

Several neonatal seizures inhibit brain growth

The metabolic response of the immature brain to seizures is quite different from the adult's. Immature rats have a cerebral metabolic rate 10–20 fold lower than the adult, but the relative increase of cortical metabolic rate during seizures is probably as high (two- to fivefold) (Fujikawa et al., 1989). Several factors contribute to imposing a very high risk for metabolic complications (Younkin et al., 1986) during neonatal seizures. In some types of experimental seizures, a profound mismatch develops between metabolic needs and cerebral blood flow (Fujikawa et al., 1989). Seizures inhibit DNA and protein synthesis (Dwyer et al., 1986) imposing severe metabolic stress on the growing brain. The healthy neonate's brain may obtain as much as one third of its energy from ketone bodies, which become unusable if there is anoxia during seizures, since the oxidation of ketone bodies requires molecular oxygen. Thus, anoxia associated with seizures enhances the dependence of the brain on glucose. The neonatal brain has sizable reserves of glycogen, but very low concentrations of phosphorylase, phosphoglucomutase, and cyclic AMP, which are needed to activate protein kinase A and to transform phosphorylase B into its active form, permitting mobilization of those glycogen reserves. The maximal rate of glucose transport across the immature blood–brain barrier has been estimated to be only one fifth of the adult rate in the rat, probably as a result of lower capillary density in the neonatal brain. This transport rate appears to be lower than the maximal glycolytic rate in cortex, and becomes rate-limiting for the metabolic response of the brain to seizures. As a result, even when blood glucose is in normal range, brain glucose falls rapidly during sustained seizures in newborn rats, rabbits, and marmoset monkeys (Fujikawa et al., 1989). By contrast, lactate accumulation is not a major problem during status epilepticus in the immature brain, because of its ability to carry lactate across the blood–brain barrier, out of brain and into the circulation of suckling animals.

Effect of seizures on brain mitotic activity

The adult brain is largely a postmitotic organ. Neurons become incapable of mitotic activity by 18 days postnatal in rat cerebellum, 20 days in rat forebrain, and 1 year in human cerebellum. Experimental seizures in infant rats inhibit mitotic activity (Suga & Wasterlain, 1980), resulting in a reduction in number of cells (Table 2) in the brain region where seizures occur (Wasterlain & Plum, 1973; Wasterlain, 1976; Wasterlain et al., 1990). A single bout of seizures can inhibit cerebral and cerebellar cell division for several days (Suga & Wasterlain, 1980). The result is a reduction of the number of brain cells (Fig. 2). In brain regions which still have a large mitotic potential (e.g. the cerebellum of a 4-day-old rat undergoing seizures) this deficit can be made up by later acceleration of cell division (Fig. 2). However, in brain regions where seizures occur at the tail end of the growth curve for mitotic activity (e.g. forebrain of a 4-day-old rat) seizures can, even in the total absence of histological lesions or cell necrosis, permanently reduce the number of cells in that brain region (Fig. 1).

Table 2. *Effects of neonatal seizures on brain growth*

	Control	Experimental	Differences
Body weight, g	61.5 ± 4.3	61.5 ± 4.4	n.s.
Brain weight, g	1.0824 ± 0.0299	0.9851 ± 0.0289	$P < 0.01$
Brain DNA, µg	1576 ± 68	1289 ± 45	$P < 0.01$
Brain cells no. $\times 10^{-6}$	254 ± 11	208 ± 7	$P < 0.01$

Experimental rats received two electroconvulsive seizures daily between the ages of 2 and 11 days. Food intake was adjusted to maintain similar body growth. Rats were sacrificed at 30 days, when cell multiplication has stopped and reductions in cell numbers are permanent. Seven control and seven experimental animals were used.

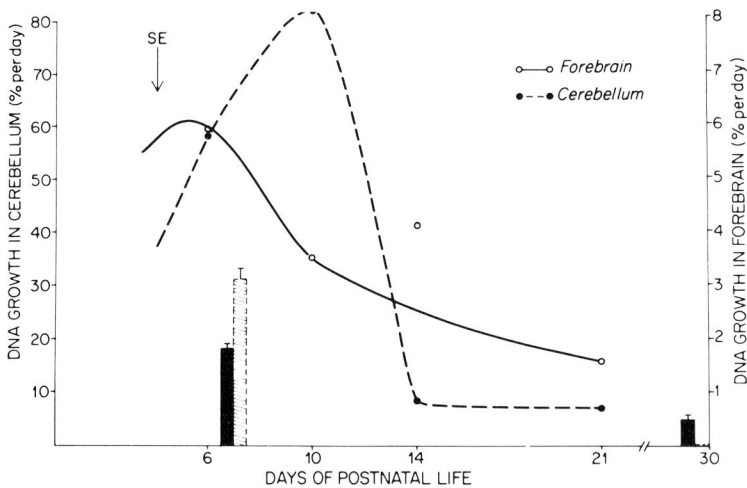

Fig. 2. *Relationship between brain growth and reversibility of seizure-induced deficits. On top, velocity curves of DNA accumulation illustrate the decline after day 4 in forebrain while cerebellum peaks at 10–12 days. Vertical bars (bottom) indicate the seizure-induced reduction in cell number, which represented a deficit of 16.8 per cent (F) and 18 per cent (C) at 7 days and of 4 per cent (F) and 2 per cent (C) at 30 days. The large cerebellar deficit observed 3 days after SE is erased by 30 days of age, whereas in forebrain a significant deficit remains permanently.*

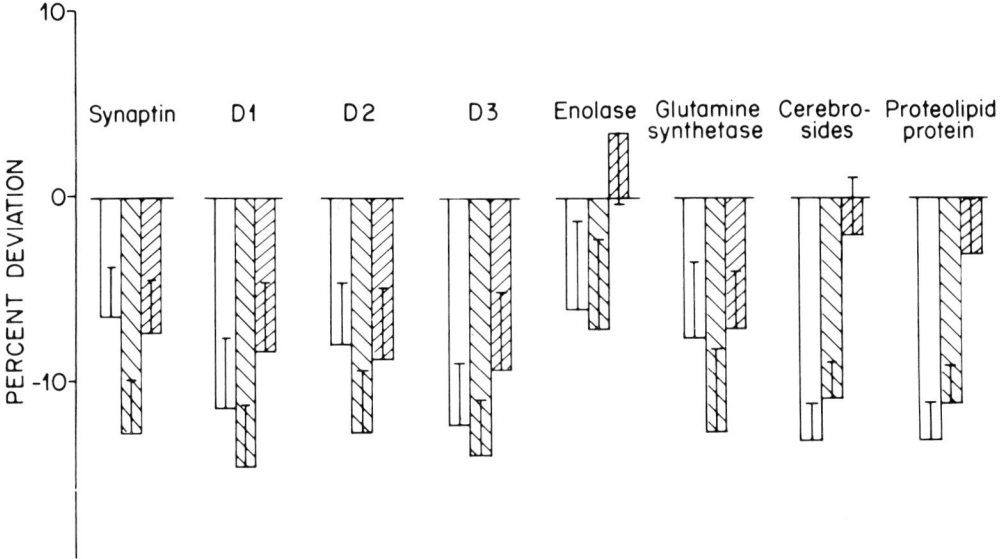

Fig. 3. This figure shows, in seizure-treated rats, the percentage of deviation from paired control littermates in the forebrain content of some synaptic protein markers (Synaptin, D1, D2, D3), of a neuronal cell body marker (enolase), of a glial protein (glutamine synthetase), and of myelin-enriched lipids. Rats were subjected to daily electroconvulsive seizures between the ages of 2 and 11 days (left columns), 9 and 18 days (middle columns), and 19 and 28 days (right column) and sacrificed at the age of 30 days. Reductions of synaptic, glial, and myelin markers in the first two groups suggest a curtailment of neuronal processes and their support cells (from Jorgensen et al., 1980).

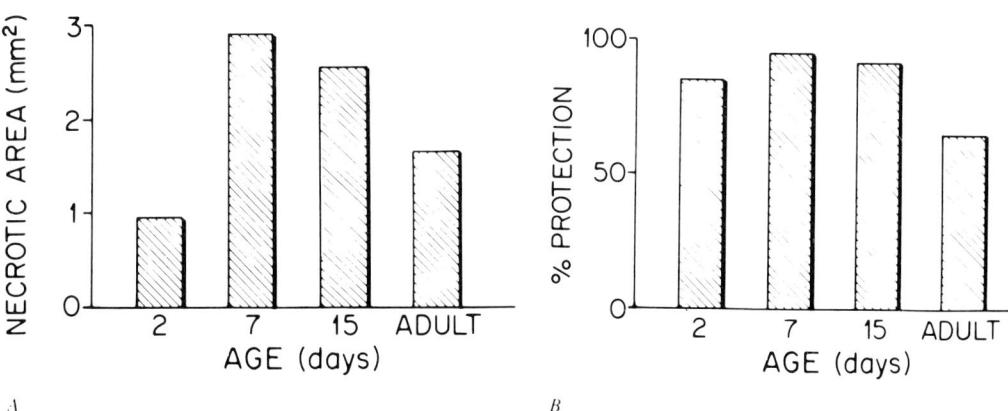

Fig. 4. A: NMDA-induced neurotoxicity is assessed by measuring the surface of the necrotic area (ordinate) induced by NMDA injected into the rat cerebral cortex at various ages. B: MK–801 neuroprotective efficacy (ordinate) is expressed as the percent reduction of the surface of the NMDA-induced necrotic area by co-injected MK–801. Sprague–Dawley rats at various ages (n = 4–5) underwent microinjection of 50 nmol of NMDA with or without 50 nmol of MK–801 into the parietal cortex. Animals were perfusion-fixed with buffered formaldehyde 3 days later. Serial coronal sections of 8 μm thickness were cut and stained with hematoxylin and eosin. Maximal necrotic areas were measured using an image analyser.

Seizures and the establishment of cell to cell connections

The establishment of synaptic connections requires active growth cones, and large amounts of neurotransmitters liberated by seizures can influence the competition for field of innervation by axons from different populations, and the programmed elimination of excess synaptic terminals. Seizures occurring thoroughout the period of active myelination in the rat brain result in a selective and permanent deficit in myelin-specific lipids, without a similar reduction of lipids which are general components of membranes (Dwyer & Wasterlain, 1982). A concomitant reduction of many synaptic markers in the absence of reduction of markers of neuronal cell bodies is also observed (Fig. 3). This suggests that seizures occurring during critical periods of axonal and dendritic growth can result in a permanent curtailment of cell to cell connections (Jorgensen et al., 1980). Neonatal seizures not only slowed brain growth but also delayed the appearance of behavioural milestones (Fig. 4). The effect of seizures on indices of myelination and synaptic development has never been studied in the human brain, but effects similar to those observed in the rat could be responsible for the developmental arrest and behavioural regression observed with certain seizure types in the immature brain. In recent years, however, a considerable amount of indirect evidence suggests that inhibitory effects of seizures on brain growth should be expected. For example, in the Helisoma neuron B19, both a calcium ionophore (Mattson & Kater, 1987) and neurotransmitter-induced calcium influx into the growth cones (Cohan et al., 1987) inhibit neurite outgrowth (Haydon et al., 1984). In cultured rat hippocampal pyramidal neurons, glutamate causes a sustained elevation of intracellular calcium (Krnjevic et al., 1986; Kudo & Ogura, 1986; Kudo et al., 1987). This also inhibited the outgrowth of dendrites (Mattson et al., 1988). Calcium channel blockers prevented this inhibition of growth of dendrites and a calcium ionophore reproduced it (these effects should not be confused with the radically different action of calcium in tumour cell lines, see Reboulleau, 1986). Phorbol esters and activators of protein kinase C mediated through quisqualate receptors also inhibit growth cones (Mattson et al., 1988). Thus the extreme activation of both NMDA and non-NMDA receptors by seizures could have potentially deleterious effects on brain development.

Excitotoxicity in the developing brain

In the adult brain, EAAs liberated during status epilepticus kill neurons through actions on specific NMDA and non-NMDA receptors. In the immature brain, this situation is quite different and the net outcome of seizures is controversial. Vulnerability to stimulation of NMDA and AMPA receptors is enhanced at key ages in the immature brain, but vulnerability to kainate receptor stimulation is extremely low, and the immaturity of the presynaptic machinery limits the amount of EAAs liberated from the presynaptic apparatus during seizures, with two consequences: some seizure types do not seem to produce any histological damage at all in the immature brain, and other seizure types may produce damage in an anatomical pattern totally different from that seen in the adult.

Toxicity of NMDA and AMPA receptor stimulation

Microinjection of NMDA into the striatum of the rat produces far more damage in the neonate than in the adult brain (McDonald et al., 1988; Yang et al., 1989). We confirmed this age-dependent enhancement of excitotoxicity by microinjection of NMDA into the neocortex and hippocampus of rats (Yang et al., 1989) and showed that toxicity is transiently enhanced in the first and second weeks of life (Fig. 4), and that the neuroprotective efficacy of blocking NMDA channels also peaks at the same ages (McDonald et al., 1987, 1989b; Olney et al., 1989; Yang et al., 1989). Ibotenate, a mixed EAA agonist, is also toxic to the neonatal hippocampus at doses considerably less than required to produce comparable cell loss in the adult rat brain (Cook & Crutcher, 1986). Quisqualate and AMPA toxicity is also transiently overexpressed in the immature brain (Silverstein et al., 1986, 1987; Ferriero et al., 1989). These results demonstrate that the overexpression of NMDA and AMPA receptors in the immature brain is capable of leading to cell injury and to cell death and that the receptors are fully coupled to the cellular machinery needed to express excitotoxicity (Table 3).

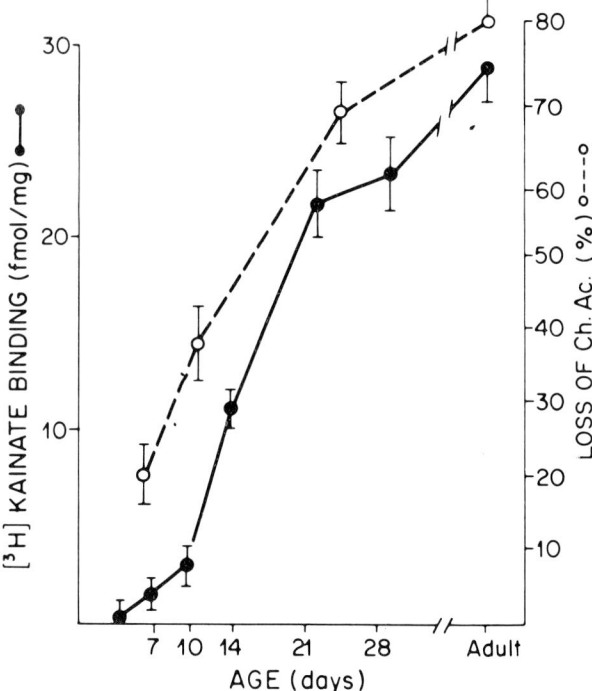

Fig. 5. Development of specific binding (glutamate displaceable) of [3H]-kainate (50 nM) in striatal membrane preparations is compared to development of kainate neurotoxicity, measured by the loss of the neuronal enzyme choline acetyltransferase 2 days following injection of 10 nmol of kainate into striatum. Note the parallelism of the curves. Data from Campochiaro & Coyle (1978).

Table 3. *Neurotransmitter and seizure-induced excitotoxicity in the immature brain*

Neurotransmitter	Receptor class	Ca_i	Neuronal injury	Peak toxicity at age	Peak receptor expression in
L-glutamate	NMDA	⇑	Widespread	7 days	7 days
	AMPA	⇑	+	7 days	7 days
	Kainate	⇑	Local*	Adult	Adult
	ACPD	Bound → Free	?		
GABA	$GABA_A$ †	⇑	?	?	1st week
Acetylcholine	Muscarinic	Bound → Free	?	?	?

These data derive from experiments performed in the rat.
*Kainate induces focal (e.g. CA3) damage by direct action, widespread damage by secondary activation of NMDA receptor.
†In the immature brain, most $GABA_A$ receptors depolarize neurons, while in the adult they usually hyperpolarize them. The excitatory effects of GABA receptors are greatest early in life; total receptor concentrations peak in adulthood.

Resistance of the developing brain to kainate toxicity

In contrast to NMDA and AMPA, the immature rat brain is quite resistant to neuronal damage from kainate, which is an important neurotoxin in the adult (Campochiaro & Coyle, 1978; Zaczek & Coyle, 1982; Nadler et al., 1981; Nitecka et al., 1984). The late development of kainate receptors in the immature brain and the marked regional differences in the cell types using such receptors provide a partial explanation for the resistance of the brain to kainate-induced damage (Fig. 5). Suprisingly, kainate in spite of the paucity of its specific receptors does induce seizures in developing rodents. In the adult, a dose of kainate of 3 mg/kg IP in the rat produces little histological damage, while 10 mg/kg produces extensive neuronal necrosis. In neonates, 3 mg/kg of kainic acid IP in the rat produces seizures but no damage, and higher doses are invariable fatal, precluding the use of doses of kainate which produce damage reliably in the adult. Since our current understanding of the mechanism of damage suggests that both seizures and damage are the result of receptor occupancy, it is not clear why the two can be dissociated, and further studies of neuronal firing frequencies, metabolic rates, ATP depletion, and extracellular glutamate concentration have yet to be carried out in these models.

Can neonatal seizures cause neuronal necrosis?

In neonates, experimental seizures induced by kainic acid (Velíšek *et al.*, Chapter 13, this volume), pilocarpine (Cavalheiro *et al.*, 1987), and bicuculline (Soderfeldt *et al.*, 1990) failed to produce neuronal necrosis in any brain region. However, preliminary results in our laboratory using electrical stimulation of the perforant path at the angular bundle showed that 2 h of recurrent seizure-like stimulation results in loss of paired pulse inhibition, a phenomenon associated in the adult with damage to hilar interneurons.

Histological examination reveals damage to the inner granule cells of the dentate gyrus, and to some hilar interneurons, suggesting that some seizure types can cause neuronal necrosis in 14–16-day-old rats. At the same time, there is remarkable sparing of CA1 pyramidal cells and a considerable sparing of the CA3 neurons, which often show severe injury following repeated perforant path stimulation in the adult. The pattern of neuronal necrosis seen after perforant path stimulation in immature rats would be unlikely to lead to Ammon's horn sclerosis, and calls into question the hypothesis that hippocampus sclerosis and Ammon's horn sclerosis can result from complicated febrile seizures or from status epilepticus in infancy or childhood.

Conclusions

The transient overexpression of some EAA receptors in the immature brain accounts for both plasticity and excitotoxicity early in life. At the same time, other EAAs systems develop late, and the immature brain is quite resistant to the type of brain damage usually induced in the adult through those receptors. A straightforward explanation for these age-locked, paradoxical effects of the EAA system on development and survival of neurons would see mild, physiological levels of excitation as facilitating plasticity and development of synaptic connections, while the overexcitation brought about by seizures could, by opening certain ligand-gated ionic channels, cause neuronal injury and curtail neurite growth and the establishment of synaptic connections. We have yet to examine the effect of EAAs released during neonatal seizures on programmed neuronal death, which depending on circumstances they could either cause or prevent. The net result of the complex interaction between EAA systems during seizures in the developing brain is just beginning to be explored, but we can hope that further understanding of this important area could prevent many of the adverse effects of seizures and their metabolic complications in the developing brain.

Acknowledgements

This study was supported by Research Grant NS13515 from NINDS, by the Research Service of the VA, and by the Epilepsy Foundation of America.

References

Adler, J., Erba, G., Winston, K.R., Welch, K. & Lombroso, C.T. (1991): Results of surgery for extratemporal partial epilepsy that began in childhood. *Arch. Neurol.* **48**, 133–140.

Aicardi, J. (1986): Consequences and prognosis of convulsive status epilepticus in infants and children. *Jpn J. Psychol. Neurol.* **40**, 283–290.

Aicardi, J. & Baraton, J. (1971): A pneumonencephalographic demonstration of brain atrophy following status epilepticus. *Dev. Med. Child Neurol.* **13**, 660–667.

Aicardi, J. & Chevrie, J.J. (1970): Convulsive status epilepticus in infants and children. A study of 239 cases. *Epilepsia* **11**, 187–197.

Aicardi, J., Chevrie, J.J. (1983): Consequences of status epilepticus in infants and children. *Adv. Neurol.* **34**, 115–125.

Aruffo, C., Ferszt, R., Hildebrandt, A.G. & Cervos-Navarro, J. (1987a): Low doses of L-monosodium glutamate promote neuronal growth and differentiation *in vitro*. *Dev. Neurosci.* **9**, 228–239.

Aruffo, C., Ferszt, R., Hildebrandt, A.G. & Cervos-Navarro, J. (1987b): *In vitro* neuronal plasticity triggered by subtoxic doses of monosodium glutamate. *Prog. Clin. Biol. Res.* **253**, 229–237.

Barca, M.A. & Toledano, A. (1982): Histochemical electron microscopic study of the enzyme glutamate dehydrogenase (GD) in post-natal developing cerebellum. *Cell. Mol. Biol.* **28**, 187–195.

Barks, J.D., Silverstein, F.S., Sims, K., Greenamyre, J.T. & Johnston, M.V. (1988): Glutamate recognition sites in human fetal brain. *Neurosci. Lett.* **84**, 131–136.

Baudry, M., Arst, D., Oliver, M. & Lynch, G. (1981): Development of glutamate binding site and their regulation by calcium in rat hippocampus. *Dev. Brain Res.* **1**, 37–48.

Ben Ari, Y., Cherubini, E. & Krnjevic, K. (1988): Changes in voltage dependence of NMDA currents during development. *Neurosci. Lett.* **94**, 88–82.

Berger, M.L., Tremblay, E., Nitecka, L. & Ben Ari, Y. (1984): Maturation of kainic acid seizure-brain damage syndrome in the rat. III. Postnatal development of kainic acid binding sites in the limbic system. *Neuroscience* **13**, 1095–1104.

Brewer, G.J. & Cotman, C.W. (1989): NMDA receptor regulation of neuronal morphology in cultured hippocampal neurons. *Neurosci. Lett.* **99**, 268–273.

Campochiaro, P. & Coyle, J.T. (1978): Ontogenic development of kainate neurotoxicity: correlates with glutamatergic innervation. *Proc. Natl. Acad. Sci. USA* **75**, 2025–2029.

Cavalheiro, E.A., Silva, D.F., Turski, W.A., Calderazzo, F.L., Bortolotto, Z.A. & Turski, L. (1987): The susceptibility of rats to pilocarpine-induced seizures is age-dependent. *Brain Res.* **465**, 43–58.

Choi, D.W. (1985): Glutamate neurotoxicity in cortical cell culture is calcium-dependent. *Neurosci. Lett.* **58**, 293–297.

Choi, D.W. (1987): Ionic dependence of glutamate neurotoxicity. *J. Neurosci.* **7**, 369–379.

Choi, D.W., Koh, J.Y. & Peters, S. (1988): Pharmacology of glutamate neurotoxicity in cortical cell cultures: attenuation by NMDA antagonists. *J. Neurosci.* **8**, 185–196.

Choi, D.W., Maulucci-Gedde, M. & Kriegstein, A.R. (1987): Glutamate neurotoxicity in cortical cell culture. *J. Neurosci.* **7**, 357–368.

Chugani, H.T. & Engel, J.Jr. (1986): PET in intractable epilepsy. In: *Intractable epilepsy: experimental and clinical aspects*, eds. D. Schmidt & P.L. Morselli, pp. 119–128. New York: Raven Press.

Chugani, H.T., Shewmon, D.A., Peacock, W.J., Shields, W.D., Mazziotta, J.C. & Phelps, M.E. (1988): Surgical treatment of intractable neonatal-onset seizures: the role of positron emission tomography. *Neurology* **38**, 1178–1188.

Chugani, H.T., Shields, W.D., Shewmon, D.A., Olson, D.M., Phelps, M.E. & Peacock, W.J. (1990): Infantile spasms: I. PET identifies focal cortical dysgenesis in cryptogenic cases for surgical treatment. *Ann. Neurol.* **27**, 406–413.

Cline, H.T., Debski, E.A. & Constantine-Paton, M. (1987): N-methyl-D-aspartate receptor antagonist desegregates eye-specific stripes. *Proc. Natl. Acad. Sci. USA* **84**, 4342–4345.

Cohan, C.S., Conner, J.A. & Kater, S.B. (1987): Electrically and chemically mediated increases in intracellular calcium in neonatal growth cones. *J. Neurosci.* **7**, 3588–3599.

Collingridge, G.L. & Bliss, T.V.P. (1987): NMDA receptors – their role in long-term potentiation. *Trends Neurosci.* **10**, 288–293.

Cook, T.M. & Crutcher, K.A. (1986): Intrahippocampal injection of kainic acid produces significant pyramidal cell loss in neonatal rats. *Neuroscience* **18**, 79–92.

Coopersmith, R. & Leon, M. (1984): Enhanced neural response to familiar olfactory cues. *Science* **225**, 849–851.

Corsellis, J.A.N. & Bruton, C.J. (1983): Neuropathology of status epilepticus in humans. In: *Status epilepticus: mechanisms of brain damage and treatment*, eds. A.V. Delgado-Escueta, C.G. Wasterlain, D.M. Treiman & R.J. Porter, pp. 129–139. New York: Raven Press.

Cunningham, T.J. (1982): Naturally occurring neuron death and its regulation by developing natural pathways. *Int. Rev. Cytol.* **74**, 163–186.

Currie, S., Heathfield, W.G., Henson, R.A. & Scott, D.F. (1971): Clinical course and prognosis of temporal lobe epilepsy – a survey of 666 patients. *Brain* **94**, 173–190.

Cusami, R., Dulac, O. & Diebler, C. (1988): Lesions focales dans les spasmes infantiles. *Neurophysiol. Clin.* **18**, 235–241.

Dodrill, C.B. & Wilensky, A.J. (1990): Intellectual impairment as an outcome of status epilepticus. *Neurology* **40** (Suppl. 2), 23–27.

Dunn, D.W. (1988): Status epilepticus in children: etiology, clinical features, and outcome. *J. Child Neurol.* **3**, 167–173.

Dwyer, B.E., Donatoni, P. & Wasterlain, C.G. (1982): A quantitative autoradiographic method for the measurement of local rates of brain protein synthesis. *Neurochem. Res.* **7**, 563–576.

Dwyer, B.E. & Wasterlain, C.G. (1982): Electroconvulsive seizures in the immature rat adversely affect myelin accumulation. *Exp. Neurol.* **78**, 616–628.

Dwyer, B.E., Wasterlain, C.G., Fujikawa, D.G. & Yamada, L. (1986): Brain protein metabolism in epilepsy. In: *Basic mechanisms of the epilepsies. Molecular and cellular approaches (Advances in neurology)*, Vol. 44, eds. A.V. Delgado-Escueta, A.A. Ward, D.M. Woodbury & R.J. Porter, pp. 903–918. New York: Raven Press.

Egebjerg, J., Bettler, B., Harmans-Borgmeyer, I. & Heinemann, S. (1991): Cloning of a cDNA for a glutamate receptor subunit activated by kainate but not AMPA. *Nature* **351**, 745–750.

Engel, J.Jr. & Shewmon, D.A. (1991): Impact of the kindling phenomenon on clinical epileptology. In: *Kindling and synaptic plasticity. The legacy of Graham Goddard*, pp. 195–210. Boston: Birkhauser.

Fagg, G.E. & Foster, A.C. (1983): Amino acid neurotransmitters and their pathways in the mammalian central nervous system. *Neuroscience* **9**, 701–719.

Falconer, M.A. (1972): Temporal lobe epilepsy in children and its surgical treatment. *Med. J. Aust.* **1**, 1117–1121.

Ferriero, D.M., Simon, R.P. & Soberano, H.Q. (1989): The quisqualate analogue α-amino-3-hydroxy-5-methyl-4-isoxazole propionate is neurotoxic to neonatal rat striatum. *Ann. Neurol.* **26**, 445.

Fonnum, F. (1984): Glutamate: a neurotransmitter in mammalian brain. *J. Neurochem.* **42**, 1–11.

Foster, A.C. & Wong, E.H.F. (1987): The novel anticonvulsant MK-801 binds to the activated state of the *N*-methyl-D-aspartate receptor in rat brain. *Br. J. Pharmacol.* **91**, 403–409.

Fujikawa, D.G. Intraamygdala injections of 2-amino-7-phosphoheptanoic acid protects against neuronal necrosis from fully developed pilocarpine-induced seizures. *Neurosci. Lett.* in press.

Fujikawa, D.G., Dwyer, B.E., Lake, R.R. & Wasterlain, C.G. (1989): Local cerebral glucose utilization during status epilepticus in newborn primates. *Am. J. Physiol.* **256** (*Cell Physiol.* 24), C1160–C1167.

Fujiwara, T., Ishida, S., Miyakoshi, M. *et al.* (1979): Status epilepticus in the childhood: a retrospective study of initial convulsive status and subsequent epilepsies. *Folia Psychiatr. Neurol. Jpn.* **33**, 337–344.

Greenamyre, T., Penney, J.B., Young, A.B., Hudson, C., Silverstein, F.S. & Johnston, M.V. (1987): Evidence for transient perinatal glutamatergic innervation of globus pallidus. *J. Neurosci.* **7**, 1022–1030.

Hammon, B. & Heinemann, U. (1988): Developmental changes in neuronal sensitivity to excitatory amino acids in area CA1 of the rat hippocampus. *Dev. Brain Res.* **38**, 286–290.

Harris, K.M. & Teyler, T.J. (1984): Developmental onset of long-term potentiation in area CA1 of the rat hippocampus. *J. Physiol.* **346**, 27–48.

Haydon, P.G., McCobb, D.P. & Kater, S.B. (1984): Serotonin selectively inhibits growth cone dynamics and synaptogenesis of specific identified neurons. *Science* **226**, 561–564.

Jensen, I. & Vaernet, K. Temporal lobe epilepsy. Follow-up investigation of 74 temporal lobe resected patients. *Acta Neurochir.* **37**, 173–200.

Jorgensen, O.S., Dwyer, B.E. & Wasterlain, C.G. (1980): Synaptic protein after electroconvulsive seizures in immature rats. *J. Neurochem.* **35**, 1235–1237.

Kass, I. & Lipton, P. (1982): Mechanisms involved in irreversible anoxic damage to the *in vitro* rat hippocampal slice. *J. Physiol.* (Lond) **332**, 459–479.

Kirino, T., Tamura, A. & Sano, D. (1981): Delayed neuronal death in the rat hippocampus following transient forebrain ischemia. *Acta Neuropathol.* **64**, 139–147.

Kishimoto, H., Simon, J.R. & Aprison, M.H. (1991): Determination of the equilibrium dissociation constants and number of glycine binding sites in several areas of the rat central nervous system using a Na-independent system. *J. Neurochem.* **37**, 1015–1024.

Kornhuber, J., Mack-Burkhardt, F., Konradi, C., Fritze, J. & Riederer, P. (1989): Effect of antemortem and postmortem factors on [3H]MK-801 binding in the human brain: transient elevation during early childhood. *Life Sci.* **45**, 745–749.

Kotagal, P., Rothner, D., Erenberg, G., Cruse, R.P. & Wyllie, E. (1987): Complex partial seizures of childhood onset. A five-year follow-up study. *Arch. Neurol.* **44**, 1177–1180.

Krnjevic, K. Morris, M.D. & Ropert, N. (1986): Changes in free calcium ion concentration recorded inside hippocampal pyramidal neurons in situ. *Brain Res.* **374**, 1–11.

Kudo, Y., Ito, K., Miyakawa, H., Izumi, Y., Ogura, A. & Kato, H. (1987): Cytoplasmic calcium elevation in hippocampal granule cell induced by perforant path stimulation and L-glutamate application. *Brain Res.* **407**, 168–172.

Kudo, Y. & Ogura, A. (1986): Glutamate-induced increase in intracellular Ca2+ concentration in isolated hippocampal neurons. *Br. J. Pharmacol.* **80**, 191–198.

Kvamme, E., Svenneby, G., Torgner, I.A.A., Drejer, J. & Schousboe, A. (1985): Postnatal development of glutamate metabolizing enzymes in hippocampus from mice. *Int. J. Dev. Neurosci.* **3**, 359–364.

Letourneau, P.C., Kater, S.B. & Macagno, E.R. (1991): *The nerve growth cone.* New York: Raven Press.

Lincoln, J., Coopersmith, R., Harris, E.W., Cotman, C.W. & Leon, M. (1988): NMDA receptor activation and early olfactory leaning. *Dev. Brain Res.* **39**, 309–312.

Lindsay, J., Glaser, G., Richards, P. & Ounsted, C. (1984a): Developmental aspects of focal epilepsies of childhood treated by neurosurgery. *Dev. Med. Child Neurol.* **26**, 574–587.

Lindsay, J., Ounsted, C. & Richards P. (1979a): Long-term outcome in children with temporal lobe seizures. I. Social outcome and childhood factors. *Dev. Med. Child Neurol.* **21**, 285–298.

Lindsay, J., Ounsted, C. & Richards, P. (1979b): Long-term outcome in children with temporal lobe seizures. II. Marriage, parenthood and sexual indifference. *Dev. Med. Child Neurol.* **21**, 433–440.

Lindsay, J., Ounsted, C. & Richards, P. (1979c): Long-term outcome in children with temporal lobe seizures. III. Psychiatric aspects in childhood and adult life. *Dev. Med. Child Neurol.* **21**, 630–636.

Lindsay, J., Ousted, C. & Richards, P. (1984b): Long-term outcome in children with temporal lobe seizures. V. Indications and contra-indications for neurosurgery. *Dev. Med. Child Neurol.* **26**, 25–32.

Lucas, D.R., Newhouse, J.P. (1956): The toxic effects of sodium L-glutamate on the inner layers of the retina. *Arch. Opthalmol.* **58**, 193–201.

MacLennan, H. (1983): Receptors for the excitatory amino acids in the mammalian central nervous system. *Progr. Neurobiol.* **20**, 251–271.

Mattson, M.P., Dou, P. & Kater, S.B. (1988): Outgrowth-regulating actions of glutamate in isolated hippocampal pyramidal neurons. *J. Neurosci.* **8**, 2087–2100.

Mattson, M.P. & Kater, S.B. (1987): Calcium regulation of neurite elongation and growth cone motility. *J. Neurosci.* **7**, 4034–4043.

Mattson, M.P., Murrain, M., Guthrie, P.B. & Kater, S.B. (1989): Fibroblast growth factor and glutamate: opposing roles in the generation and degeneration of hippocampal neuroarchitecture. *J. Neurosci.* **9**, 3728–3740.

Maytal, J., Shinnar, S., Moshé, S.L. & Alvarez, L.A. (1989): Low morbidity and mortality of status epilepticus in children. *Pediatrics* **83**, 323–331.

McDonald, J.W., Johnston, M.V. & Young, A.B. (1989a): Ontogeny of the receptors comprising the NMDA receptor complex. *Soc. Neurosci. Abstr.* **15**, 198.

McDonald, J.W., Silverstein, F.S. & Johnston, M.V. (1987): MK-801 protects the neonatal brain from hypoxic-ischemic damage. *Eur. J. Pharmacol.* **140**, 359–361.

McDonald, J.W., Silverstein, F.S. & Johnston, M.V. (1988): Neurotoxicity of N-methyl-D-aspartate is markedly enhanced in developing rat central nervous system. *Brain Res.* **459**, 200–203.

McDonald, J.W., Silverstein, F.S. & Johnston, M.V. (1989b): Neuroprotective effects of MK-801, TCP, PCP and CPP against N-methyl-D-aspartate induced neurotoxicity in an *in vivo* perinatal rat model. *Brain Res.* **490**, 33–40.

Minc-Golomb, D., Levy, Y., Kleinberger, N. & Schramm, M. (1987): D-[3H]Aspartate release from hippocampus slices studied in a multiwell system: controlling factors and postnatal development of release. *Brain Res.* **402**, 255–263.

Monaghan, D.T. & Cotman, C.W. (1985): Distribution of N-methyl-D-aspartate-sensitive l 3H-glutamate-binding sites in rat brain. *J. Neurosci.* **5**, 2909–2919.

Moriyoshi, K., Masu, M., Ishii, T. & Shigemoto, R. (1991): Molecular cloning and characterization of the rat NMDA receptor. *Nature* **354**, 31–37.

Nadler, J.V., Evenson, D.A. & Cuthbertson, G.J. (1981): Comparative toxicity of kainic acid and other acidic amino acids toward rat hippocampal neurons. *Neuroscience* **6**, 2505–2517.

Nitecka, J.V., Tremblay, E., Charton, G., Bouillot, J.P. Berger, M.L. & Ben Ari, Y. (1984): Maturation of kainic acid seizure-brain damage syndrome in the rat: II. Histopathological sequelae. *Neuroscience* **3**, 1073–1094.

Olney, J.W. (1969): Brain lesions, obesity and other disturbances in mice treated with monosodium glutamate. *Science* **164**, 719–721.

Olney, J.W. (1978): Neurotoxicity of excitatory amino acids. In: *Kainic acid as a tool in neurobiology*, eds. E.G. McGeer, J.W. Olney & P.L. McGeer, pp. 96–107. New York: Raven Press.

Olney, J.W. (1986): Inciting excitotoxic cytocide among central neurons. *Adv. Exp. Med. Biol.* **203**, 631–645.

Olney, J.W., Ikonomidou, C., Mosinger, J.L. & Frierdich, G. (1989): MK–801 prevents hypobaric-ischemic neuronal degeneration in infant rat brain. *J. Neurosci.* **9**, 1701–1704.

Penix, L.P., Mansouri, F., Morin, A.M. & Wasterlain, C.G. (1991): Neuroprotection from excitotoxic damage in a rat model of status epilepticus. *Soc. Neurosci. Abstr.* **17**, 68.1.

Peterson, C., Neal, J.H. & Cotman, C.W. (1989): Development of N-methyl-D-aspartate excitotoxicity in cultured hippocampal neurons. *Dev. Brain Res.* **48**, 187–195.

Rauschecker, J.P. & Hahn, S. (1987): Ketamine-xylazine anaesthesia blocks consolidation of ocular dominance changes in kitten visual cortex. *Nature* **326**, 183–185.

Rebolleau, C.P. (1986): Extracellular calcium-induced neuroblastoma differentiation: invlovement of phosphatidylinositol turnover. *J. Neurochem.* **46**, 820–930.

Represa, A., Tremblay, E. & Ben-Ari, Y. (1989): Transient increase of NMDA-binding sites in human hippocampus during development. *Neurosci. Lett.* **99**, 61–66.

Reynolds, E.H. (1981): Biological factors in psychological disorders associated with epilepsy. In: *Epilepsy and psychiatry*, eds. E.H. Reynolds, M.R. Trimble, pp. 264–290. Edinburgh: Churchill Livingston.

Reynolds, I.J., Murphy, S.N. & Miller, R.J. (1987): 3H-labeled MK–801 binding to the excitatory amino acid receptor complex from rat brain is enhanced by glycine. *Proc. Natl. Acad. Sci. USA* **84**, 7744–7748.

Rothe, F., Schmidt, W. & Wolf, G. (1983): Postnatal changes in the activity of glutamate dehydrogenase and aspartate aminotransferase in the rat nervous system with special reference to the glutamate transmitter metabolism. *Dev. Brain Res.* **11**, 67–74.

Rothman, S. (1984): Synaptic release of excitatory amino acid neurotransmitter mediates anoxic neuronal death. *J. Neurosci.* **4**, 1884–1891.

Rothman, S.M. & Olney, J.W. (1986): Glutamate and the pathophysiology of hypoxic-ischemic brain damage. *Ann. Neurol.* **19**, 105–111.

Rothman, S.M., Thurston, J.H. & Hauhart, R.E. (1987): Delayed neurotoxicity of excitatory amino acids *in vitro*. *Neuroscience* **22**, 471–480.

Schmidt, W. & Wolf, G. (1988): High-affinity uptake of L-[3H]glutamate and D-[3H]aspartate during postnatal development of the hippocampal formation: a quantitative autoradiographic study. *Exp. Brain Res.* **70**, 50–54.

Shewmon, D.A. & Erwin, R.J. (1988): Focal spike-induced cerebral dysfunction is related to the after-coming slow wave. *Ann. Neurol.* **23**, 242–247.

Shields, W.D., Shewmon, D.A., Chugani, H.T. & Peacock, W.J. (1990): The role of surgery in the treatment of infantile spasms. *J. Epilepsy* **3** (Suppl), 321–324.

Shields, W.D. (1991): Infantile spasms and developmental delay: cause versus effect. *Epilepsia* **32** (Suppl 3), 60.

Silverstein, F.S., Chen, R. & Johnston, M.V. (1986): The glutamate analogue quisqualic acid is neurotoxic in striatum and hippocampus of immature rat brain. *Neurosci. Lett.* **71**, 13–18.

Silverstein, F.S., Torke, L., Bark, J. & Johnston, M.V. (1987): Hypoxia-ischemia produces focal disruption of glutamate receptors in developing brain. *Brain Res.* **431**, 33–39.

Sloviter, R.S. & Dempster, D.W. (1985): Epileptic brain damage is replicated qualitatively in the rat hippocampus by central injection of glutamate or aspartate but not by GABA or acetylcholine. *Brain Res. Bull.* **15**, 39–60.

Soderfeldt, B., Fujikawa, D.G. & Wasterlain, C.G. (1990): Neuropathological changes during status epilepticus in newborn monkeys. In: *Neonatal seizures*, eds. C.G. Wasterlain & P. Vert, pp. 91–98. New York: Raven Press.

Suga, S. & Wasterlain, C.G. (1980): Effects of neonatal seizures or anoxia on cerebellar mitotic activity in the rat. *Exp. Neurol.* **67**, 573–580.

Till, K. (1967): Hemispherectomy for infantile hemiplegia. *Dev. Med. Child Neurol.* **9**, 773–774.

Tremblay, E., Roisin, M.P., Represa, A., Charriaut-Marlangue, C. & Ben Ari, Y. (1988): Transient increased density of NMDA binding sites in the developing rat hippocampus. *Brain Res.* **461**, 393–396.

Tsumoto, T., Hagihara, K., Sato, H. & Hata, Y. (1987): NMDA receptors in the visual cortex of young kittens are more effective than those of adult cats. *Nature* **327**, 513–514.

Verdoorn, T.A., Burnashev, N., Monyer, H., Seebur, P.H., Sakmann, B. (1991): Structural determinant of ion flow through recombinant glutamate receptor channels. *Science* **252**, 1715–1718.

Vinters, H.V., Fisher, R.S., Corford, M.E., Peacock, W.J. & Shields, W.D. (1990): Neuropathologic substrates of infantile spasms: a study based on surgical resected cortical tissue. *Epilepsia* **31**, 652.

Wasterlain, C.G. (1976): Effects of neonatal status epilepticus on rat brain development. *Neurology* **26**, 975–986.

Wasterlain, C.G., Fujikawa, D.G., Dwyer, B.E., Vannucci, R.C., Schwartz, P.H. & Morin, A.M. (1990): Brain damage in the neonate: multiple periods of selective vulnerability each reflect discrete molecular events resulting from normal brain development. In: *Neonatal seizures*, eds. C.G. Wasterlain & P. Vert, pp. 69–82. New York: Raven Press.

Wasterlain, C.G. & Plum, F. (1973): Retardation of behavioural landmarks after neonatal seizures in rats. *Arch. Neurol.* **29**, 38–45.

Watkins, J.C. & Evans, R.H. (1983): Excitatory amino acid transmitters. *Ann. Rev. Pharmacol. Toxicol.* **21**, 165–204.

Watkins, J.C. & Olvermann, H.J. (1987): Agonists and antagonists for excitatory amino acid receptors. *Trends Neurosci.* **10**, 265–272.

Werner, P., Voig, M., Keinanen, K., Wisden, W. & Seeburg, P.H. (1991): Cloning of putative high-affinity kainate receptor expressed predominantly in hippocampal CA3 cells. *Nature* **351**, 742–744.

Whittle, I.R., Ellis, H.J. & Simpson, D.A. (1981): The surgical treatment of intractable childhood and adolescent epilepsy. *Aust. NZ J. Surg.* **51**, 109–196.

Wieloch, T. (1985): Neurochemical correlates to selective neuronal vulnerability. *Prog. Brain Res.* **63**, 69–85.

Wong, E.H., Kemp, J.A., Priestley, T., Knight, A.R., Woodruff, G.N. & Iversen, L.L. (1986): The anticonvulsant MK–801 is a potent *N*-methyl-D-aspartate antagonist. *Proc. Natl. Acad. Sci. USA* **83**, 7104–7108.

Woodruff, M.L. (1974): Subconvulsive epileptiform discharge and behavioural impairment. *Behav. Biol.* **11**, 431–458.

Yang, C.X., Morin, A.M., Fujikawa, D.G., Schwartz, P.H., Hattori, H. & Wasterlain, C.G. (1989): Ontogenesis of NMDA-mediated excitotoxicity. *Neurology* **39** (Suppl. 1), 373.

Younkin, D.P., Delivoria-Papdopouos, M., Maris, J. *et al.* (1986): Cerebral metabolic effects of neonatal seizures measured *in vivo* ^{31}P NMR spectroscopy. *Ann. Neurol.* **20**, 513–519.

Zaczek, R. & Coyle, J.T. (1982): Excitatory amino acid analogues: neurotoxicity and seizures. *Neuropharmacology* **21**, 15–26.

Author Index

Albrecht, D.	99	von Haebler, D.	99
Avanzini, Giuliano	29, 107	Llinas, Rodolfo R.	79
Avoli, Massimo	51	Mecarelli, Oriano	89
Beck, H.	99	Moshé, S.L.	121
Bendotti, C.	67	Monno, A.	67
Buzio, S.	107	Mutani, Roberto	5
Cantello, Roberto	5	Nixdorf, B.	99
Cherubini, Enrico	115	Panzica, F.	107
Civardi, Carlo	5	Paré, Denis	79
Curtis, Marco de	79	Prince, David A.	17
Fariello, R.G.	41	Rizzi, M.	67
Feo, Maria Rita de	89	Samanin, R.	67
Ficker, E.	99	Sancini, G.	107
Franceschetti, S.	107	Sankar, Raman	135
Frassoni, Carolina	59	Sperber, E.F.	121
Galli, A.	67	Spreafico, Roberto	59
Gianelli, Maria	5	Stabel, J.	99
Heinemann, U.	99	Velíšek, L.S.	121
Hwa, Granger G.C.	51	Vezzani, A.	67
La Grutta, V.	1	Wasterlain, Claude G.	135

Subject Index

action potentials, juvenile nervous tissue — 99
adenosine (A-1) receptors, hippocampus,
    blockade — 20
afterdischarges
    role in kindling — 122–123
    threshold — 93
allylglycine, systemic administration to
    immature animals — 90
α_1-adrenoceptors, in hippocampal kindling — 75
alumina
    GABAergic inhibition blocking studies — 6
    modelling partial seizures — 8
amino-hydroxymethyl-isoxazolopropionate (AMPA),
    excitotoxicity — 144
amino-hydroxymethyl-isoxazolopropionate
    (AMPA) receptors — 139
    development — 140
amino-hydroxymethyl-isoxazolopropionate-type
    channels,
    opening, neuronal necrosis — 138
2-amino-5-phosphonovaleric acid (APV), effect
    on EAA-induced
    EPSP in neocortex — 110–111, 112
4-aminopyridine (4AP), interictal
    epileptiform activity — 54
Ammon's horn, sclerosis — 146
amygdala
    kindling
        electrical ontogenetic studies — 93
        vs hippocampus — 122–123
    neonatal rats, penicillin application — 92
amygdaloid seizures, cat — 8
anatomy
    antiepileptic drug action — 46–47
    neocortex, development — 59–65
animal epilepsies — 45
animal models — 5–11
anoxia, *see also* hypoxic cell death
    neonatal brain — 141
anticonvulsants, vs antiepileptic drugs — 41–42
Antiepileptic Drug Development Program — 43
antiepileptic drugs, *see also* specific drugs
    mechanisms of action — 41–47
antiperoxidant agents — 9
apamine, work on rhythmic bursting, thalamic reticular
    nucleus — 35
AP-5 (NMDA receptor antagonist)
    effect on brain development — 141
    effect on evoked giant depolarizing potentials — 118
area tempesta — 2
    effect of GABA-elevating drugs — 6–7
arousal, effect on spike-and-wave discharges — 30–31
artificial cerebrospinal fluid — 108
aspartate
    as cortical neurotransmitter — 64
    work on rhythmic bursting, thalamic
        reticular nucleus — 35
astrocytes, development — 101
A-type potassium currents, maturation
    in hippocampal cells — 103
axon growth, projecting neurons vs local
    circuit neurons — 64
axotomy, sodium channels — 19

baboons, photosensitive myoclonic seizures — 45
baclofen, effect on hippocampus — 20
bicuculline
    effect on EAA-induced EPSP in neocortex — 111
    effect on $GABA_A$ receptors in neonate — 116
    systemic administration — 10
        immature animals — 90
bicuculline-induced convulsion test — 45
blood, intracortical injection — 8
bromide — 42
burst-after-hyperpolarization, role in rhythmic
    spike-and-wave discharges — 33
burst generation, cortical neurons — 18–19
bursting discharges, CA3 subfield, hippocampus — 80
BZP, effect on $GABA_A$ receptor — 46

CA3 neurons, immature, hippocampus,
    effect of GABA — 115–119
CA3 subfield
    maturation — 115–116
    pyramidal neurons, hippocampus — 80
cadmium, work on rhythmic bursting, thalamic reticular
    nucleus — 35–37
calcium, low calcium-induced epileptogenesis — 102
calcium influx
    effect on neuron growth — 144
    neuronal necrosis — 138
    neuron growth retardation — 141
cAMP accumulation, measurement in
    kindling experiment — 69, 70–71, 75

SUBJECT INDEX

carbamazepine 21
cascade effect, postsynaptic excitation 20–21
catecholamines, effects on kindling 126
caudate nucleus, in hippocampal epilepsy 1
cell to cell connections, effect of seizures 144
cellular changes, kindling 125–127
centrencephalic system 31
cerebral hemiatrophy 136
cerebral vesicles, human embryo 59
cerebrospinal fluid, artificial 108
chemo-affinity theory (Sperry et al.) 63
chloride conductance, effect of strychnine 7
cholinergic agents, potentiation of kindling 126
cholinergic transmission, enhancement studies, animal models 7
cobalt
  GABAergic inhibition blocking studies 6
  modelling partial seizures 8
congenital deafness, incidence of abnormal EEG 95
convulsant drugs
  causing kindling 121
  immature animals
    systemic administration 90–91
    topical application 91–92
convulsions 41
corpus callosum 9, 10
cortex
  foci, spike-and-wave pattern, animal models 9
  GABA mechanisms 51–54
  immature rats, penicillin application 92
  neurons, burst generation 18–19
cortical plate 61
cortical self-sustained afterdischarges, ontogenetic studies 93
cortico-reticular seizures 31
cortico-subcortical structures, spike-and-wave pattern, animal models 10
6-cyano-7-nitroquinoxaline-2,3-dione (CNQX)
  effect on EAA-induced EPSP in neocortex 110
  effect on hippocampal neurons 118

deafness, congenital, incidence of abnormal EEG 95
delayed cell death, glutamate 137
delayed rectifier currents, maturation in hippocampal cells 103
dentate gyrus
  granule cells, potassium currents 104
  hippocampal epilepsy 86
  horizontal cells 104
  post-traumatic recurrent excitatory connections 20–21
  temporal lobe epilepsy 80–81
depolarization
  GABA-mediated 53–54
  glial cells 100–101
designer drugs 44
diazepam 42
differentiation, neuronal 62
disinhibition, in focal epileptogenesis 19–20
Drosophila spp., potassium channels, genetic absence 24

electrode placement 81
  immature animals 89
electrolytes, in pacemaker activity 19
electroshock, ontogenetic studies 93

electroshock thresholds, drug testing 42, 44–45
encephalopathies, epileptic 29, 30
entorhinal cortex, temporal lobe epilepsy 81
enzyme changes, kindling 127
ephaptic interactions 21
epilepsy
  incidence 1
  spontaneous, kindled kittens 128
epileptic syndromes, with developmental effects 136–137
epileptiform activity, guinea-pig hippocampus, stages of development 82–86
epinephrine, effects on kindling 126
ethosuximide 37, 42
evoked synaptic activity, hippocampal neurons 116–117
excitatory amino acid antagonists 2
excitatory amino acid pathways 139–141
  ontogeny 140–141
excitatory amino acids
  effect on N-methyl-D-aspartate receptors 19
  enhancement studies, animal models 7–8
  postnatal development of EAA-mediated excitation 107–113
excitatory postsynaptic potentials 20–21
  CA3 hippocampal neurons 115
  effects of EAA 110–111
excitatory systems, enhancement studies, animal models 7–8
excitotoxic hypothesis 137–139
excitotoxicity, developing brain 135–146
extracellular space, immature nervous tissue 101–102
exuberance mechanism 63

fast inhibitory postsynaptic potentials, CA3 hippocampal neurons 115–116
feline generalized penicillin epilepsy 31
ferrous/ferric compounds, intracortical injection 8
focal epilepsy
  antiepileptic drug action 46–47
  hippocampal, experimental model 1
focal epileptogenesis 17–24
free radicals 9

GABA-activated channels, migrating neurons 65
GABA agonists, spike-and-wake patterns, animal models 10
$GABA_A$ receptor 46, 117
  vs $GABA_B$ receptors 54
  substantia nigra 127
$GABA_B$ receptors 53
GABAergic system 51–57
  history of theories 43–44
  inhibition
    blocking studies in animal models 6–7
    neocortex 54–57
  neurons, development 116
  neurotransmission
    maturation 108
    proconvulsant 6
GABA release, hippocampal kindling 75
GABA transaminase, effect of sodium valproate 46
γ-aminobutyric acid, see also under GABA
  depolarization of neonatal neurons 117
  effect on immature CA3 hippocampal neurons 115–119

effects on kindling	126	kindling	121–129
role in neuronal growth	118–119	immature brain, epileptogenicity	100
γ-D-glutamylglycine, reduction of hypoxic damage	137	infantile spasms	136–137
		inhibitory postsynaptic potentials	52–53
γ-vinyl-GABA	6	CA3 hippocampal neurons	115–116
gap junctions	21	juvenile nervous tissue	99
generalized absence epilepsy in rats from Strasbourg (GAERS)	29	inhibitory systems, blocking studies in animal models	6–7
thalamo-cortical connections in SWD generation	31	inside-outside sequence, neuronal migration	61–62
generalized epilepsy, ontogenetic models	90	interictal epileptogenesis	18–21
generalized epileptogenesis	29–37	convulsant drugs	54
genetic animal models	94–95	interictal-ictal transitions	22–23
giant depolarizing potentials (GDP), CA3 hippocampal neurons	116–117	interictal spikes	17
		microelectrode correlate	6
glial cells	100–102	intermediate zone, cortex	61
potassium redistribution	100–101	in vitro slice preparations, cortex	55–57
globus pallidus, in hippocampal epilepsy	1–2	inward rectifying currents, adult hippocampal cells	103
glucose levels, neonatal seizures	141–142	iron hypothesis, post-traumatic epilepsy	8–9
glutamate	7	isoforms, $GABA_A$ receptors, substantia nigra	127
as cortical neurotransmitter	64		
effect on neocortex	109	jacksonian epilepsy, animal models	8
neuron growth promotion	141	juvenile myoclonic epilepsy (Janz syndrome)	29, 30
toxicity	139		
work on rhythmic bursting, thalamic reticular nucleus	35	kainate	7
		effect on hippocampus	121
glutamate/aspartic acid	7	immature rats	92
glutamate receptors, changes leading to recurrent excitatory connections	21	neurons	118
		excitotoxicity	145–146
		systemic administration	10
glycine, effect on hippocampal neurons	118	to immature animals	90–91
glycine binding sites, NMDA receptor complex	139–140	work on rhythmic bursting, thalamic reticular nucleus	35
		kainate receptors	7, 139
glycine-mediated inhibition, blocking studies in animal models	7	development	140
		kainate-type channels, opening, neuronal necrosis	138
granule cells, dentate gyrus, potassium currents	104	ketone bodies, as fuel for neonatal brain	141
GVG (Vigabatrin)	46	kindling	10–11, 67
		antagonism	128
Haber-Weiss reactions	9	immature animals	121–129
Helisoma neuron B19, calcium influx, effect on neuron growth	144	permanence	127–128
		rates	124
heme compounds, intracortical injection	8	significance for human epilepsy	128–129
hemiatrophy, cerebral	136	lactate accumulation, neonatal brain	142
hippocampus		lamotrigine	7, 46
vs amygdala, kindling	122–123	learning	
CA2-CA3 area, bursting neurons	19	cortical	140–141
CA3 neurons, immature, effect of GABA	115–119	effect of epileptic syndromes	136
GABA-mediated synchronous potential	54	Lennox-Gastaut syndrome	136–137
immature, potassium	99–115	lesion experiments, thalamic reticular nucleus, GAERS rats	35
immature rats, kainic acid application	92	limbic seizures, guinea pig model	79–86
kindling		lipid membranes, peroxidation	9
electrical ontogenetic studies	93–94	local anaesthetics	46
noradrenergic and peptidergic neurotransmission	67–76	local circuit neurons, cortex	63, 64
		long-term potentiation	125
sclerosis	146	hippocampus, electrical ontogenetic studies	93
stereo-electro-encephalography	79–80	vs kindling	11
threshold stimulation	1	low calcium-induced epileptogenesis	102
history, antiepileptic treatments	42–45	low magnesium-induced epileptogenesis	102–103
horizontal cells, dentate gyrus	104		
hyperpolarization, GABA-mediated	53	magnesium	
hypoxic cell death, due to synaptic activity	137	blockade of NMDA channel	112, 115
		low magnesium-induced epileptogenesis	102–103
immature animals		reduction of hypoxic damage	137
epilepsy	89–95	marginal zone, neocortex, human embryo	59
		matrix cells, neocortex, human embryo	59

SUBJECT INDEX

medial septal nucleus, GABAergic control via caudate nucleus	1
mental deterioration, epileptic syndromes	136
minimal threshold tests, vs supramaximal tests, antiepileptic drugs	42
mitotic activity, neonatal brain	142
monkey, jacksonian epilepsy	8
mossy fibre sprouting	21
motor phenomena, kindling in rats	123–125
myelination	126
seizures during	144
myoclonus epilepsies, progressive	30
Na-K-ATPase, juvenile nervous tissue	99, 100
neocortex	
bursting neurons	19
development	
functional	107–108
morphology	59–65
GABAergic inhibition	54–57
immature, disinhibition	20
neonatal epilepsy, brain growth inhibition	141
Nernst equation	100–101
neuronal free regions, developing neocortex	60
neuronal migration	61–62
neuronal necrosis, role of neonatal seizures	146
neurotransmitter studies	2
N-methyl-D-aspartate	
as cortical neurotransmitter	64–65
effect on neocortex	109–110
excitotoxicity	144
responses in immature neocortex	112–113
work on rhythmic bursting, thalamic reticular nucleus	35
N-methyl-D-aspartate blockers, protective effect	137–138
N-methyl-D-aspartate receptor antagonists, effect on evoked giant depolarizing potentials	118
N-methyl-D-aspartate receptors	7, 44, 139–140
activation	
cortex	20
interictal-ictal transitions	22
development	
human	140
rat hippocampus	140
effect of excitatory amino acids	19
juvenile nervous tissue	100
modulation of giant depolarizing potentials	117–118
role in kindling	68
noradrenergic neurotransmission, hippocampus, kindling	67–76
norepinephrine	
effects on kindling	126–127
kindling antagonism	128
measurement of release in kindling experiment	69
oligodendrocytes, maturation	102
ontogenetic models of epilepsy	89–95
opiates, effects on kindling	126
orthodromic stimulation, potassium levels	100
oscillatory circuit, reticular thalamic nucleus, Wistar rats	29
osmotic minipumps, in kindling experiment	69–70
pacemaker activity	19

pacemaker groups of neurons	21
paired-pulse inhibition, CA1 area of hippocampus	117
Papio papio baboons, photosensitive myoclonic seizures	45
pars compacta, substantia nigra	2
antiepileptic drug action	47
pars reticulata, substantia nigra	2
partial seizures	
animal models	8
antiepileptic drugs, development	45
ontogenetic models	90–91
PCP receptors, development	140
PCP/sigma receptors, decrease in kindling	127
penicillin	
cortico-subcortical structures, spike-and-wave pattern	10
GABAergic inhibition blocking studies	6
immature animals, topical application	92
systemic administration	10
pentylenetetrazol	
drug testing	42
systemic administration to immature animals	90
peptidergic neurotransmission, hippocampus, kindling	67–76
perforated synapses vs non-perforated synapses, kindling	125
perfusion of brain preparations	81
peroxidation, lipid membranes	9
perspective layer I, cortex	61
petit mal	29
animal models	9
phenobarbital	42
phenytoin	21, 42
GABAmimetic properties	46
phosphatidylinositol (PI) turnover, measurement in kindling experiment	69, 71–72, 75
phospholipase C, hippocampal activation	75
phospholipid membranes, peroxidation	9
photosensitive myoclonic seizures, Papio papio baboons	45
pilocarpine, systemic administration to immature animals	91
positron emission tomography	137
postsynaptic cortical GABA mechanism	51–53
postsynaptic inhibition, cortex	19–20
post-traumatic epilepsy, animal models	8-9
potassium	
effect on neurons	100
extracellular	21
immature hippocampus	99–115
in pacemaker activity	19
potassium channels, Drosophila, genetic absence	24
potassium currents, maturation in hippocampal cells	103–104
prefrontal lesions, and kindling	126
preprosomatostatin, hippocampal kindling	72–73
presynaptic cortical GABA mechanism	51
primordial plexiform layer (PPL)	60–61
progabide	44
progressive epileptogenic encephalopathies	30
progressive myoclonus epilepsies	30
projecting neurons, cortex	63
pyramidal neurons, CA3 subfield, hippocampus	80
pyridoxine	
deficiency	55

dependency	30	effect of GABA-elevating drugs	6–7
		and kindling	127
quinolate	7	succinic-semialdehyde dehydrogenase, effect of sodium	
quisqualate		valproate	46
blockade by cyano-nitroquinoxaline-dione	118	superfusion experiments, calcium- and magnesium-free	
effect on neocortex	109	solutions	101–102
excitotoxicity	144	supramaximal tests, vs minimal threshold tests,	
work on rhythmic bursting, thalamic reticular		antiepileptic drugs	42
nucleus	35	surgery, psychosocial functioning	
quisqualate receptors	7	focal lesions	137
		temporal lobe epilepsy	136
rapidly recurring hippocampal seizures, electrical		surround inhibition	19–20
technique	94	sustained repetitive firing, effect of	
rat, neuronal differentiation	62	antiepileptic drugs	46
recruiting, vs spike-and-wave discharges	30	synapses	
recurrent excitatory connections	20	development and kindling	126
refractory periods, kindling stimuli in immature rats	125	effect of seizures	144
respiration, neonatal brain	141	formation, cortical development	64
reticular thalamic nucleus, Wistar rats	29	synaptic vesicles, kindling, redistribution	125, 128
electrical stimulation	9	synchronization, mechanisms	21
rhythmic spike-and-wave discharges	32–37		
rhythmogenic thalamic mechanisms, spike-and-wave		temporal evolution, epileptiform activity, guinea-pig	
discharges	32–37	hippocampus	82–86
		temporal lobe epilepsy	
screening, antiepileptic drugs	44	animal models	8
second messenger systems, interictal-ictal transitions	23	GABAergic neuron alterations	6
slice preparations, cortex	55–57	surgery, psychosocial functioning	136
slow inhibitory postsynaptic potentials, CA3		tetraethylammonium	
hippocampal neurons	115–116	effect on delayed rectifier currents	103
slow negative field potentials	102	work on rhythmic bursting, thalamic reticular	
sodium channels		nucleus	33–34, 35
antiepileptic drugs	21, 46	tetrodotoxin	
axotomy	19	effect on rat thalamus	33, 35
sodium valproate, on GABA metabolism	46	modification of convulsants on hippocampal	
somatostatin		neurons	118
effect of kindling on synthesis and release	67	thalamic nuclei, cat, electrical stimulation	9
in hippocampal kindling	73–74, 75–76	thalamic reticular nucleus,	
measurement of release in kindling experiment	69, 70	see reticular thalamic nucleus	
spike-and-wave discharges		thalamus, spike-and-wave discharges	29, 31–33
generalized, animal models	9	therapeutic index	44
thalamus	29, 31–33	Timm-Haug silver stain, study of kindling	128
spiking	1, 17	trauma	
spontaneous synaptic activity, CA3 hippocampal		antiperoxidant agents	9
neurons	116	cortex	20
status epilepticus		two-locus model, juvenile myoclonic epilepsy	30
animal models	10	tyrosine hydroxylase, decrease in kindling	127
long-term effects in rats	91		
mental deterioration	136	undershoots, potassium levels	102
stereo-electro-encephalography, hippocampus	79–80	unidirectional loop organization, hippocampus	80
stereotactic apparatus, immature animals	89		
steroid hormones, and kindling	127	ventricular zone, neocortex, human embryo	59
stimulation parameters, kindling experiments	122–123	veratridine, effects of kindling on aspartate and	
strychnine		glutamine	
glycine-mediated inhibition blocking studies	7	release	126
immature animals, topical application	91	Vigabatrin	46
subplate, cortex	61	vitamin B6, see pyridoxine	
substantial high frequency discharge, penicillin			
application	92		
substantia nigra	2		
antiepileptic drug action	47	wet dog shakes	124